Tumors of the Spinal Canal

Simon Hanft • Paul C. McCormick
Editors

Tumors of the Spinal Canal

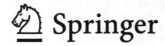 Springer

Editors
Simon Hanft
Department of Neurological Surgery
Rutgers Robert Wood Johnson Medical School
New Brunswick, NJ
USA

Paul C. McCormick
Department of Neurosurgery
New York-Presbyterian/Columbia University
New York, NY
USA

Department of Neurosurgery
Westchester Medical Center and New York Medical College
Valhalla, NY
USA

ISBN 978-3-030-55098-1   ISBN 978-3-030-55096-7   (eBook)
https://doi.org/10.1007/978-3-030-55096-7

This Springer imprint is published by the registered company Springer Nature Switzerland AG
The registered company address is: Gewerbestrasse 11, 6330 Cham, Switzerland

To my parents, Flora and Adam, who have done everything imaginable to support my career; "And so it was I entered the broken world/ To trace the visionary company of love": to my wife, Michelle, for whom I have a true green light love and whose dedication to our twin daughters, Hollace and Daphne, is limitless; and to Rick Komotar, who may be shocked to find his name in a book involving the spine, but whose ongoing mentorship and enthusiasm for neurosurgery have been the most important touchstones in my career.

—Dr. Simon Hanft

To Paul Jr., Kyle Lindsey, and Kaleigh.
You have grown into outstanding individuals who will accomplish so much more.

—Dr. Paul C. McCormick

Foreword

Tumors of the Spinal Canal, edited by Simon Hanft and Paul McCormick, is a superb treatise on the treatment of intradural extra- and intramedullary spine tumors by true experts in the field. The book provides not only technical pearls for resection of these often-complicated tumors, but also provides a thoughtful rationale for preoperative, intraoperative, and adjuvant decision-making. This book delves into the nuances of treatment and answers important questions that have not been specifically addressed in the literature, such as: When does one operate on VHL-associated hemangioblastomas or giant extradural schwannomas? What is the risk-benefit of resecting a benign schwannoma or meningioma from the vertebral artery? When do tumors require instrumented fusion? What are the radiation options for residual or unresectable disease? With the discovery of molecular drivers, can targeted therapies impact outcomes for these tumors? The authors provide clear expert opinions on the most complicated aspects of intradural tumor management. This book will make your proverbial decision-making fork in the road into a straight line.

Mark Bilsky, MD
Memorial Sloan Kettering Cancer Center
Weill Cornell Medical College
New York, NY, USA

Preface

To break the pentameter, that was the first heave
—Pound, The Pisan Cantos

When we set out to put together a book dedicated to tumors of the spinal canal, we had a basic goal in mind: make it new. The realities of writing a neurosurgical text are largely inescapable—room must be made for facts and stats. But our hope was to make it more pragmatic and drawn from personal experience. The emphasis, therefore, was on the authors and their individual surgical approaches to these tumors. Each chapter could be subtitled "how we do it": specific cases are the linchpin and illustrate how these operations are conducted on a fundamental technical level. We wanted to provide a window into operating rooms across the country. Multiple perspectives are represented here—some new voices admixed with those of the pantheon.

This book deals with tumors in the intradural space. It does not venture into primary and metastatic tumors impacting the vertebral column. We felt that in surveying the existing literature, there was no book dedicated to tumors occupying the spinal canal. Indeed the pathologies discussed here are included in more expansive volumes on spinal oncology, but it was our mission to make these tumors the star of the show. We sought emphasis on the actual surgical encounter, and even more so, guidance regarding the management of residual and recurrent disease. Even more quotidian concerns, such as when to order surveillance MRIs, are largely glossed over in the general literature, lacunes that we hoped this book would identify and fill.

Each tumor type constitutes its own chapter. And a few additional chapters focus on more novel trends in the field, namely radiotherapy and minimally invasive approaches. We wanted the book to answer two basic questions: how do these neurosurgeons go about removing these tumors? And when the surgery falls short of a cure, where can the neurosurgeon turn?

It is our hope that *Tumors of the Spinal Canal* is soon regarded as a practical reference for both the surgical and nonsurgical management of these tumors. Despite the advances in modern neurosurgery, there is still a major role for traditional approaches to these tumors, and we believe this volume effectively bridges those two worlds. It is forward-looking but with a firm foundation in the past, "one arc synoptic of all tides below" to borrow from Hart Crane. Our sincerest hope is that the ultimate benefit will be realized by the patients who bear the burden of these diagnoses.

New Brunswick, NJ, USA   Simon Hanft, MD
New York City, NY, USA   Paul C. McCormick, MD

Acknowledgments

We would like to thank a few individuals who either knowingly or unknowingly contributed to the composition of this text. Dr. Hanft would like to single out his colleagues, in particular Dr. Shabbar Danish, who has been essential in developing the tumor program at Rutgers and the Cancer Institute of New Jersey with his incredible energy and vision; Filipe Feiteiro, who has dedicated many hours in caring for these patients and stands as the most committed caregiver our department has ever known; Dr. Michael Nosko, who as the patriarch of our current department established a distinguished yet unassuming tradition of high quality neurosurgical care; and Dr. Robert Aiken, who has been a leader in the field of neuro-oncology and partnered with us in the treatment of many of these patients. To resident alumni who were in the trenches for many of these operations and whose assistance was vital: Drs. John Quinn, Rachid Assina, Brian Fernholz, Michael Cohen, Celina Crisman, Ahmed Meleis, David Slottje, Irene Say, Nick Hernandez, Arthur Carminucci, and Yehuda Herschman. A special level of gratitude goes to Dr. Nitesh Patel for his help with this publication, and for many others—"I greet you at the beginning of a great career, which yet must have had a long foreground somewhere."

To the dedicated people of Rutgers Robert Wood Johnson Hospital: operating room staff (Danielle Falgiano, Maria Fernandez-Pazos, Jeff Manuola, Wendy Maurizio, Nick Meo, and Stephanie Osman); Heidi Kaufman and the neuromonitoring team whose excellent technical knowledge was critical to the success of these operations and preparation of this text; Chris Fjotland, neuro-anesthesiologist for many of these cases; nurses of the PACU, neuro ICU, and 7 tower; office staff, including Mahreen Quadeer and Cathy Furnbach, Kiki Campbell, Tiara Owens, Kim Jacobs, Amanda Guerrero, and Siobhan DaSilva; social workers (Kereecha Thomson) and physical therapists; MRI technicians; physician assistants (John Kauffmann, Jessica McElroy, Danielle Morris, Jesse Pannell); and fellow medical school faculty. These are people who continue to provide the best care possible to these and many other patients— often in the shadows, without ever getting the recognition they deserve.

We would also like to thank the hardworking physicians of New Jersey who have been instrumental in diagnosing these often difficult to pinpoint masses. They continue to provide wonderful care to these patients long after they've made it through these operations: Drs. Roger Behar, Tejas Deliwala, Bruno Fang, Kevin Gall, Jeff Greenberg, Sam Gupta, Josh Hersh, Qasim

Husain, Samantha Kanarek, Jeffrey Miller, Stacey Miller-Smith, Mike Nissenblatt, Dipak Pandya, Haodong Song, Li Sun, Matthew Terranova, Manish Viradia, and Scott Yager.

Dr. McCormick would like to acknowledge his chairman, Dr. Robert Solomon, and his colleagues in the Department of Neurosurgery at Columbia University College of Physicians and Surgeons who have supported and advanced his career in the evaluation and treatment of patients with disorders of the spine and spinal cord, especially spinal cord tumors. He is especially grateful to Bennett M. Stein, MD, who served as both a teacher and role model.

And to the patients themselves, who in the harrowing days after being told they have a tumor, found the strength to put their trust in us. We try to be better surgeons because of them.

Contents

Part IV   New Age Surgical Approaches

Contributors

John Bruckbauer, MD Candidate Department of Neurological Surgery, Thomas Jefferson University Hospital, Philadelphia, PA, USA

Mychael Delgardo, BS Department of Neurosurgery, Neurological Institute of New York/Columbia University, New York, NY, USA

Ryan G. Eaton, MD Department of Neurological Surgery, The Ohio State University Wexner Medical Center, Columbus, OH, USA

John C. Flickinger, MD University of Pittsburgh School of Medicine, Departments of Radiation Oncology, Pittsburgh, PA, USA

University of Pittsburgh School of Medicine, Departments of Neurological Surgery, Pittsburgh, PA, USA

Peter C. Gerszten, MD, MPH University of Pittsburgh School of Medicine, Departments of Radiation Oncology, Pittsburgh, PA, USA

University of Pittsburgh School of Medicine, Departments of Neurological Surgery, Pittsburgh, PA, USA

Simon Hanft, MD Department of Neurological Surgery, Rutgers Robert Wood Johnson Medical School, New Brunswick, NJ, USA

Department of Neurosurgery, Westchester Medical Center and New York Medical College, Valhalla, NY, USA

James Harrop, MD Department of Neurological Surgery, Thomas Jefferson University Hospital, Philadelphia, PA, USA

Roger Härtl, MD Neurological Surgery, Weill Cornell Brain and Spine Center, New York-Presbyterian Hospital, Weill Cornell Medicine, New York, NY, USA

R. Nick Hernandez, MD Neurosurgery, Rutgers New Jersey Medical School, Newark, NJ, USA

Dominique M. O. Higgins, MD, PhD Department of Neurosurgery, Neurological Institute of New York/Columbia University, New York, NY, USA

Kevin Hines, MD Department of Neurological Surgery, Thomas Jefferson University Hospital, Philadelphia, PA, USA

Meng Huang, MD Department of Neurosurgery, University of Miami, Miami, FL, USA

George I. Jallo, MD Institute for Brain Protections Sciences, Johns Hopkins All Children's Hospital, Saint Petersburg, FL, USA

Sertac Kirnaz, MD Neurological Surgery, Weill Cornell Brain and Spine Center, New York-Presbyterian Hospital, Weill Cornell Medicine, New York, NY, USA

M. Benjamin Larkin, MD, PharmD Neurosurgery, Baylor College of Medicine, Houston, TX, USA

Allan D. Levi, MD, PhD Department of Neurosurgery, University of Miami, Miami, FL, USA

Russell R. Lonser, MD Department of Neurological Surgery, The Ohio State University Wexner Medical Center, Columbus, OH, USA

Glen R. Manzano, MD Department of Neurosurgery, University of Miami, Miami, FL, USA

Paul C. McCormick, MD Department of Neurosurgery, Neurological Institute of New York/Columbia University, New York, NY, USA

Ahmed M. Meleis, MD Neurological Surgery, University of Texas MD Anderson Cancer Center, Houston, TX, USA

Hima B. Musunuru, MD University of Pittsburgh School of Medicine, Departments of Radiation Oncology, Pittsburgh, PA, USA

Mohammad Hassan A. Noureldine, MD, MSc Department of Neurosurgery, Johns Hopkins University School of Medicine/Johns Hopkins All Children's Hospital, Saint Petersburg, FL, USA

Stephanie Perez, MD Candidate Department of Neurological Surgery, Thomas Jefferson University Hospital, Philadelphia, PA, USA

Victor Sabourin, MD Department of Neurological Surgery, Thomas Jefferson University Hospital, Philadelphia, PA, USA

Franziska Schmidt, MD Neurological Surgery, Weill Cornell Brain and Spine Center, New York-Presbyterian Hospital, Weill Cornell Medicine, New York, NY, USA

Nir Shimony, MD Institute of Neuroscience, Geisinger Medical Center, Geisinger Commonwealth School of Medicine, Danville, PA, USA

Johns Hopkins University School of Medicine, Institute for Brain Protection Sciences, Johns Hopkins All Children's Hospital, Saint Petersburg, FL, USA

Anthony Stefanelli, MD Department of Neurological Surgery, Thomas Jefferson University Hospital, Philadelphia, PA, USA

Claudio E. Tatsui, MD Neurosurgery, University of Texas MD Anderson Cancer Center, Houston, TX, USA

Joseph P. Weiner, MD Rutgers Cancer Institute of New Jersey, Department of Radiation Oncology, New Brunswick, NJ, USA

Part I
Extramedullary Tumors

Schwannoma

1

Simon Hanft

Introduction

Schwannomas of the spinal canal represent, in many ways, the ideal subject for neurosurgical care. These intradural, extramedullary lesions are benign, slow growing entities that can be removed through low risk approaches that confer significant, often complete, symptom relief. It is one of the true circumstances in our field where an operation alone is the definitive, curative step. Obviously there are more complicated versions of these growths: size, location, extent of cord compression, adherence to adjacent nerve roots, vascularity, and origin from an important functioning nerve root are all factors that can increase the complexity of the operation. Unlike their cranial counterparts, which often require arduous skull base approaches with fairly high and lasting morbidity, schwannomas of the spinal canal can be addressed through standard approaches with a far greater risk-benefit profile. They remain nearly exclusively surgical entities—upfront radiation, even if delivered in stereotactic fashion, is often outweighed by the benefits of surgical resection.

Our goal in this chapter is slightly different than the traditional effort put forth in most other pedagogic treatments of this tumor type. The hope is that the neurosurgeon reading this will develop a deeper understanding of how to appropriately counsel patients regarding this tumor. In addition, surgical techniques discussed here will equip the surgeon to better manage these tumors. We also believe that discretion and judgment can be gleaned from this chapter: not only should neurosurgeons develop a better sense of the goals of surgery and how aggressive to be, but they should be able to recognize what schwannomas they can comfortably remove and what ones should be handed off to a specialist in this domain. Therefore, the emphasis here is on the unique anatomy and behavior of this tumor along with a discussion of surgical techniques and nuances.

The chapter is divided into three sections: purely intradural schwannomas, intradural-extradural schwannomas (including the dumbbell subtype), and purely extradural schwannomas. We do not discuss purely extraforaminal schwannomas, which can be regarded as its own disease entity, as these often require multi-disciplinary surgical approaches depending on location. The goal here is to address the most commonly encountered schwannomas by a practicing neurosurgeon, and that category is overwhelmingly dominated by tumors exclusively within the canal and those with foraminal extension. This is done using illustrative cases of each schwannoma subtype from our institutional experience.

S. Hanft (✉)
Department of Neurological Surgery, Rutgers Robert Wood Johnson Medical School,
New Brunswick, NJ, USA

Department of Neurosurgery, Westchester Medical Center and New York Medical College,
Valhalla, NY, USA
e-mail: simon.hanft@wmchealth.org

© Springer Nature Switzerland AG 2021
S. Hanft, P. C. McCormick (eds.), *Tumors of the Spinal Canal*,
https://doi.org/10.1007/978-3-030-55096-7_1

The Basics

Schwannomas represent roughly one-third of all primary tumors involving the spinal canal [1]. They arise from the Schwann cell which makes up the myelin sheath of the nerve root. Approximately 95% of schwannomas are solitary and sporadic, with the small remaining percent associated with neurofibromatosis type 2 (NF2) or schwannomatosis [2, 3]. Schwannomas in NF2 are regarded as more aggressive as they adhere to adjacent nerves and lead to a higher rate of postoperative deficits. Schwannomatosis is considered the third form of neurofibromatosis and applies to patients older than 30 without NF2 and with at least two schwannomas—it has been a diagnosis in use for roughly 20 years [4]. The vast majority of spinal schwannomas are classified as conventional; other variants include cellular, plexiform, and melanotic [5, 6]. Conventional schwannomas have exceedingly low potential for malignant transformation, whereas their more rare counterparts, the cellular and melanotic forms in particular, have a higher tendency to transform. Histologic characterization of these schwannomas is predicated on the Antoni A and B patterns, with Antoni A showing hypercellularity. As is the case across all CNS tumor types, the ki67 index is now routinely reported and roughly correlates to recurrence potential [7].

Around 70% of schwannomas are purely intradural, with 15% purely extradural and 15% both intra- and extra-dural. Intramedullary schwannomas represent less than 1% and are so exceedingly rare that we do not address them in this chapter [8].

Neurofibromas are not given separate treatment in this chapter, though a case of neurofibroma is presented. Clinically and radiographically, they can be indistinguishable from schwannomas. Their growth pattern is invasive into multiple fascicles of a nerve, whereas schwannomas displace adjacent fascicles and remain encapsulated. The surgical implication for neurofibromas is that the parent nerve needs to be taken in order to achieve gross total removal.

The potential for malignant transformation, though low, is higher than conventional schwannomas at 5–10%, which prompts consideration of adjuvant radiation in the case of subtotal resection [1–4].

How Schwannomas Work

Schwannomas are well-encapsulated tumors, classically demarcated by an afferent nerve rootlet (nerve ENTERING the tumor) and efferent nerve rootlet (nerve EXITING the tumor) (Fig. 1.1). The tumor grows eccentric to the rootlet and essentially splays the rootlet over its surface. Though the rootlet nearly always blends beyond recognition into the tumor capsule/substance, there are occasions where this attenuated rootlet, or even fascicles of the rootlet, can be identified in continuity on the tumor surface. Identification and stimulation of the afferent and efferent nerve rootlets are fundamental steps in the surgical treatment of these tumors.

Each exiting spinal nerve (e.g. C5 or L3) comprises multiple nerve rootlets. These rootlets arise from the ventral (motor) and dorsal (sensory) aspect of the spinal cord before joining as one exiting nerve [9]. It is from one of these individual rootlets that a schwannoma develops (Fig. 1.2). Schwannomas preferentially grow off sensory nerve rootlets as opposed to pure motor nerves, the latter of which accounts for 2–5% of spinal schwannomas [1, 10]. This sensory origin allows for complete removal of the tumor and its associated nerve rootlet in the majority of cases— there are no meaningful deficits associated with taking a sensory nerve. Even in cases of motor nerve root origin, typically the motor nerve rootlet itself can be sacrificed along with the tumor in order to achieve gross total resection without causing a neurologic deficit [10–14]. This is often the case for a number of proposed reasons:

1. *Myotomal overlap*—the concept that there is a degree of plasticity such that adjacent motor nerves take over for the compromised nerve

a   b

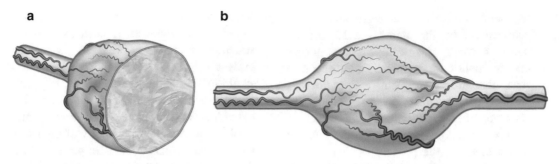

Fig. 1.1 Schwannoma. (**a**) Schwannoma in cross section. (**b**) Lateral view of a schwannoma showing an afferent rootlet entering the tumor mass and an efferent rootlet exiting. The corkscrew vessels both on the nerve rootlets and tumor surface are characteristic findings. Typically, the afferent nerve rootlet has more dilated vessels due to congestion from tumor compression

Fig. 1.2 Dorsal and ventral nerve rootlets. Cross section of the spinal cord revealing the exiting nerve rootlets from both the ventral and dorsal regions. A small schwannoma is shown arising from a dorsal nerve rootlet in the canal before the rootlet coalesces into the dorsal nerve root that then merges with the ventral nerve root as the exiting spinal nerve. As this schwannoma grows, it will first compress the adjacent dorsal rootlets before impacting the ventral nerve rootlets and ultimately the spinal cord. This is a simplified view of one type of schwannoma growth pattern

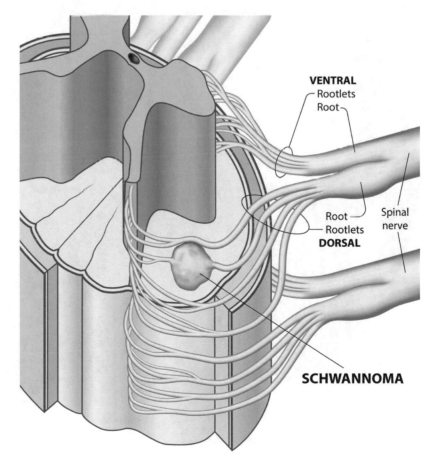

(e.g. an L3 motor nerve schwannoma is compensated for by the uninvolved L2 and L4 motor nerves); this compensatory theory mainly applies to the patient's preoperative state, though we do believe that there is plasticity and new motor coding that can occur after motor nerve rootlet sacrifice as well.

2. *Chronic silencing*—in conjunction with the above concept, the process of deactivating the involved motor nerve by the slow growth of the tumor through chronic compression and possible devascularization; this incremental process allows for adjacent motor nerves to take over the involved nerve function [15].

3. *Nerve rootlet redundancy*—a concept borrowed from engineering, analogous to the structural redundancy seen in suspension bridges (Fig. 1.3)—the tumor arises from a single rootlet among the many that comprise the full exiting nerve, and so sacrifice of this individual rootlet should not significantly weaken the overall conductivity of the nerve with so many other rootlets in place, even if the involved rootlet shows electrical activation during surgery (Fig. 1.3).

These concepts often explain why patients either have no postoperative motor deficits or temporary deficits that improve with time after schwannoma removal with nerve root sacrifice

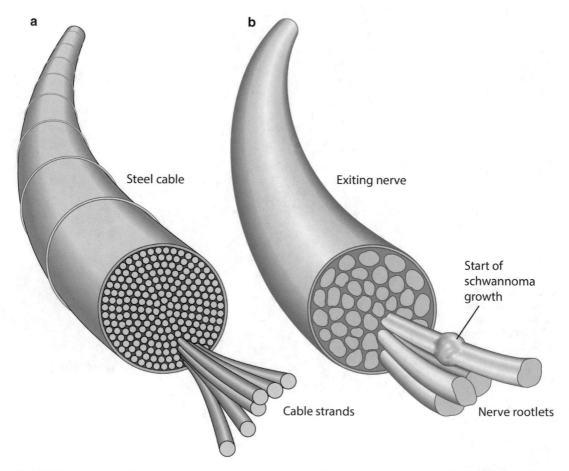

Fig. 1.3 Suspension cable and exiting nerve. (**a**) The single main cable for a suspension bridge contains numerous individual steel cables. This intrinsic redundancy will retain the overall cable strength even if one or more individual cables weaken and snap. (**b**) In analogous fashion, the exiting nerve comprises multiple individual nerve rootlets. Disconnecting one of these rootlets in the process of surgically removing a schwannoma leaves enough of the remaining rootlets intact to maintain connectivity and downstream muscle activation

[14, 15]. To be certain, there are cases of schwannoma resection where a permanent motor deficit is induced, so sacrificing the nerve should be avoided where possible if the afferent and/or efferent components of the involved nerve rootlet stimulate during surgery. We will discuss the importance of this intra-operative decision point later in this chapter. Though these three concepts are meant to account for why patients can often tolerate complete nerve root sacrifice in these operations, they are not a license to take the involved nerve with impunity.

Presentation

Nearly all purely intradural *lumbar* schwannomas present with severe pain, a particularly debilitating kind of radiating, sciatic pain. Patients may often point out low back pain as well, but that is just likely the origin of the radiating pain (as opposed to a mechanical issue), and the radicular symptoms are nearly always the major complaint. There can be accompanying paresthesias and numbness. Weakness is uncommon as are bowel/bladder changes. Typically the growth of these masses is so chronic, that when they reach a critical mass the pain complaints are so significant that rarely do patients escape medical attention to the point where weakness and bowel/bladder function appear compromised. Extradural schwannomas, intriguingly, are nearly always incidentally found. These masses, likely due to slow growth and the fact that the traversing nerve roots in the canal are not compressed, do not present with the raging radicular symptoms that accompany purely intradural schwannomas. In fact, these extradural schwannomas typically need to grow to such a large size so that they invade the canal and then contact the traversing nerves, in which case the patient will start to develop symptoms typical of the purely intradural schwannoma variety [16].

Although the same types of symptoms are associated with *cervical and thoracic schwannomas*, the important difference is that these tumors, due to spinal cord compression, cause a myelopathic clinical picture. Therefore, patients with schwannomas in the cervical and thoracic region do often present with weakness of one or more extremities, numbness, and imbalance with fairly obvious gait changes. Of note, thoracic schwannomas may escape radiographic detection for long periods due to the relative rarity of compressive pathology in the thoracic spine. This can lead to significant symptom decline before an astute clinician orders a thoracic MRI. Lumbar nerve roots have more physical and electrical capacity to absorb compression, so extradural lumbar schwannomas can go undetected until they reach large sizes. In fact, we have encountered barely symptomatic or even asymptomatic lumbar schwannomas with near complete canal obliteration, scalloping of the vertebral body, and other chronic bony changes, such as foraminal widening. Indeed the amount of tolerance the lumbar nerve roots have for compression is remarkable in some instances. The penultimate case presented in this chapter demonstrates this phenomenon well.

MRI Features

Typical MRI characteristics of schwannomas include: T1 iso-to-hypointensity (roughly 75% isointense and 25% hypointense), T2 hyperintensity (often mixed signal), and enhancement with contrast. There are some variations in the post-contrast appearance: though most schwannomas show homogeneous enhancement, there can be heterogeneous and even rim enhancement. These latter appearances are likely related to internal hemorrhage and cystic degeneration [17].

Evidence of foraminal widening and scalloping of the vertebral body are strong indicators of slow growth associated with schwannomas. Pedicle erosion can be identified as well [18]. If these findings are encountered on the MRI, a schwannoma is the very likely diagnosis—meningiomas are not associated with these characteristics. In fact, searching for evidence of foraminal widening is recommended for preoperative planning, as it may indicate a degree of instability that might warrant upfront instrumentation. If there is any question of foraminal involvement, we often obtain a preoperative CT to better delineate the pattern of bony changes.

Intradural Schwannomas

The distinction between a purely intradural schwannoma and one with an extradural component can sometimes be made on a preoperative MRI. Especially in the case of larger schwannomas, it can be difficult to differentiate how much of the resulting spinal cord compression, or spinal nerve root compression, is from an intradural mass versus an extradural mass compressing the thecal sac and its contents, or both. Classification schemes have been proposed for characterizing these various schwannoma growth patterns [19, 20]. The neurosurgeon must be prepared to deal with both intradural and extradural components in all of these operations and should have a plan of action before going in.

As a general rule, intradural schwannomas are more often symptomatic than tumors that are primarily extradural. An intradural tumor comes to clinical attention typically at a smaller size than their extradural counterparts due to proximity to, as well as compression of, neighboring nerve roots. Since these tumors are circumscribed within the spinal canal, these symptoms are more likely to occur.

Here we present three operative cases with each representing a purely intradural schwannoma arising from the cervical, thoracic, and lumbar regions. Table 1.1 lists the points of emphasis when counseling a patient about the risks of surgery and likelihood of recurrence. This is in the context of intradural schwannomas but can be slightly modified for tumors with extradural extension, depending on tumor size and location—these are not one-size-fits-all criteria [7, 21]. Another note is that we present cases in which a traditional laminectomy is performed, though we recognize the widespread use of laminotomy/laminoplasty, hemilaminectomy, interlaminar and MIS approaches for these tumors.

Table 1.1 Preoperative surgical counsel—intradural schwannomas

1.	Sensory deficit 10–20%, either new or exacerbation of preoperative symptom
2.	Motor deficit 5%, either new or exacerbation of preoperative symptom
3.	Infection <5%
4.	CSF leak/pseudomeningocele <5%
5.	Epidural hematoma 1–2%
6.	Spinal instability requiring reoperative fusion in the future 1–2%
7.	Urinary/fecal incontinence <1%
8.	Recurrence rates:
	1% if the nerve root sacrifice accompanies resection
	5% if subtotal resection/intracapsular resection
	5–10% if subtotal resection w/elevated ki67 > 5%, and adjuvant radiation may be recommended

Case 1: Lumbar Schwannoma, Intradural

Presentation/Imaging A 44-year-old female presenting with 2–3 months of progressive low back pain that now radiates down both legs, right greater than left. She denies weakness, numbness, and bowel/bladder issues. MRI of the lumbar spine was ordered revealing a 2 cm mass occupying the entire canal at the level of the L4 body (Fig. 1.4). The mass demonstrated peripheral rim enhancement and was severely compressing the cauda equina nerve roots.

Operation The patient underwent a partial L3 and L4 laminectomy with midline dural opening for removal of the tumor. Our practice is to perform as central a laminectomy as possible, which is done in an effort to preserve the facets and, therefore, avoid long-term instability. We achieve epidural space hemostasis with floseal/surgiflo and try to avoid leaving cottonoids in the lateral gutters which can make dural reflection less effective. Prior to dural opening, transdural ultrasound can be utilized to localize the underlying mass and confirm that the appropriate extent of laminectomy was performed [22].

The dura is initially opened using a tenting 4-0 nurolon stitch with an 11-blade to make the small initial durotomy. The goal is to preserve the

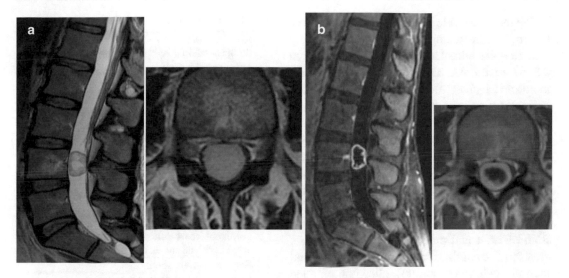

Fig. 1.4 (**a**) Sagittal and axial T2 images showing the mass centered at L4. Note the degree of circumferential nerve root displacement on the axial image. (**b**) Sagittal and axial T1 post contrast images showing peripheral rim enhancement with a central area of necrotic/hemorrhagic tissue

arachnoid layer, thereby limiting CSF egress. If the arachnoid is violated during the dural opening, which is common, the CSF egress can be rapid, thereby inducing bleeding from the epidural space. There also can be nerve root herniation in the case of larger tumors, so, ideally, the arachnoid layer is opened separately with a sharp nerve hook and microscissors. The dura itself is opened one of two ways: a blunt nerve hook, cocked back at a 45° angle, can extend the durotomy for the duration of the desired opening; or a dental tool with an 11-blade, similar to how the brain dura is opened, can achieve the durotomy in an albeit slower fashion. We tent the dura typically in three spots (depending on the length of the durotomy, this can be two or even four locations) with 4-0 nurolon sutures to the paraspinal muscles. This paraspinal suture optimizes the amount of dural reflection which increases the exposure of the intradural space, as opposed to simply hanging the sutures out of the wound to clamps. This approach can also reduce epidural venous bleeding [23].

A word about the arachnoid opening: the arachnoid, immediately encountered upon opening the dura, should be opened with a combination of a sharp nerve hook and microscissors. This will facilitate visualization of the tumor. But attention must be paid to another arachnoid layer that is more directly adherent to the tumor surface. We strongly recommend spending the time to dissect this arachnoid layer off the tumor, thereby exposing the actual tumor capsule. Once the surgeon is working on the tumor capsule directly, it is easier to mobilize the tumor and identify adjacent nerve roots that can be dissected away from the capsule. In fact, the ventral nerve root can share the same arachnoid sheath. Therefore, if the tumor is entered into without dissecting this arachnoid layer, the ventral nerve runs the risk of being damaged [23].

After the dura and arachnoid were opened in this case, the consistency of the mass was soft, fleshy, and brown-pink in coloration. It was immediately visible between the cauda equina nerve roots. After safely reflecting and insulating the surrounding nerve roots, the tumor surface was cauterized using non-stick bipolars and opened with a pair of microscissors. Specimen was grasped with tumor forceps and sent for frozen and permanent section. A combination of suction, tumor forceps, and ultrasonic aspiration with the CUSA (Cavitron ultrasonic surgical aspirator, Integra Lifesciences) was utilized to debulk the tumor internally.

We then were able to identify an afferent nerve feeding into the tumor. This was stimulated using a monopolar stimulation probe anywhere from 0.3 mA to 1.5 mA. The muscle groups routinely monitored include: quadriceps, anterior tibialis, gastrocnemius, peroneus longus, and the anal sphincter. Since there was no stimulation of these muscle groups even at the higher currents, we considered the afferent nerve clinically silent and, therefore, safe for sacrifice. The efferent nerve extending from the caudal aspect of the tumor was identified and stimulated in similar fashion, also leading to no muscle contractions. Both afferent and efferent nerve rootlets were, therefore, cauterized using the bipolars and incised with microscissors, allowing en bloc removal of the remaining tumor. The dura was closed using a 4-0 silk suture in running, locked fashion. We prefer a silk to nurolon suture as the silk stitch frays less over the course of a complete running dural closure. A Valsalva maneuver is then performed to 40 mm Hg for 10 seconds; if there is CSF leakage, an interrupted stitch is placed, occasionally buttressed with a small piece of paraspinal muscle if the defect is larger than a pinhole. If there is no leakage, we then cover the suture line with Adherus AutoSpray ET (extended tip applicator) dural sealant and use a small 1 in × 3 in duragen as an additional layer above the dural sealant after it solidifies. Muscle, fascia, and dermis are closed in standard fashion. For the skin (epidermis), we utilize a running, non-locked 2-0 nylon suture, which we feel provides additional strength and, when adequately spaced, a relatively pain-free removal in the office. Postoperative MRI confirmed gross total resection and final pathology confirmed WHO Grade I schwannoma.

For lumbar schwannomas, here are some of our technical observations summarized in Table 1.2:

1. *Stimulation spread*: When using a stimulation probe on the afferent nerve, there can be current spread to adjacent nerve rootlets, especially in a congested region of the canal (either closer to the conus, or simply due to large tumor size and resultant nerve root compres-

Table 1.2 Surgical pearls

1.	*Arachnoid dissection* – Ensure you have removed deeper arachnoid layer so you are working on the tumor capsule itself.
2.	Look for *congested vessels* on the surface to help identify the afferent nerve of origin.
3.	Surgical removal proceeds by *internal debulking* and progressive delivery of tumor contents into the developing resection cavity.
4.	Section the *dentate ligament* and rotate the cord if the tumor is primarily ventral.
5.	If the schwannoma is presumed intradural/extradural, *start by resecting extradural* as there may be no intradural extent
6.	Consider leaving a small plug of tumor at the nerve root sleeve during extradural resection to avoid CSF leak and an oft challenging repair.
7.	Nerve root stimulation:
	Range between 0.3 and 2.0 mA
8.	*Stimulate capsule before entering* as functioning fascicles may be on the tumor surface.
9.	*Isolate afferent nerve*—insulate spinal cord or traversing nerves with a cotton pattie to limit spread of current and false positives; elevate the afferent nerve and tumor slightly out of the canal to reduce contact with adjacent nerves.
10.	Sphincter stimulation is a contraindication for nerve root sacrifice.

sion). This can lead to stimulation of muscle groups that suggest the afferent nerve is active, when, in fact, this is due to spread/crossover. It is, therefore, important to isolate the afferent nerve as completely as possible. This can be done by insulating adjacent nerves with a small cottonoid, or by gently lifting the afferent nerve up towards the dura and away from the traversing nerves. We also recommend using lower stimulation currents, such as 0.3 mA, in these situations, as higher levels can induce the spread effect. Some would argue that such a low stimulation threshold may fail to activate a compressed and damaged nerve by the schwannoma, leading to false negatives. So there is a bit of a balancing act involved. Isolate, stimulate, and if silent, then cut—it is the closest a neurosurgeon gets to the feel of defusing a bomb.

2. *Stimulation* via *adherent nerves*: If, while stimulating the afferent or efferent nerves, there is reproducible stimulation of a muscle

group, then the surgeon must thoroughly inspect the tumor capsule in all dimensions. This is most likely due to the attachment of a traversing nerve to the tumor capsule and, if identified, this rootlet should be carefully dissected off the tumor and the afferent nerve restimulated. This dissection is usually accomplished with a microdissector, sharp incision of arachnoid adhesions with microscissors, and a sharp nerve hook. Bipolar cauterization should be avoided for the obvious reason of damaging the active nerve. If the functional rootlet cannot be safely dissected away, or if the afferent nerve continues to stimulate despite successful clearance of all evident traversing rootlets, you should commit the patient to a subtotal resection. Though the patient will likely tolerate traditional sectioning of the afferent and efferent nerves with complete schwannoma extrication, we find it difficult to recommend this maneuver if you are reliably producing muscle contractions with your stimulator probe. The surgeon should factor in patient age, co-morbidities, and amount of residual tumor at the end of the surgery when making the decision on nerve root sacrifice, in order to ensure gross total resection.

3. *Stimulation adequacy*: Another consideration, if there is still stimulation of the afferent nerve, is to stimulate the unaffected nerves in the canal. If, for example, there is robust stimulation of the same muscle group that the focused stimulation of the afferent nerve induced, one can argue for afferent rootlet sacrifice on the assumption that there are enough remaining intact nerve rootlets providing requisite activation of that muscle group. Alternatively, if there is no successful stimulation of the muscle group in question via the traversing rootlets, then the afferent nerve likely represents the primary connection to this muscle and should be spared. There is no established baseline threshold of activation that would guide this intraoperative decision. But, conceptually, it makes sense, so we do endorse its consideration as a factor in deciding whether to sacrifice the afferent

nerve. This goes back to the "nerve rootlet redundancy" idea—the afferent nerve can be taken since there are enough remaining rootlets to adequately supply the target myotome.

4. *Save the sphincter*: If there is any meaningful stimulation of the anal sphincter muscle via the afferent nerve, we strongly recommend to preserve the rootlet and consider a subtotal resection. The possible functional implications are so significant that we do not find it worth the risk of diminishing the nerve supply to this region.

Case 2: Thoracic Schwannoma, Intradural

Presentation/Imaging The patient is a 24-year-old male who has relatively recent onset weakness in the left leg. It has become worse over a three-week period to the point where he is having considerable difficulty ambulating. He was admitted to the hospital for further evaluation, where a thoracic MRI revealed a nearly 3 cm in cranio-caudal extent intradural extramedullary mass from T1-3 (Fig. 1.5). There is homogeneous contrast uptake and severe displacement of the spinal cord to the right. The mass appears dorsolateral in the canal and completely intradural with no evidence of foraminal involvement. Differential diagnosis included meningioma, less likely schwannoma, given its appearance within the canal and lack of extension into the foramen.

Operation The patient was positioned in a Mayfield three-pin headclamp with a Wilson Frame on a regular OR table, keeping the patient's head in a military chin-tuck position. Localization was done with a C-arm machine and neurophysiology monitoring with MEPs and SSEPs. We utilize MEP and SSEP monitoring in schwannomas involving the spinal cord, along with direct monopolar probe nerve rootlet stimulation. For lumbar schwannoma cases that don't involve the spinal cord, only the monopolar probe is utilized. A midline dural opening was made. The tumor was encountered immediately upon dural/arachnoidal incision. The spinal cord was noted to be severely attenuated and positioned to the right and ventrally. We began by cauterizing the tumor

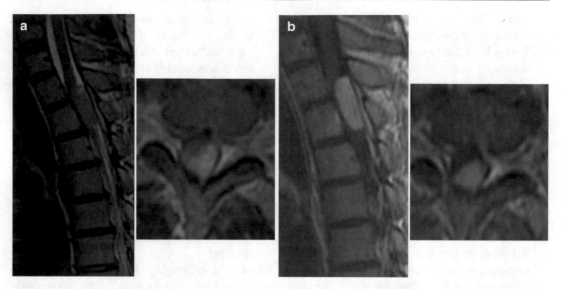

Fig. 1.5 (a) Sagittal and axial T2 images showing an oblong mass extending from T1-3. On the axial projection, there is severe rightward displacement of the spinal cord with very little visible cord substance. (b) Sagittal and axial T1 post contrast images show homogeneous enhancement within the mass. There is no obvious dural tail to suggest meningioma

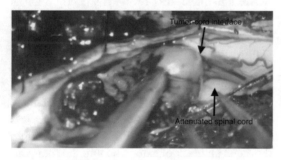

Fig. 1.6 Intraoperative photo (rostral to the left, caudal to the right) showing the schwannoma peeling away from the spinal cord at its caudal pole

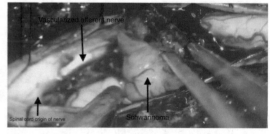

Fig. 1.7 Intraoperative photo (same alignment) now showing the rostral pole of the tumor coming away from the spinal cord with a clear view of a vascularized afferent nerve rootlet originating very close to the spinal cord substance

surface, opening the capsule using microscissors, and debulking the mass internally with tumor forceps and ultrasonic aspiration. We were able to develop a neat plane between the medial edge of the tumor and the spinal cord interface (Fig. 1.6). We were then able to identify the caudal pole of the tumor, which we grasped and mobilized into our field. The same was ultimately done for the rostral pole, which had a clear attachment to what appeared to be a vascularized nerve (Fig. 1.7). Stimulation of this tissue at multiple currents from 0.3 mA to 2 mA resulted in no muscle firing. It was, therefore, sacrificed with bipolar cauterization and microscissors. The same process was followed for what appeared to be the efferent nerve. This allowed en bloc removal of the mass. Postoperative MRI showed gross total resection and pathology confirmed a WHO Grade I schwannoma.

Case 3: Cervical Schwannoma, Intradural

Presentation/Imaging The patient is a 60-year-old male with 2 years of paresthesia involving

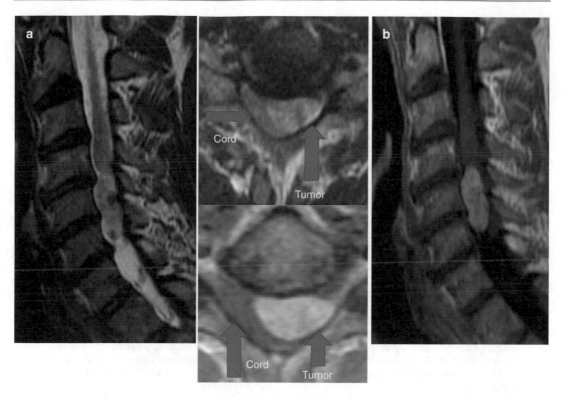

Fig. 1.8 (**a**) Sagittal and axial T2 images showing heterogeneous signal within an ovoid mass in the left aspect of the canal from C5-6. The axial image shows severe rightward displacement of the spinal cord. (**b**) Sagittal and axial T1 post contrast images show a homogenously enhancing mass causing severe spinal cord compression. The mass lies lateral and ventral to the spinal cord

the shoulders, trunk, and hands. These symptoms have become progressively worse and, more recently, have been accompanied by numbness in both legs and imbalance. A cervical MRI revealed a nearly 3 cm craniocaudal mass in the intradural extramedullary compartment causing severe spinal cord compression with rightward displacement (Fig. 1.8). The mass enhances homogeneously and does appear to slightly conform to the exiting nerve root region, but there is no foraminal extent or bony widening of the foramen. The mass is clearly circumscribed within the canal, leaving schwannoma and meningioma as the most likely diagnoses.

Operation Patient positioning was the same here as in Case 2. The patient underwent a C4-6 laminectomy, with complete laminectomies at C4-6 and a partial laminectomy at C7. Again, great care is taken to preserve the facets, as

long-term instability is a potential issue, especially in a three or more level laminectomy. The dura was opened in the midline utilizing a blunt nerve hook and reflected with three nurolon sutures bilaterally. The arachnoid was preserved upon dural opening and then opened with a sharp nerve hook. The mass was immediately encountered. It appeared to be between the exiting C5 and C6 nerve roots (Fig. 1.9). The process of surgical removal involved debulking the tumor internally with ultrasonic aspiration, then grasping and mobilizing the portion ventral to the cord and nerve roots into our window between the C5 and C6 nerve roots for further debulking. This was done systematically until we identified a small afferent branch from C5 and an even smaller efferent branch, both of which were so attenuated that they appeared almost as arachnoid bands/adhesions (Fig. 1.10). These were cauterized and incised, allowing en

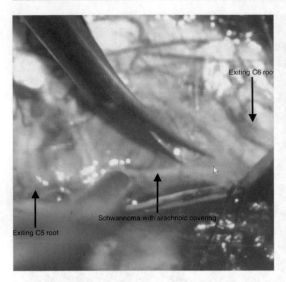

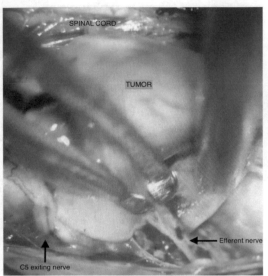

Fig. 1.9 Intraoperative photograph (rostral to the left, caudal to the right) showing the exiting C5 and C6 nerve roots, between which is located the schwannoma. Microscissors are being used to open the arachnoid layer above the tumor prior to entering the tumor for debulking purposes. Small individual nerve rootlets also appear to be flowing over the tumor capsule—these were sacrificed without effect

Fig. 1.10 Intraoperative photograph (same alignment) showing the majority of the remaining tumor now reflected dorsal to the cord. There is a very attenuated efferent nerve, mimicking an arachnoid adhesion, that is ultimately cauterized and taken. The spinal cord is above the tumor in the picture, which is anatomically to the right within the canal

bloc removal. Closure was performed as described above and the patient had no postoperative deficits and already noticed sensory improvements.

The key surgical principle in these cases is to utilize the corridor made by the tumor. In this case, though the majority of the tumor was ventral to the spinal cord itself, we kept a narrow corridor between the exiting C5 and C6 nerve roots, through which we patiently and progressively debulked the tumor. By using tumor forceps to then grasp the ventral component of the mass and bring it into our newly cleared field, we were able to ultimately visualize and remove all of the tumor without any manipulation of the cord or roots. Towards the end, around 30–40% of the tumor was removed as one piece from in front of the cord as we had debulked enough tumor. Often this satisfying en bloc removal awaits the surgeon demonstrating patience in gradually debulking the mass in stepwise fashion. Postoperative MRI showed no residual tumor and pathology revealed a Grade I schwannoma.

Intradural/Extradural Schwannomas (Dumbbell)

The so-called "dumbbell" schwannoma is a unique entity that effectively straddles the intradural and extradural compartments. In Case 4, we discuss a traditional dumbbell schwannoma, and in the subsequent cases we discuss variations on that theme—schwannomas with more intradural than extradural involvement and vice versa. A true dumbbell schwannoma, equally intra- and extradural, is most common in the cervical region [24, 25].

Case 4: Cervical Dumbbell Schwannoma

Presentation/Imaging The patient is a 23-year-old female who presents with a combination of neck pain, left arm tingling with weakness, and progressive imbalance. MRI of the cervical spine reveals a large, mainly homogeneously enhancing mass, 4 cm in its greatest dimension located behind the C2 and C3 bodies with near extension to the level of C1 causing dramatic cord compression and shift of the cord to the left (Fig. 1.11).

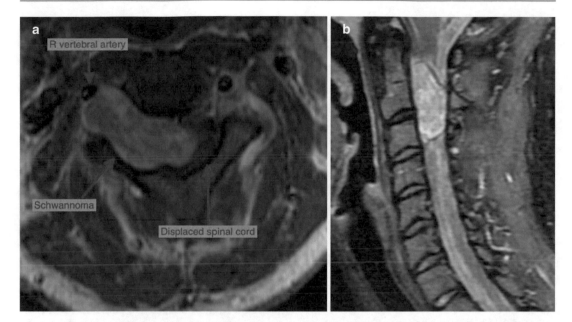

Fig. 1.11 (a) Axial T1 postcontrast MRI. Large dumb-bell schwannoma in cross-section showing displacement of the right vertebral artery and spinal cord to the left. (b) Sagittal T1 postcontrast MRI showing 4 cm craniocaudal extent of the tumor

The mass clearly exits and widens the C2-3 foramen and reaches and even displaces the vertebral artery on the right. A preoperative CT (Fig. 1.12) confirms the extent of foraminal widening, relationship to the vertebral artery (which is patent), and also shows attenuation of the C2 pars, which will render it difficult to cannulate for instrumentation purposes.

Preoperative Considerations The goal of the operation in this young patient is, first and foremost, to achieve decompression of the spinal cord. This will involve removal of the intradural component. The question then becomes, how aggressive should the surgeon be regarding the extradural component? Given this patient's young age, the size of the extradural component, and the resulting bony remodeling and destruction already accomplished by the tumor, we proceeded with the goal of a complete resection in mind. This does elevate the risk of vertebral artery injury, persistent CSF leakage (removal of the tumor on both sides of the dura can lead to a challenging closure of the expanded nerve root sleeve), and will mandate the use of instrumentation for stabilization. But it is critical to note, in this case, that the tumor itself has

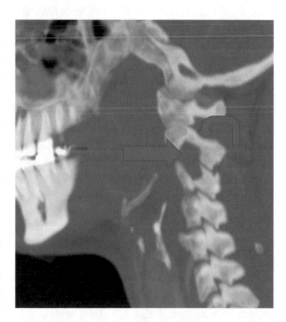

Fig. 1.12 Sagittal CT noncontrast. Block arrow pointing to widened C2-3 foramen. Curved arrow pointing to attenuated C2 pars

caused significant structural changes to the bone such that even a limited attempt at tumor removal from the canal itself would likely necessitate the use of instrumentation. Accordingly, the patient was counseled preoperatively about the high likelihood of a fusion as part of the operation.

Operation The patient is positioned prone in Mayfield head clamp with a Wilson frame in the military chin-tuck position. Neuromonitoring for SSEPs, EMGs, and MEPs is performed. An incision is made from the suboccipital bone down to C5. The C2 lamina was so thinned out by the tumor that the tumor itself was visible above and below the lamina to the right. A C2-3 laminectomy was performed revealing a significant amount of extradural tumor. We debulked this with a combination of bipolar cauterization, ultrasonic aspiration and tumor forceps. Ultimately, this allowed decompression and more complete visualization of the thecal sac. We then performed a midline durotomy and exposure of the intradural component in standard fashion. Typically we do not favor T-shaped dural incisions as these can be difficult to close in watertight fashion and are more relevant for tumors with fairly minimal extradural extent, though many advocate their use for all dumbbell tumors. The spinal cord was identified and severely compressed by an intradural mass located in the right aspect of the canal. We began to cauterize and debulk the tumor and, at an early stage, the afferent C3 nerve root was identified, stimulated (and shown to be silent), and then cauterized and incised. We ultimately removed the entire intradural tumor, following it out into the extradural space through a significantly dilated nerve root sleeve. This presented one of the challenging aspects of the surgery, closure of this opening, which we returned to later.

After the intradural tumor was removed, we flapped the dura back over the dural opening, thereby revealing the extradural compartment again. We continued to cauterize and debulk the tumor. We removed the C2 pars, which was already significantly thinned by the tumor, as well as the superior aspect of the C3 facet. This was done with both matchstick drill and Kerrison rongeur. Bipolar cauterization of the compressed foraminal veins, along with occasional use of SurgiFlo, is an important intermittent maneuver in this surgery, as the bleeding can be brisk [26]. As we continued to debulk

the tumor and follow it outside of the foramen, we encountered the vertebral artery, which was densely adherent to the tumor capsule. Careful bipolar cauterization, with the tips preferentially along the tumor so as not to stenose the artery, and sharp dissection with microscissors were the method of mobilizing the artery away from the mass. In this fashion, we were able to completely disconnect the tumor from the vertebral artery. We then rolled this portion of the tumor towards the canal for further debulking and removal. Gross total resection was accomplished.

We now addressed the dural closure with three 4-0 silk interrupted stitches through the intradural nerve sleeve opening, supplemented by the same number of stitches on the extradural side. A standard running locked 4-0 silk stitch was done for the midline durotomy. Even with the inside/outside nerve root closure technique, there was still minimal CSF leakage upon Valsalva maneuver, which prompted us to leave a lumbar drain in place at the end of the operation.

Inspection of the bony elements revealed complete obliteration of the C2 pars on the right, near complete loss of the right C3 superior facet, and an intact C1 ring and lateral mass. The requirement for instrumentation was obvious. We were able to place lateral mass screws in standard fashion at C3 on the right, as well as the left C3 and bilateral C4 lateral masses. The right C2 screw was mainly left in the C2 body as very little C2 pars and pedicle remained. A longer screw was placed (26 mm) to allow the screw head to line up with the C3-4 lateral mass screws. Though this kept the screw threads visible on the C2 screw, it was the best compromise given the amount of bony destruction. A standard C2 pars screw was placed on the left. Postoperative CT shows the final position of the hardware (Fig. 1.13). Closure proceeded in standard fashion, followed by lumbar drain placement.

The patient recovered well with no neurologic deficits. She did have persistent headaches, likely due to CSF leakage from the canal, which lasted for 1–2 months after the operation, but ultimately normalized. The wound was never threatened. Postoperative MRI (Fig. 1.14) showed gross total resection. Final pathology

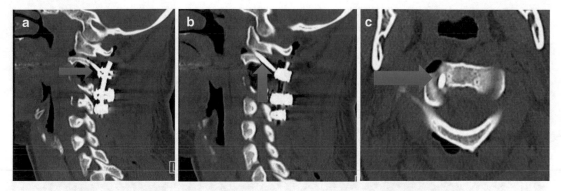

Fig. 1.13 (a) Sagittal CT noncontrast. Block arrow pointing to hybrid C2 pedicle/body screw and widened C2-3 foramen. (b) Sagittal CT noncontrast. Next cut showing C2 screw traveling into C2 body. (c) Axial CT noncontrast. C2 screw shown terminating in the C2 body with slight rostral violation above C2

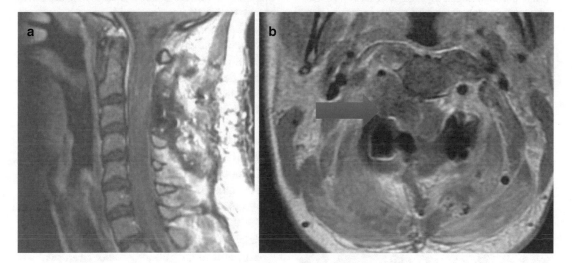

Fig. 1.14 (a) Sagittal T1 postcontrast. No evidence of residual enhancing tumor. (b) Axial T1 postcontrast. Block arrow points to extraforaminal region now filled with CSF and blood. No enhancement to suggest residual tumor. Patent vertebral artery

revealed WHO Grade I schwannoma. Nearly 5 years from surgery, there has been no tumor recurrence and the hardware remains well positioned.

Case 5: Cervical Schwannoma, Mainly Intradural

Presentation/Imaging The patient is a 56-year-old female with 2–3 months of worsening numbness in the hands and paresthesias from the elbows down. She does have pain in the same distribution, but no weakness. MRI of the cervical spine reveals a 1.5 cm homogeneously enhancing mass, ventral to the spinal cord at C4-5, with severe cord compression. There is extension of the mass rostrally out through the C3-4 foramen on the right—the mass has traveled from the C4 nerve root a level down into the canal (Fig. 1.15). There is clear widening of the right C3-4 foramen on CT that clearly establishes the foraminal-extraforaminal extent of this mass (Fig. 1.16).

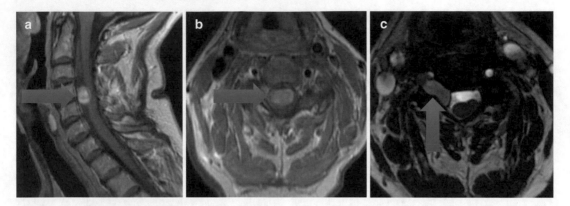

Fig. 1.15 (**a**) Sagittal T1 postcontrast. Block arrow points to enhancing intradural mass behind the C4-5 disc with cord compression. (**b**) Axial T1 postcontrast. Block arrow points to enhancing mass with a challenging ventral location. (**c**) Axial T2. Block arrow points to extraforaminal tumor extending out through the C3-4 foramen, one level above the intradural tumor location, and contacting the vertebral artery

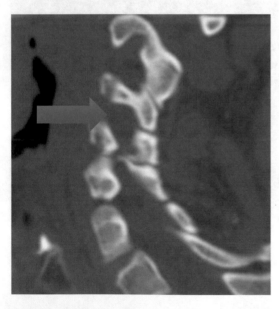

Fig. 1.16 Sagittal CT noncontrast. Block arrow points to widened C3-4 foramen on the right consistent with remodeling from schwannoma growth

Preoperative Considerations This case raises interesting questions for surgical management. It is obvious that the intradural portion of the tumor requires open surgical resection, given the patient's symptoms and degree of cord compression. But what about the extraforaminal tumor? This portion of the tumor is almost certainly clinically silent. We can confidently ascribe the patient's symptoms to the intradural mass as opposed to this smaller amount of extradural

growth. So should we resect this portion? In general, our practice has been to leave this extradural portion behind for multiple reasons, all of which contribute to increased surgical morbidity without improvement in preoperative symptoms:

1. Increase in overall surgical time and blood loss.
2. Complicated lateral dural closure increasing the chance of CSF leak and associated symptoms.
3. Facet destabilization necessitating upfront or delayed cervical fusion; in order to access the extraforaminal tumor, facet removal is required and most likely leaves the patient with gross or at least subtle instability that will worsen over time.
4. Vertebral artery injury.

We often find that this extradural portion does not even grow over the long term and, if it does, the growth tends to be very slow and responsive to focused radiation. So, in the end, our practice is to leave the extradural tumor in place, monitor for growth with annual surveillance MRI, and then to treat with stereotactic radiosurgery (SRS) if there is growth. The exception here is if the pathology does show a higher grade schwannoma (e.g. melanotic or cellular subtype) or neurofibroma, in which case we do believe adjuvant radiation is appropriate [27–29]. Please refer to Table 1.3 for a summary of this management approach.

Table 1.3 To chase or not to chase?

Factors impacting whether to resect foraminal and extraforaminal extent
1. Patient criteria: Age, co-morbidities
2. Tumor proximity to vertebral artery
3. Need for stabilization which accompanies facet removal
4. More complicated dural closure with higher rate of CSF leak
5. Spinal level—If the nerve is functionally important, sacrifice can induce deficit
6. Increased OR time with attendant risks including blood loss
7. Ominous possibility of still failing to achieve gross total resection
8. Longer recovery with possible longstanding issues related to nerve injury and fusion
9. More recent data showing SRS as an effective salvage for residual tumor

Operation This case involved standard positioning for a cervical laminectomy, as described in multiple cases in this chapter. Here, a full C4-5 laminectomy was performed with a standard midline durotomy. Upon opening the arachnoid, the tumor was not immediately visible. This was due to its ventral location in the canal. Therefore, we identified the dentate ligament in the right aspect of the canal between the spinal cord and the dura. The dentate was incised in two locations and then sutured with a 5-0 prolene to the contralateral paraspinal muscles. This safely reflected the spinal cord and allowed us to visualize the mass. There was a rather prominent rootlet along the surface of the mass likely representing a sensory C4 nerve rootlet. It was stimulated at 0.3–0.5 mA with no associated muscle firing and, therefore, was sacrificed. This allowed us direct access to the tumor surface which was cauterized and incised. Debulking was performed with ultrasonic aspiration and bipolar cauterization, with the tumor being progressively mobilized into the right aspect of the canal for continued resection. We were then able to identify the afferent nerve, also located ventral in the canal, which likely represented a C4 motor nerve rootlet. When stimulated with our monopolar probe, it was silent. Interestingly, we had an excellent view of the exiting C5 nerve below, and stimu-

lated this with clear firing of the deltoid muscle, a sort of intraoperative positive control for our probe. We therefore cauterized and cut the afferent C4 nerve. We could easily see the remaining tumor exiting out through the nerve root sleeve. It was also visible as we closed the dura, but again the decision was made, consistent with our preoperative discussion and goals, to leave this segment behind.

The patient did have slight deltoid weakness (4/5) postoperatively that completely improved by her 6 month follow-up visit. Her preoperative symptoms completely improved with no residual deficits. Postoperative MRI showed complete removal of the intradural mass with the residual foraminal mass in place (Fig. 1.17). Final pathology confirmed Grade I schwannoma. This patient has been monitored with annual MRIs for nearly 4 years—the intradural compartment shows no recurrent tumor and the extradural mass is unchanged in size (Fig. 1.18). In the event of clear growth, we will proceed to stereotactic radiotherapy.

Case 6: Cervical Schwannoma, Mainly Intradural

Presentation/Imaging This case is similar to Case 5 and we are including a brief treatment of it here as another example of how we recommend managing these lesions. This patient is 54 years old and presenting with months of worsening neck pain only. Her examination is completely benign. MRI of the cervical spine shows a nearly homogeneously enhancing mass situated behind C2 and C3, more than 3 cm in craniocaudal dimension, causing severe spinal cord compression (Fig. 1.19). There is a small portion extending out through the C2-3 foramen to the right.

Preoperative Considerations This case is slightly different than Case 5 in that more than 90% of the overall tumor volume occupies the intradural compartment, whereas in the prior case roughly 70–80% of the tumor volume was intradural. Since an intradural resection alone would represent a near total resection in this case, should we even remotely consider "chas-

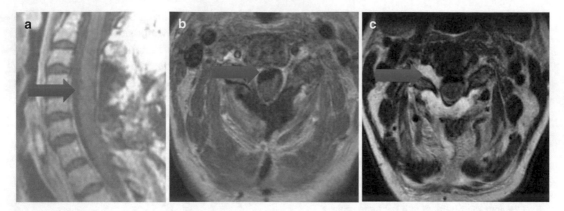

Fig. 1.17 (a) Sagittal T1 postcontrast. Block arrow points to resection site. Note slight persistent deformation of the spinal cord. No residual enhancement to suggest remaining tumor. (b) Axial T1 postcontrast. Block arrow points to resection cavity with same persistent spinal cord deflection. (c) Axial T2. Block arrow points to postoperative residual foraminal/extraforaminal tumor

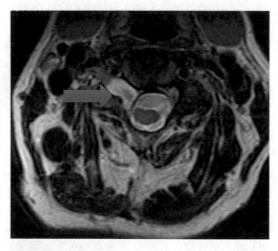

Fig. 1.18 Axial T2. MRI over 3 years from surgery shows unchanged size of the extradural schwannoma

Operation/Follow-Up The operation proceeded in similar fashion to Case 5, with the important exception being that the tumor was visible upon opening the dura. It therefore did not require sectioning of the dentate ligament and rotation of the spinal cord. There were no issues removing the entire intradural tumor after identifying and sectioning the silent afferent nerve rootlet (Fig. 1.20). Postoperatively, there was ultimately complete improvement in preoperative neck pain. Immediate postoperative MRI confirmed complete removal of the intradural portion. Pathology was Grade I schwannoma. We also present an MRI from 2 years later that shows no change to the residual extradural tumor, which we will continue to monitor for growth (Fig. 1.21).

ing" the foraminal tumor? The vertebral artery is less in play here than above, and perhaps enough of the right C2-3 facet can be preserved to avoid fusion. Obviously the patient's young age and high performance status influence us to consider the benefit of a complete resection. In the end, we applied our basic principle of removing the intradural portion and leaving the foraminal portion behind in keeping with the rationale laid out in Case 5.

Case 7: Cervical Neurofibroma, More Extradural than Intradural

Presentation/Imaging The patient is a 46-year-old female with 3 months of progressive symptoms. Initially, she noticed pain in the neck radiating down the left arm into the hand, accompanied by tingling in the hand as well. Over the past month, she has noticed weakness in the left arm as well as the left leg, with occasional stumbling. Her ambulation from the left leg weakness became so acutely

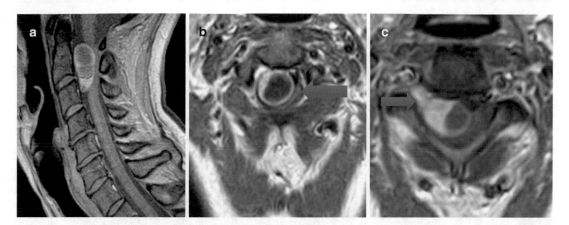

Fig. 1.19 (**a**) Sagittal T1 postcontrast. Large intradural mass with some heterogeneity causing significant cord compression. (**b**) Axial T1 postcontrast. Rim enhancement and spinal cord deflection to the left. The block arrow points to the extremely attenuated spinal cord. (**c**) Axial T1 postcontrast. Block arrow points to the extradural tumor traveling out through the right C2-3 foramen

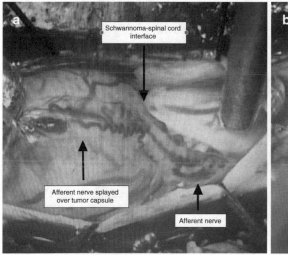
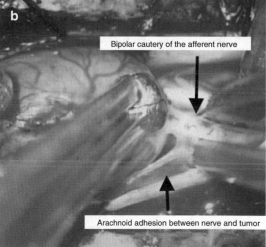

Fig. 1.20 (**a**) Intraoperative photo showing the intradural schwannoma and its afferent nerve. The spinal cord is deflected. Note the continuation of the afferent nerve along the tumor surface, though severely attenuated and splayed. Also note the hyper-vascularity of the afferent nerve surface. (**b**) Bipolar cauterization of the afferent nerve as a precursor to disconnection and subsequent tumor removal

severe that she was admitted through the ER. MRI of the cervical spine revealed a large heterogeneously enhancing mass at C6-7 with a rim-enhancing intradural component, a non-enhancing foraminal component, and a large enhancing component with cystic elements extending extraforaminal into the scalene musculature of the neck (Fig. 1.22). There is clear spinal cord compression and expansion of the left C6-7 foramen.

Preoperative Considerations This is a uniquely complicated mass. We think it is fairly obvious that the effort to achieve a gross total resection of this is not worth the morbidity. The tumor extent into the neck musculature would require a separate anterior approach (jointly with an ENT head and neck surgeon) and likely would involve nerve root sacrifice with possible postoperative deficits.

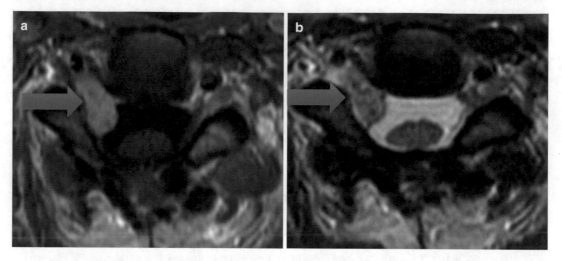

Fig. 1.21 (**a**) Axial T1 postcontrast. Block arrow points to residual enhancing extradural tumor in the right C2-3 foramen. Unchanged in size compared to the initial post-operative MRI. (**b**) Axial T2. Block arrow points to the same residual tumor

To re-emphasize, the source of this patient's symptoms is mainly from spinal cord compression. Removing the intradural component is therefore the goal, though in this case, the intradural component represents less of the overall tumor volume than its extradural counterpart. This will decompress the spinal cord, likely alleviate symptoms, and provide a diagnosis. The effort to remove the foraminal and extraforaminal portions was regarded as too morbid in this case.

Operation The positioning and approach were standard in this case, which included a C6-7 laminectomy and midline durotomy. The tumor did have multiple sensory nerve rootlets draped over it. We stimulated these to confirm lack of motor response and cauterized and incised them. As we debulked the tumor, we identified a thicker exiting nerve rootlet caudal to the mass that did have multiple rootlets entering into it. We stimulated this root at a low setting with the monopolar probe, from 0.3 to 0.5 mA, with clear and reproducible activation of the left brachioradialis and hand muscles (opponens pollicis and flexor digiti minimi). This nerve was therefore preserved and the resection completed. Interestingly, we were able to angle our tumor forceps out through the exiting sleeve and a decent amount of additional

tumor was removed in this fashion. We did not pursue the extradural tumor which was not readily visible in the canal and would have required facet removal for exposure as anticipated.

Postoperatively, the patient did well with near complete resolution of arm and leg strength as well as the radicular pain. There remained residual neck pain even 1 year after surgery. Postoperative MRI showed removal of the intradural component with partial removal of the foraminal component (Fig. 1.23). Pathology revealed a neurofibroma with a focally high ki67 index of 10%. Given the significant amount of residual tumor, the patient's young age, and the final pathology of neurofibroma with high ki67, we recommended adjuvant fractionated radiation in this case, which the patient tolerated well [30].

Extradural Schwannomas (with Significant Foraminal Extent)

In this last section, we present three cases of schwannomas that are purely extradural in location, but with invasion into the spinal canal and foramen. As noted earlier, it is this growth into the canal with resulting compression of spinal cord and/or nerve roots that leads to symptoms. This accounts for why purely extraforaminal

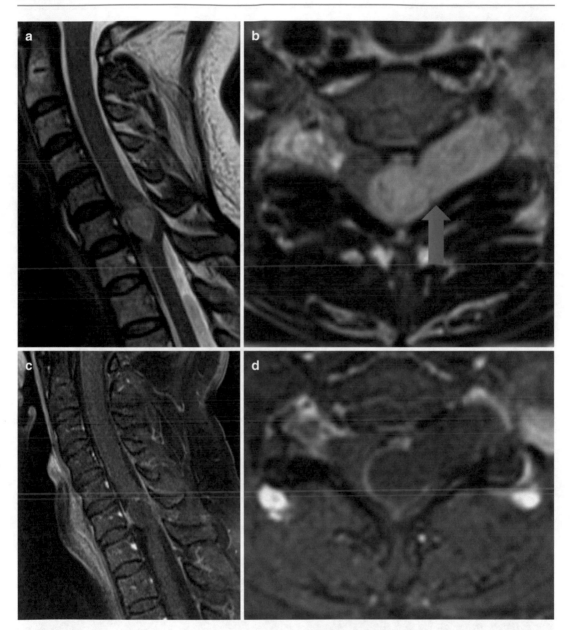

Fig. 1.22 (a) Sagittal T2. Hyperintense mass (intradural component) causing spinal cord deformation mainly behind the C6 body. (b) Axial T2. Spinal cord compression and deflection to the right. Hyperintense mass visualized in the intradural compartment, extending through the foramen. There appears to be a "waist" which is indicated by the block arrow and likely delineates the intra from extradural portion. (c) Sagittal T1 postcontrast. The intradural portion is seen with faint rim-enhancement. (d) Axial T1 postcontrast. The rim enhancement is best seen on the right aspect of the tumor along the spinal cord interface. The foraminal component shows no clear enhancement. (e) Axial T1 postcontrast. Block arrow points to the avidly enhancing extraforaminal component that has extended into the neck muscles. (f) Axial T1 post-contrast. Another view of the extraforaminal component. Here the block arrow indicates a cystic portion of the tumor and its farthest reach into the neck muscles

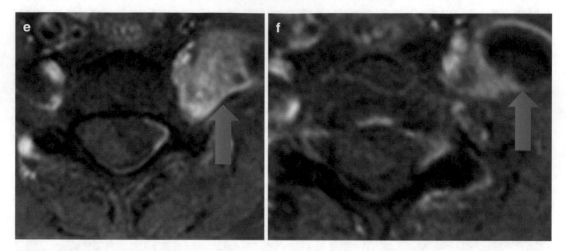

Fig. 1.22 (continued)

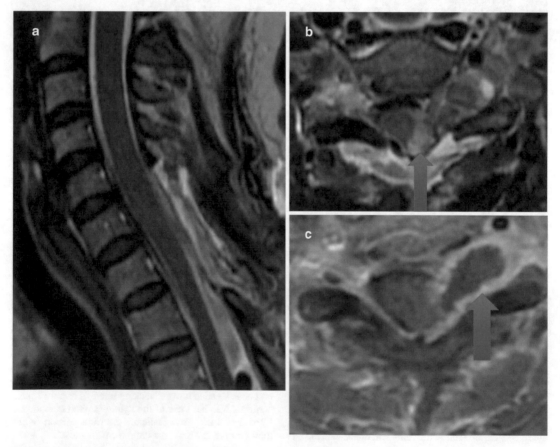

Fig. 1.23 (a) Sagittal T2. Postoperative MRI shows evacuation of the intradural mass. (b) Axial T2. Block arrow points to resection cavity. (c) Axial T1 postcontrast. Block arrow points to removal of tumor within the fora-men that was accomplished by reaching out through the nerve root sleeve. This was done to reduce the overall tumor burden for anticipated radiation planning

schwannomas, which are not covered in this chapter, can become incredibly large before reaching clinical attention, if ever. It also accounts for why most intraforaminal schwannomas are clinically silent, and if discovered in the setting of low back pain and/or sciatica, should be very carefully endeavored upon as the mass is most likely NOT the source of the symptom.

Case 8: Cervical, Extradural

Presentation/Imaging The patient is a 56-year-old female presenting with a primary symptom of neck pain ongoing for many months. More recently, over the course of weeks, she has developed imbalance secondary to right leg and foot weakness. MRI of the cervical spine reveals a large 3.2 cm heterogeneously enhancing mass at C1-2 causing severe spinal cord compression and deflection to the right. There is a dumbbell shape to this mass as it partially exits and expands the left C1-2 foramen (Fig. 1.24).

Operation The positioning and approach were standard in this case, involving an incision from the suboccipital region to just below C2. Even before a C1-2 laminectomy was performed, the tumor was visible. We began to debulk the extra-dural tumor with bipolar cauterization and ultra-sonic aspiration. Initially, we could not visualize the dura. We continued to debulk the tumor, which allowed us to identify the exiting C3 nerve root inferiorly, followed by the portion of C2 nerve (the efferent nerve) exiting the tumor far laterally. Ultimately, enough tumor was removed to identify the dura medially. We then mobilized the remaining tumor, which remained ventral and lateral to the dura, further laterally and identified the afferent C2 nerve exiting from the dura itself. There was a 1 cm segment of normal afferent C2 nerve between the dura and the tumor. We did not stimulate the nerve as it was the C2 nerve which could be sacrificed with no motor and likely only minimal sensory deficit. This allowed us to place

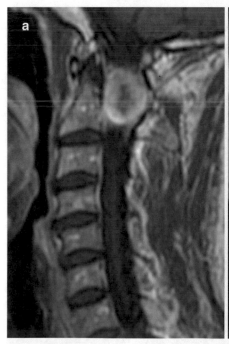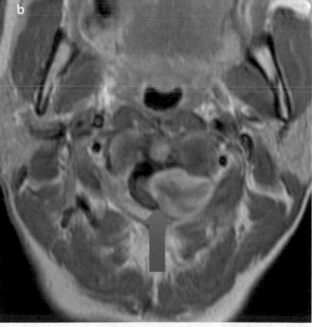

Fig. 1.24 (**a**) Sagittal T1 postcontrast. Large heterogeneously enhancing mass at C1-2. (**b**) Axial T1 postcontrast. Block arrow points to the mass-spinal cord interface. There is attenuation of the spinal cord as it is shifted to the right. The mass abuts the lamina on the left and exits into the foramen, though it stops well short of the vertebral artery. It is difficult to differentiate how much of the mass is intradural vs. extradural from this MRI, but a clue is the extent to which the borders of the mass go beyond the presumed circumference of the dura within the canal. The fact there is foraminal extension and laminar contact are also indicators of a primarily extradural location

two separate 2-0 silk ties between the origin of the tumor and the exit of the afferent C2 nerve. Cutting between the ties thus freed the tumor and we completed its extrication from the extradural/foraminal compartment for a gross total resection. We did not open the dura and search for more tumor, given the clear demarcation between the afferent nerve and the mass. Be aware of brisk bleeding in this C1-2 location from the vertebral venous plexus and compressed foraminal veins–SurgiFlo and gelfoam are often more helpful than bipolar cauterization.

Postoperatively, the patient complained of persistent neck pain, but there was interval improvement of her leg weakness and balance. Immediate postoperative MRI confirmed complete tumor removal (Fig. 1.25). Final pathology revealed a schwannoma but with some neurofibroma elements. Given the patient's age and gross total resection, we opted for annual surveillance MRIs as opposed to adjuvant radiation.

Case 9: Thoracic, Extradural

Presentation/Imaging The patient is a 61-year-old female who had 2–3 years of occasional numbness traveling down the right hip and leg region. This has become worse over the past few months and is now accompanied by flank pain radiating from the left mid-back region around into the trunk below the breast. These symptoms prompted an outpatient thoracic MRI, revealing a large 3 cm homogeneously enhancing mass at T6 with a dumbbell shape and extension out through the left T6 foramen. The spinal cord is severely pancaked along with deflection anteriorly and to the right. There is a strong suggestion of the mass being purely extradural, as there is capping of the dorsal epidural fat (Fig. 1.26).

Operation Standard prone positioning on an open Jackson table was performed. A midline incision was made allowing visualization of the

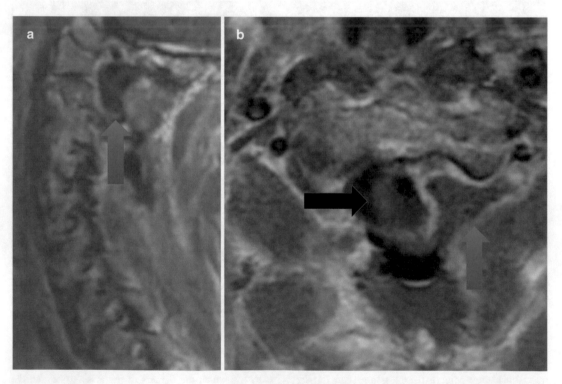

Fig. 1.25 (**a**) Sagittal T1 postcontrast. Block arrow points to the resection cavity. (**b**) Axial T1 postcontrast. Black block arrow points to a slightly re-expanded spinal cord. Blue block arrow points to resection cavity with no residual enhancement

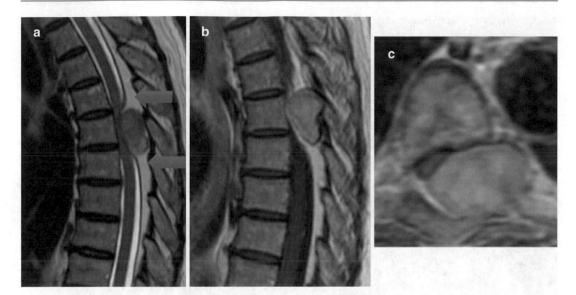

Fig. 1.26 (**a**) Sagittal T2. Large hyperintense mass causing severe spinal cord compression at T6. Arrows point to epidural fat capping above and below the tumor indicative of an extradural location. (**b**) Sagittal T1 postcontrast. Mass with homogeneous enhancement. (**c**) Axial T1 post-contrast. Dumbbell shape with dramatic spinal cord flattening and extension of the mass into the extraforaminal zone as well (beyond the lateral edge of the T6 vertebral body)

T5-7 spinous processes and subsequent T6 laminectomy with partial T5 and T7 laminectomies. The tumor was immediately visible in the spinal canal. The same technique of bipolar cauterization of the surface and internal debulking with suction, tumor forceps, and ultrasonic aspiration was performed. We then removed the inferior aspect of the T6 facet along with the superior aspect of the T7 facet on the left to increase exposure of the tumor in the foramen. The inferior extent of the tumor was encountered earliest, followed by the superior plane up against the T6 pedicle and remaining facet. We then reflected the tumor away from the dura. The exiting T6 nerve root feeding into the tumor was identified, cauterized, and incised. We intentionally left a plug of residual tumor at the exiting nerve root sleeve so as not to cause a CSF leak that is typically challenging to repair.

The lateral border was then approached and there appeared to be some adhesions between the tumor capsule and the pleura, as well as rib head. These were easily dissected away with a Rhoton microdissector and then the remaining tumor was lifted out en bloc.

We did perform a small intradural exploration for any additional tumor. The durotomy was created in standard fashion. We were able to explore the zone of the exiting T6 nerve root by gently retracting the arachnoid and spinal cord with a microdissector. There did appear to be a small amount of intradural tumor that we incised away from the afferent nerve and subsequently cauterized. Again we left a plug of tumor within the nerve root sleeve to avoid the increased morbidity of a protracted lateral dural closure and CSF leak.

Postoperatively, the patient experienced symptom improvement across the board, though it did take 4–6 months. She did always complain of occasional incisional soreness. Final pathology showed Grade 1 schwannoma. Immediate postoperative MRI showed a gross total resection and there has been no recurrence on surveillance MRIs for 4 years (Fig. 1.27). We did not recommend upfront fusion here despite disarticulating the T6-7 facet complex on the left due to the location of the mass in the mid-thoracic region and

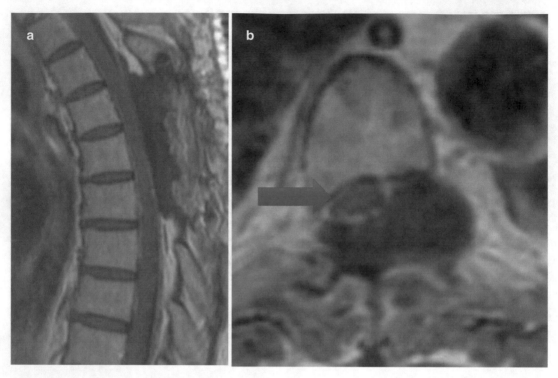

Fig. 1.27 (**a**) Sagittal T1 postcontrast. Resection cavity demonstrated with no residual enhancement. (**b**) Axial T1 postcontrast. Block arrow points to partially re-expanded spinal cord. No evidence of residual tumor in the resection cavity

the belief that a unilateral facet disruption would not lead to long-term instability. The patient, though, was counseled about this in advance and was aware that a future stabilizing surgery, such as a percutaneous pedicle screw construct, might be required.

Case 10: Lumbar, Extradural

Presentation/Imaging This is a 68-year-old female who presented a few months earlier with relatively sudden onset pain radiating down the right leg in a classic sciatic distribution. She underwent PT with significant improvement in her pain. However, her physiatrist was concerned enough by her residual pain to order an MRI. This lumbar MRI revealed a nearly 4.5 cm homogeneously enhancing mass, mainly situated at the level of L3, causing scalloping of the L3 vertebral body with extension out through the L3 foramen on the right. There is near complete obliteration of the thecal sac. Its appearance was strongly suggestive of a giant schwannoma (Fig. 1.28). We ultimately recommended surgery, despite her relative lack of symptoms, due to its impressive size, the patient's high level of current functional independence, her relatively young age, and the degree of nerve root compression. The plan was for tumor resection accompanied by L2-4 fusion given the amount of right L3 pedicle and right L2-3 facet destruction.

Operation Standard prone positioning on an open Jackson table was performed. A midline incision over the L2-4 spinous processes was performed. A complete L2 and L3 laminectomy was done with a partial L4 laminectomy. We also removed the right inferior L2 and superior L3 facets at this stage. The tumor was immediately visible in the right aspect of the canal, though there was some of the thecal sac stretched over the dorsal aspect of the tumor that we swept to the left using microdissectors. This allowed an unobstructed corridor to the tumor. We debulked

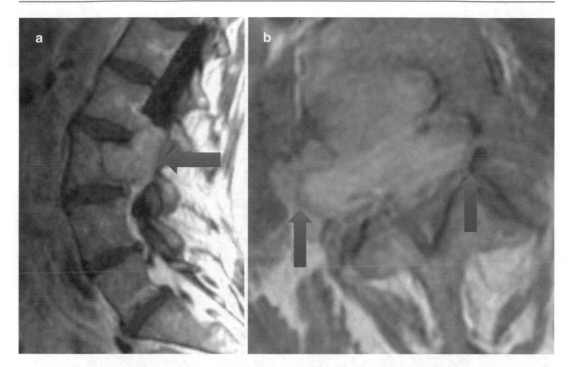

Fig. 1.28 (**a**) Sagittal T1 postcontrast. Block arrow points to large homogeneously enhancing mass with scalloping of the L3 vertebral body. (**b**) Axial T1 postcontrast. Block arrows point to the lateral limits of the mass. The thecal sac cannot be visualized and can therefore be regarded as obliterated. The mass extends into the L3 vertebral body and out through the foramen as well

the tumor progressively, using ultrasonic aspiration as the main tool. The major initial steps were to progressively mobilize and roll the ventral portions of the tumor into our resection cavity at various points during the debulking. We then were able to identify what appeared to be the L2 nerve root exiting under the right L2 pedicle, but we later realized this was just the L3 nerve root dramatically displaced rostrally by the mass. Monopolar stimulation did NOT lead to any muscle activity, indicating its electrophysiologic silence.

Soon we identified the tumor takeoff from the lateral aspect of the thecal sac, which had been violated during our dissection and was already leaking CSF. There was no evidence of intradural tumor extension as we cleared the exiting nerve root sleeve vicinity. There was a clear afferent nerve extending, perhaps from the axilla itself, into the tumor. This was stimulated, noted to be silent, and taken. The L3 nerve that had been identified earlier was re-stimulated and sacrificed as well. This was a key decision, as it completely opened up our working corridor at the possible price of postoperative L3 weakness despite the lack of muscle contraction with stimulation. We then were able to foist the remaining tumor out of the foramen and extraforaminal compartment using an upgoing curette and tumor forceps. A large piece was thus removed en bloc for a gross total resection.

We were able to use a portion of the incised L3 nerve root as a patch for the lateral dural closure using 4-0 silk suture in three interrupted sites. No CSF was encountered after Valsalva maneuver. We then proceeded to insert robot-guided pedicle screws at L2-4 on the left and L2 and L4 on the right, skipping L3, given the pedicle erosion.

Immediate postoperative MRI showed gross total resection with the implants in appropriate position (Fig. 1.29). Grade 1 schwannoma was the final pathology. The patient had a very mild

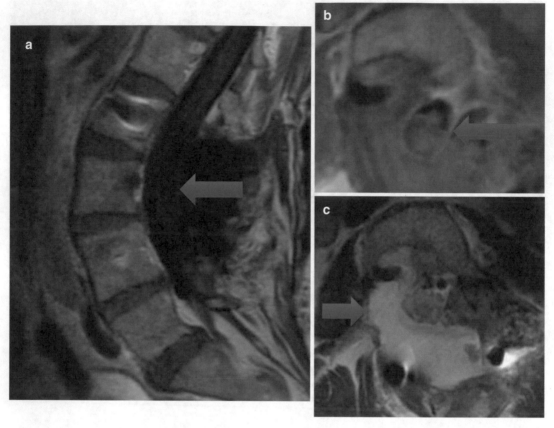

Fig. 1.29 (**a**) Sagittal T1 postcontrast. Block arrow points to resection cavity with no residual enhancement to suggest tumor. (**b**) Axial T1 postcontrast. Block arrow points to re-expanded thecal sac with now visible cauda equina nerve roots. Also no evidence of residual enhancement. (**c**) Axial T2. Block arrow points to fluid-filled resection cavity with re-expanded thecal sac

quadriceps weakness on the right, but was already independently ambulatory at her one-month postoperative visit. Subsequent MRIs out to 3 years show no tumor recurrence. She complains of persistent low back soreness, but her right leg strength is normal and there have been no episodes of her original radiating pain.

Extradural Schwannomas: Additional Considerations

In this section, we want to discuss considerations for fusion and the intracapsular technique for extradural schwannoma removal. Also included is a brief discussion of asymptomatic tumors and strategies for treating residual and recurrent schwannomas.

The Question of Upfront Fusion

Case 10 presented a giant schwannoma which is admittedly a very rare phenomenon. What we do see more frequently, and almost always incidentally, are extradural schwannomas in the lumbar region (less so thoracic) involving the foramen with varying degrees of extraforaminal extent. These are mainly intraforaminal tumors. The process of removing these schwannomas always involves the decision of whether to perform an upfront instrumented fusion. Typically, fusion is performed because adequate visualization of the foraminal portion involves removing the facet, which is often regarded as a destabilizing maneuver, even on a unilateral basis. Facetectomy of equal to or more than 50% is the general threshold for fusion. Upfront instrumentation is ultimately the surgeon's choice and, if not initially pursued, can be easily salvaged with a future operation, perhaps via minimally invasive percutaneous pedicle screw fixation [31–33].

Of note, minimally invasive (MIS) approaches with tubular retractor systems have gained traction over recent years [34]. Especially for purely extraforaminal schwannomas, the facet can be completely spared, thereby obviating the need for instrumentation. The major limitation with this approach is that nerve stimulation and monitoring can be very challenging. For those neurosurgeons comfortable with these approaches, they should be considered for symptomatic and/or growing extradural lumbar schwannomas. Lateral retroperitoneal approaches have also become an option in the lumbar region for schwannoma resection, as the more common XLIF/DLIF operation has become more widely adopted for degenerative spine pathology [35]. Please refer to Chap. 10 where MIS approaches are described in detail.

Intracapsular Approach

Now the issue of whether to sacrifice the involved lumbar nerve root, especially in the lower lumbar region (L3-S1), can be a source of great concern for surgeon and patient as well. Though, as noted above, sacrificing the entire involved nerve is unlikely to lead to a significant deficit, the mere possibility of a major deficit can be quite ominous. Ergo, the oft adopted approach of tumor "enucleation," also known as an "intracapsular" approach, to schwannoma removal. Essentially, the capsule of the tumor is opened in longitudinal fashion and the schwannoma is shelled out of the capsule, often en bloc, while leaving the remainder of the nerve fascicles intact. Peripheral nerve schwannomas are often approached in this fashion. Giant spinal schwannomas, along with some purely extradural schwannomas and select intradural schwannomas, can be subjects for an intra-

capsular dissection. This approach has the disadvantage of leaving the capsule behind, which does have some neoplastic potential, albeit low [29, 36]. But the act of enucleating the tumor confers adequate symptom relief and long-term tumor control [27, 37].

Here is a case (Case 11) of a 36-year-old female with a right S1 schwannoma that appeared to correlate to symptoms of intermittent leg pain over a ten year period, worsening over the past year with about 1–2 mm growth on 6 month MRI (Fig. 1.30). We performed a right S1 hemilaminectomy and then visualized the tumor and the afferent S1 nerve feeding into it. We were also able to identify the S2 nerve at the dorsal and inferior boundary of the mass. We stimulated both nerves with clear muscle activation at low thresholds (0.3–0.5 milliamps). We also stimulated the tumor surface without any muscle activation, indicating that this was a silent fascicle and there were no active fascicles near our field. The tumor surfaced was cauterized, incised, and internal debulking proceeded. At a very early stage, we were able to use microdissectors to develop a plane superiorly and laterally between the tumor and its capsule. Then followed dissection off of the medial and inferior capsule. A complete en bloc enucleation was achieved. Re-stimulation of the S1 nerve showed no change in downstream muscle activation. Postoperative MRI showed minimal residual enhancement (likely the capsule and not actual tumor) and the patient was neurologically intact (Fig. 1.31).

Asymptomatic Schwannomas

The objective of this section is simply to point out that patients often harbor remarkably large extradural schwannomas without any evidence of symptomatology. As long as the growth is concentrated outside of the spinal canal, these masses can escape clinical detection for years. This phenomenon can be explained by the exceptionally indolent growth rates of these tumors, which collectively is around 1–3 mm per year (5% volume), and in certain tumors a growth plateau is likely reached [38, 39]. Of note, schwannomas

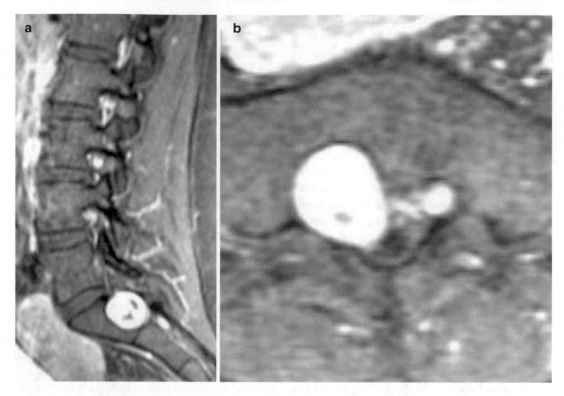

Fig. 1.30 (**a**) Sagittal T1 postcontrast. Nearly 2.5 cm right S1 mass with homogeneous enhancement and some remodeling of the sacrum. (**b**) Axial T1 postcontrast. The mass appears to abut and slightly deform the thecal sac

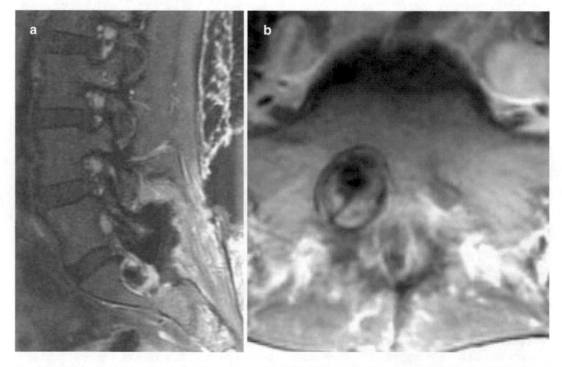

Fig. 1.31 (**a**) Sagittal T1 postcontrast. Interval enucleation of the mass with some linear residual enhancement posteriorly, most consistent with tumor capsule. (**b**) Axial T1 postcontrast. Posterior enhancement redemonstrated but >90% removal of the original enhancement/tumor

with a heterogeneous contrast pattern on MRI may have a higher tendency for growth than those with homogeneous enhancement, likely related to cyst expansion in the former [40]. The burden for offering surgery remains high in these cases: the combination of high surgical morbidity and lack of preoperative symptoms makes the risk-benefit profile difficult to accept. We do advocate CT-guided biopsy in certain cases to verify the schwannoma diagnosis. In patients with a known history of cancer, or if the lesion has some concerning MRI findings, a CT-guided biopsy is a low risk intervention that can help to establish diagnosis. Once the schwannoma diagnosis is verified, the neurosurgeon can then comfortably proceed to annual surveillance.

In general, we do not automatically proceed to surgery even if there is evidence of growth. This remains a multifactorial decision based on patient's age, desires, medical conditions, tumor size, and tumor location. Upfront radiation enters the equation for tumors that require a major operation for removal, especially in some patients who are older and have medical issues. The best available evidence is for stereotactic radiosurgery (SRS) via the CyberKnife platform [41, 42]. Symptom improve-

ment and long-term radiographic control have been reported in tumors treated with SRS alone [43]. We feel that as first-line therapy, SRS is most applicable to intraforaminal schwannomas that have demonstrated growth in patients who are less than ideal surgical candidates. Tumors circumscribed within the foramen nearly always necessitate upfront fusion, and SRS is a reasonable way of managing these lesions without putting the patient through an operation for both lesion removal and stabilization [44, 45]. Extraforaminal (or paravertebral) schwannomas, due to their greater volume on average, are often too large for single fraction or hypofractionated SRS and require a more conventional radiation scheme [46]. Please refer to Chap. 8 for more detailed considerations of radiotherapy.

To re-emphasize, if the patient does develop neurologic symptoms clearly referable to the schwannoma, then the calculus changes. Barring this, we have to resist the urge to be absolute in our indications when it comes to extradural schwannomas, and really spinal schwannomas in general. The final figure (Fig. 1.32) shows four incidentally discovered extradural schwannomas that have shown minimal to no radiographic pro-

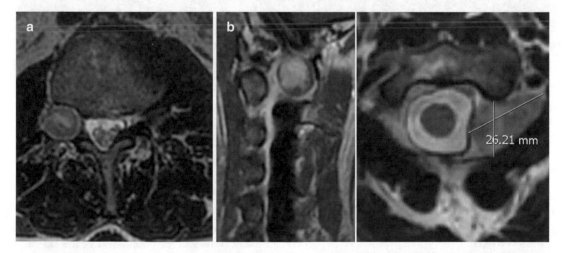

Fig. 1.32 (**a**) Axial T2. 66-year-old male presenting with sudden onset left leg pain that improved over weeks, lumbar MRI revealed a 2.5 cm R L2-3 cm extradural schwannoma, stable over 2 years. (**b**) Sagittal T1 postcontrast and axial T2. 41-year-old male with an episode of severe neck pain that improved, cervical MRI revealed a 2.6 cm L C1-2 extradural schwannoma, stable over 3 years. (**c**)

Sagittal and axial T1 postcontrast. 61-year-old male with low back pain that resolved, lumbar MRI revealed a 5.5 cm R L1-2 extradural schwannoma, stable over two years. (**d**) Sagittal and axial T2. 85-year-old male underwent lumbar MRI after a fall, revealed a 4 cm L L4 cystic schwannoma now stable over 6 years

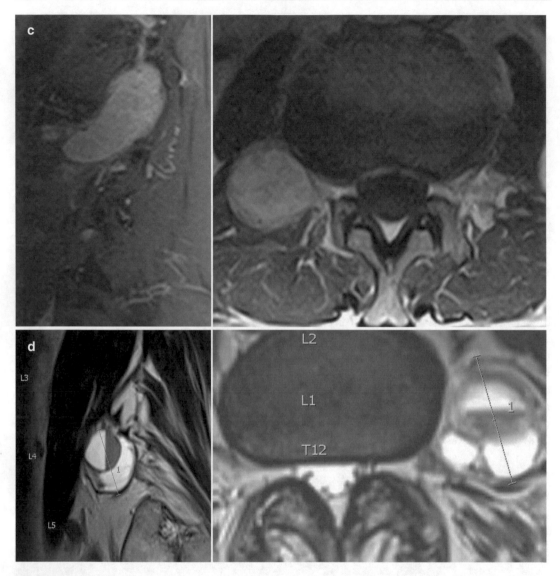

Fig. 1.32 (continued)

gression, validating the plan for continued surveillance in keeping with the logic espoused
above.

Recurrence

A brief note on the recurrence of spinal schwannomas. The collective recurrence rate for spinal
schwannomas is often regarded as around 5%,
but is clearly much lower for those tumors that
are completely removed along with their nerve

roots of origin, and higher for certain pathologic
subtypes of schwannoma as well as subtotally
resected schwannomas, including intracapsular
resections [47]. Even in subtotally resected
schwannomas, more than 70% remain stable,
but that number can be skewed based on ki67
index (>5%) and sheer volume of residual tumor
left behind at the initial surgery [7]. Adjuvant
SRS can be pursued based on pathology
(schwannoma subtype and ki67) and extent of
residual along with patient age. If adjuvant SRS
is withheld, we typically recommend surveil-

Table 1.4 Recurrent/residual schwannomas—our general guidelines

1.	Near total resection (>90%), older patient (>65), and normal ki67 (1–2%): Annual MRI
2.	Near or subtotal resection, older patient, and elevated ki67 (>5%): 6-month MRI with SRS upon progression
3.	Near total resection, young patient, normal Ki67: annual MRI
4.	Near or subtotal resection, young patient, elevated ki67: consider adjuvant SRS
5.	Residual neurofibroma and young patient: consider adjuvant SRS

lance MRIs on a 6 month basis. In those cases where a gross total resection was achieved, or a near total resection with a low ki67 on final pathology, annual surveillance MRIs are appropriate. Depending on patient age, usually a five-year surveillance window with no growth is adequate, but this can be extended based on surgeon preference. Our goal is to capture the recurrence at an early enough stage so that SRS can be considered as opposed to repeat open surgery. Please refer to Table 1.4 for a summary of our general approach to residual/recurrent tumors. There remains no medical therapy for schwannomas, though a recent case report noted the incidental regression of a spinal schwannoma in a patient being treated with a chemotherapeutic drug for multiple myeloma [48]. Perhaps there will be more serendipitous discoveries like this as immunotherapy and anti-angiogenic drugs continue to emerge.

Conclusions

Schwannomas of the spinal canal are a uniquely neurosurgical entity. Due to variations in size, location, and relationship to involved nervous structures, there are individual challenges associated with the surgical removal of these lesions. We hope that our categorical breakdown and case illustrations will help to clarify the various surgical and nonsurgical strategies at the neurosurgeon's disposal. Though schwannomas are, for the most part, forgiving tumors, we strongly recommend a restrained approach when attempting resection. Neurosurgeons must keep in mind the indolent growth pattern of this benign entity before taking unnecessary surgical risks in the name of gross total resection. Very often, the patient will experience considerable symptom relief from a significant debulking of the intradural component alone. Coupled with advances in radiosurgery platforms, these facts make it increasingly difficult to justify chasing the foraminal and extraforaminal extent of these tumors. With the proliferation of lumbar MRIs for such common symptoms as low back and sciatic pain, more incidental schwannomas will be encountered than ever. It will be the role of the neurosurgeon to regard these tumors judiciously and to resist the siren call of operating, especially given the generally straightforward and satisfying nature of these surgeries. Our patients will appreciate us for it.

References

1. Conti P, Pansini G, Mouchaty H, Capuano C, Conti R. Spinal neurinomas: retrospective analysis and long-term outcome of 179 consecutively operated cases and review of the literature. Surg Neurol. 2004;61:34–43.
2. Mautner VF, Tatagiba M, Lindenau M, Funsterer C, Pulst SM, Baser ME, Kluwe L, Zanella FE. Spinal tumors in patients with neurofibromatosis type 2: MR imaging study of frequency, multiplicity, and variety. AJR Am J Roentgenol. 1995;165:951–5.
3. Koeller KK, Shih R. Intradural extramedullary spinal neoplasms: radiologic-pathologic correlation. Radiographics. 2019;39:468–90.
4. Li P, Zhao F, Zhang J, Wang Z, Wang X, Wang B, Yang Z, Yang J, Gao Z, Liu P. Clinical features of spinal schwannomas in 65 patients with schwannomatosis compared with 831 with solitary schwannomas and 102 with neurofibromatosis type 2: a retrospective study at a single institution. J Neurosurg Spine. 2016;24:145–54.
5. Alexiev BA, Chou PM, Jennings LJ. Pathology of melanotic schwannoma. Arch Pathol Lab Med. 2018;142:1517–23.
6. Kurtkaya-Yapicier O, Scheithauer B, Woodruff JM. The pathologic spectrum of schwannomas. Histol Histopathol. 2003;18:925–34.
7. Sohn S, Chung CK, Park S-H, Kim E-S, Kim K-J, Kim CH. The fate of spinal schwannomas following subtotal resection: a retrospective multicenter study by the Korea spinal oncology research group. J Neuro-Oncol. 2013;114:345–51.

8. Kodama Y, Terae S, Hida K, Chu BC, Kaneko K, Miyasaka K. Intramedullary schwannoma of the spinal cord: report of two cases. Neuroradiology. 2001;43:567–71.

9. Saito T, Steinke H. The dorsal rootlets, ventral rootlets, spinal nerve, and rami. In: Tubbs RS, Rizk E, Shoja M, Loukas M, Barbaro N, Spinner EJ, editors. Nerves and nerve injuries: Vol 1: history, embryology, anatomy, imaging, and diagnostics. 1st ed. New York: Elsevier; 2015. p. 451–69.

10. Kim P, Ebersold MJ, Onofrio BM, Quast LM. Surgery of spinal nerve schwannoma: risk of neurological deficit after resection of involved root. J Neurosurg. 1989;71:810–4.

11. Celli P. Treatment of relevant nerve roots involved in nerve sheath tumors: removal or preservation? Neurosurgery. 2002;51:684–92.

12. Lenzi J, Anichini G, Landi A, Piciocchi A, Passacantilli E, Pedace F, Delfini R, Santoro A. Spinal nerves schwannomas: experience on 367 cases – historic overview on how clinical, radiological, and surgical practices have changed over a course of 60 years. Neurol Res Int. 2017;1:1–12.

13. Seppala MT, Haltia MJJ, Sankila RJ, Jaaskelainen JE, Heishanen O. Long-term outcome after removal of spinal schwannoma: a clinicopathological study of 187 cases. J Neurosurg. 1995;83:621–6.

14. Satoh N, Ueda Y, Koizumi M, Takeshima T, Iida J, Shigematsu K, Shigematsu H, Matsumori H, Tanaka Y. Assessment of pure single nerve root resection in the treatment of spinal schwannoma: focus on solitary spinal schwannomas located below the thoracolumbar junction. J Orthop Sci. 2011;16:148–55.

15. Hasegawa M, Fujisawa H, Hayashi Y, Tachibana O, Kida S, Yamashita J. Surgical pathology of spinal schwannoma: has the nerve of its origin been preserved or already degenerated during tumor growth? Clin Neuropathol. 2005;24:19–25.

16. Celli P, Trillo G, Ferrante L. Spinal extradural schwannoma. J Neurosurg. 2005;2:447–56.

17. Liu WC, Choi G, Lee SH, Han H, Lee JY, Jeon YH, Park HS, Park JY, Paeng SS. Radiological findings of spinal schwannomas and meningiomas: focus on discrimination of two disease entities. Eur Radiol. 2009;19:2707–15.

18. Parmar HA, Ibrahim M, Castillo M, Mukherji SK. Pictorial essay: diverse imaging features of spinal schwannomas. J Comput Assist Tomogr. 2007;31:329–34.

19. Sridhar K, Ramamurthi R, Vasudevan MC, Ramamurthi B. Giant invasive spinal schwannomas: definition and surgical management. J Neurosurg. 2001;94:210–5.

20. Sun I, Pamir MN. Non-syndromic spinal schwannomas: a novel classification. Front Neurol. 2017;8:1–9.

21. Safaee MM, Lyon R, Barbaro NM, Chou D, Mummaneni PV, Weinstein PR, Chin CT, Tihan T, Ames CP. Neurological outcomes and surgical complications in 221 spinal nerve sheath tumors. J Neurosurg Spine. 2017;26:103–11.

22. Prada F, Vetrano IG, Filippini A, Del Bene M, Perin A, Casali C, Legnani F, Saini M, DiMeco F. Intraoperative ultrasound in spinal tumor surgery. J Ultrasound. 2014;17:195–202.

23. Agrawal BM, Birch B, McCormick PC, Resnick DK. Intradural extramedullary spinal lesions. In: Benzel EC, editor. Spine surgery - techniques, complication avoidance, & management. 3rd ed. Philadelphia: Elsevier; 2012. p. 991–8.

24. Ozawa H, Kokubun S, Aizawa T, Hoshikawa T, Kawahara C. Spinal dumbbell tumors: an analysis of a series of 118 cases. J Neurosurg. 2007;7:587–93.

25. McCormick PC. Surgical management of dumbbell and paraspinal tumors of the thoracic and lumbar spine. Neurosurgery. 1996;38:67–75.

26. McCormick PC. Resection of a cervical dumbbell schwannoma with stabilization through a single stage extended posterior approach. Neurosurg Focus (suppl 2) 2014;37:Video 2.

27. Ito K, Aoyama T, Kuroiwa M, Horiuchi T, Hongo K. Surgical strategy and results of treatment for dumbbell-shaped spinal neurinoma with a posterior approach. Br J Neurosurg. 2014;28:324–9.

28. Kufeld M, Wowra B, Muacevic A, Zausinger S, Tonn J-C. Radiosurgery of spinal meningiomas and schwannomas. Technol Cancer Res Treat. 2012;11: 27–34.

29. Sowash M, Barzilai O, Kahn S, McLaughlin L, Boland P, Bilsky M, Laufer I. Clinical outcomes following resection of giant spinal schwannomas: a case series of 32 patients. J Neurosurg Spine. 2017;26:494–500.

30. Gerszten PC, Chen S, Quader M, Xu Y, Novotny J, Flickinger JC. Radiosurgery for benign tumors of the spine using the Synergy S with cone-beam computed tomography image guidance. J Neurosurg. 2012;117(suppl):197–202.

31. Sebai MA, Kerezoudis P, Alvi MA, Yoon JW, Spinner RJ, Bydon M. Need for arthrodesis following facetectomy for spinal peripheral nerve sheath tumors: an institutional experience and review of the current literature. J Neurosurg Spine. 2019;31:112–22.

32. Ahmad FU, Frenkel MB, Levi AD. Spinal stability after resection of nerve sheath tumors. J Neurosurg Sci. 2017;61:355–64.

33. Avila MJ, Walter CM, Skoch J, Abbasifard S, Patel AS, Sattarov K, Baaj AA. Fusion after intradural spine tumor resection in adults: a review of evidence and best practices. Clin Neurol Neurosurg. 2015;138:169–73.

34. Lu DC, Dhall SS, Mummaneni PV. Mini-open removal of extradural foraminal tumors of the lumbar spine. J Neurosurg Spine. 2009;10:46–50.

35. Safaee MM, Ames CP, Deviren V, Clark AJ. Minimally invasive lateral retroperitoneal approach for resection of extraforaminal lumbar plexus schwannomas: operative techniques and literature review. Oper Neurosurg (Hagerstown). 2018;15:516–21.

36. Hasegawa M, Fujisawa H, Hayashi Y, Tachibana O, Kida S, Yamashita J. Surgical pathology of spinal schwannomas: a light and electron micro-

scopic analysis of tumor capsules. Neurosurgery. 2001;49:1388–93.

37. Chang HS, Baba T, Matsumae M. Radical intracapsular dissection technique for dumbbell-shaped spinal schwannoma with intradural and extradural components. World Neurosurg. 2019;129:e634–40.

38. Lee C-H, Chung CK, Hyun S-J, Kim CH, Kim K-J, Jahng T-A. A longitudinal study to assess the volumetric growth rate of spinal intradural extramedullary tumour diagnosed with schwannoma by magnetic resonance imaging. Eur Spine J. 2015;24: 2126–32.

39. Ozawa H, Onoda Y, Aizawa T, Nakamura T, Koakutsu T, Itoi E. Natural history of intradural-extramedullary spinal cord tumors. Acta Neurol Belg. 2012;112:265–70.

40. Ando K, Imagama S, Ito Z, Kobayashi K, Yagi H, Hida T, Ito K, Tsushima M, Ishikawa Y, Ishiguro N. How do spinal schwannomas progress? The natural progression of spinal schwannomas on MRI. J Neurosurg Spine. 2016;24:155–9.

41. Dodd RL, Ryu MR, Kamnerdsupaphon P, Gibbs IC, Chang SD, Adler JR Jr. CyberKnife radiosurgery for benign intradural extramedullary spinal tumors. Neurosurgery. 2006;58:674–85.

42. Sachdev S, Dodd RL, Chang SD, Soltys SG, Adler JR, Luxton G, Choi CY, Tupper L, Gibbs IC. Stereotactic radiosurgery yields long-term control for benign intra-dural, extramedullary spinal tumors. Neurosurgery. 2011;69:533–9.

43. Gerszten PC, Burton SA, Ozhasoglu C, McCue KJ, Quinn AE. Radiosurgery for benign intradural spinal tumors. Neurosurgery. 2008;62:887–95.

44. Murovic JA, Gibbs IC, Chang SD, Mobley BC, Park J, Adler JR Jr. Foraminal nerve sheath tumors: intermediate follow-up after cyberknife radiosurgery. Neurosurgery. 2009;64:A33–43.

45. Kang HJ, Hwang YJ, Kim YH, Kim SY, Lee BH, Sohn MJ. Follow-up MR findings of spinal foraminal nerve sheath tumors after stereotactic irradiation. Jpn J Radiol. 2012;31:192–6.

46. Onimaru R, Hida K, Takeda N, Onodera S, Nishikawa Y, Mori T, Shirato H. Three-dimensional conformal fractionated radiotherapy for spinal schwannoma with a paravertebral or an intraosseous component. Jpn J Radiol. 2015;33:757–63.

47. Fehlings MG, Nater A, Zamorano JJ, Tetreault LA, Pal Varga P, Gokaslan ZL, Boriani S, Fisher CG, Rhines L, Bettegowda C, Kawahara N, Chou D. Risk factors for recurrence of surgically treated conventional spinal schwannomas: analysis of 169 patients from a multicenter international database. Spine (Phila Pa 1976). 2016;41:390–8.

48. Jomon MK, Pepper J, O'Connor N, Price R. Regression of a spinal schwannoma after Pomalidomide. Br J Neurosurg. 2020;18:1–2.

Meningioma

Meng Huang, Glen R. Manzano, and Allan D. Levi

Introduction

Gowers and Horsley first reported their success-ful diagnosis and surgical resection of a thoracic intradural extramedullary tumor found to be a meningioma in 1887 [1]. Building on their body of experience 50 years later, Cushing and Eisenhardt opined, "a successful operation for a spinal meningioma represents one of the most gratifying of all operative procedures" [2]. Since then, the management of spinal meningiomas by neurosurgeons has evolved significantly owing to advances in perioperative technology, but the core tenets of neurologic decompression, patho-logic diagnosis, and goal of oncologic cure remain consistent.

Epidemiology

Thought to arise from arachnoid cap cells like their intracranial counterparts, spinal meningio-mas originate in close proximity to the dentate ligaments and spinal rootlets and spread along the subarachnoid space [3–5]. Although they are typically slow-growing and histologically benign, their space occupying nature eventually precipi-tates symptoms secondary to neurologic com-

pression [1–4]. Spinal meningiomas are quite rare with reported incidence of 5 per million in women and 3 per million in men [6]. They repre-sent approximately 1.2–12.7% of all central ner-vous system meningiomas [2, 7, 8]. Within the spinal canal, they account for 25–46% of all intradural tumors [6, 8–10]. Spinal meningiomas are more prevalent in women with the average female to male ratio of 4:1, although some series have demonstrated a ratio as high as 10:1 [8, 11–16]. Sex hormone related receptors have been implicated in the tumorigenesis of these lesions, and there is some evidence suggestive of an asso-ciation with hormone replacement therapy in post-menopausal women [7, 17–19]. The average age range of patients at the time of diagnosis and treatment is between the fifth and sixth decade of life [7–9, 11–14, 16, 20].

Aside from spontaneous de novo growth, there are known predisposing factors for the develop-ment of spinal meningiomas. Neurofibromatosis Type 2 (NF2) is an autosomal dominant condition caused by a mutation in the NF2 gene located on chromosome 22q11 that produces the tumor sup-pressor protein *Merlin* (moesin-ezrin-radixin-like protein) [21]. Although the most common tumor in these patients are vestibular schwannomas, 67–90% of these patients harbor primary spinal tumors, and 14% of these are meningiomas [21, 22]. The average age of meningioma diagnosis for patients with NF2 is 28 years, much younger than the de novo population [21–23]. In a cohort of 40

M. Huang (✉) · G. R. Manzano · A. D. Levi
Department of Neurosurgery, University of Miami, Miami, FL, USA
e-mail: mxh1317@miami.edu

© Springer Nature Switzerland AG 2021
S. Hanft, P. C. McCormick (eds.), *Tumors of the Spinal Canal*,
https://doi.org/10.1007/978-3-030-55096-7_2

younger patients with a mean age of 34 years who underwent surgical resection of spinal meningiomas, 12.5% harbored the NF2 mutation [23].

Evidence for environmental factors associated with the development of meningiomas is strongest with exposure to ionizing radiation [17]. High-dose therapeutic radiation for treatment of head and neck cancers and low-dose therapeutic radiation for tinea capitis are well-established as risk factors with some studies reporting as much as a 9.5-fold increased risk [17, 24–26]. In a series of younger patients treated for spinal meningiomas, one patient who had two distinct tumors underwent childhood radiation for lymphoma [23]. There have also been reports of post-traumatic development of both intracranial and spinal meningiomas [23].

Location

Spinal meningiomas are located predominantly in the thoracic spine in 55–83% of cases [7–9, 11–14, 20, 23, 27]. The second most common location is the cervical spine with reported rates of 14–27% [7, 8, 11–14, 20, 23, 27]. It is notable that there is both an age and sex difference with respect to location in the spine. Younger male patients have a higher representation in the population of cervical meningiomas, while older female patients are more likely to have thoracic meningiomas [11, 23, 28]. Lumbo-sacral meningiomas are very rare with only 1.5% to 7% reported rates [7, 8, 11–14, 20, 23, 27].

In the axial plane, the occurrence of ventral, lateral, and dorsal locations are reported to be 19–55.9%, 22.5–70.5%, and 10–31%, respectively [7, 9, 11–14, 20]. This demonstrates a proclivity for spinal meningiomas to form laterally and anterior to the dentate ligament.

Spinal meningiomas do not always grow within the confines of the subarachnoid space. There are 15 reported cases in the literature of purely intramedullary spinal meningiomas [29]. Similarly, epidural meningiomas or intradural meningiomas with significant epidural extension are found in 5–14% of cases [7, 9, 12, 13, 20, 23].

Clinical Presentation

The clinical presentation of spinal meningiomas can be non-specific at symptom onset and is commonly misdiagnosed during the primary evaluation [15, 30]. Because of their slow-growing nature and the spinal cord's tolerance to chronic compression, initial symptoms are often characterized by non-specific localized back pain rather than neurologic complaints [9, 11, 15]. Due to the slow progression of symptoms, both primary care physicians and patients tend to observe the condition conservatively and delay imaging studies [30]. The rate of initial misdiagnosis thus ranges from 33% to 79% [11, 15, 30]. This is understandable, given the rarity of this pathology and lack of subtle neurologic signs that accompany what is otherwise a common complaint. Notably, patients are often first referred to orthopedic surgeons due to the apparent musculoskeletal nature of their symptoms [15]. This is associated with a significant delay in diagnosis [15, 30]. Although these statistics may unfavorably depict the diagnostic acumen of orthopedic surgeons, they likely reflect significant degrees of both selection and confirmation biases. Neurosurgeons, even though not commonly consulted for initial evaluation, have missed the diagnosis as well [15]. These incorrect diagnoses have precipitated unindicated surgeries, including microdiscectomy, knee exploration, wrong level laminectomy, ulnar nerve decompression, and cholecystectomy [11, 15]. The mean time from symptom onset to diagnosis is reported to range from 11 to 24 months [11–13, 15, 16, 30]. Not surprisingly, some patients retrospectively reported localized back pain up to two decades prior to diagnosis of spinal meningioma in the same spinal region [11]. Radicular pain can be mistaken for musculoskeletal back pain, especially in thoracic lesions, and is present in 7–21% of cases [7, 11, 12].

Gait disturbance is the next most frequent presenting symptom ranging from 49% to 83% of cases [8, 13, 20, 23]. This is more commonly reported in the younger patient population presumably because older patients are more likely to have baseline gait difficulty due to non-neurologically mediated orthopedic issues [23]. At the time of diagnosis, only 53–79% of patients are ambulatory [7, 8, 11–13, 16, 23, 27].

Signs of sphincter dysfunction, such as difficulty voiding, are present in 12–50% of patients [7, 11–13, 15, 20, 23]. Sensory disturbances are reported in 36–47% of patients [7, 9, 11–13, 20, 23]. Cohen-Gadol et al. noted a much higher prevalence of these disturbances in their younger patient population [23].

On physical examination, only 2–18% of patients present with completely intact neurological function [11, 31]. Confrontational motor weakness is demonstrated in 66–93% of cases [7, 9, 11, 15]. Most patients are still capable of ambulation with or without aid at the time of presentation and, notably, 97% of younger patients are ambulatory at presentation [23]. Long tract pyramidal signs are present in 65–87% of patients [11, 12, 15]. A sensory level is localizable in 39–72% of patients and can be associated with a Brown-Sequard sensory dissociation [11, 12, 15, 16, 20]. A small minority of patients present in extremis and are paraplegic or densely paretic [11, 12].

Radiological Diagnosis

Historically, prior to the advent and standardized implementation of Magnetic Resonance Imaging (MRI), myelography was the gold standard imaging modality for confirmatory diagnosis [11, 12, 15, 20]. Plain films were largely unhelpful because they rely on very subtle changes in bony architecture. In one series, 4 out of 78 patients harbored subtle signs of vertebral bone and pedicle erosion/thinning and these were all noted in patients with tumors involving the extradural compartment [20]. Only 1 patient had visible intraspinal tumor calcification on X-Ray [12]. Computed Tomography (CT) may be useful to detect calcifications, and extradural meningiomas notably contain flaky, highly dense calcifications in 51–57% of cases [32, 33]. The degree of calcification is useful in determining the degree of difficulty of surgical resection especially for ventral lesions. Spinal angiography has been performed routinely in historical series with the rationale of evaluating the relationship of the tumor to the anterior spinal artery as well as its vascularity, although no tumors were embolized [12].

Currently, MRI is the gold standard for diagnosis of spinal meningiomas, which exhibit typical characteristics (Figs. 2.1, 2.2, 2.3, 2.4, 2.5, 2.6, and 2.7) [33]. The advent of MRI decreased the latency to diagnosis by 6 months and, as a result, patients experience less severe neurologic symptoms and deficits at the time of treatment and have more favorable outcomes [13]. On T1-weighted imaging, spinal meningiomas

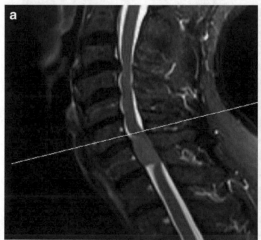
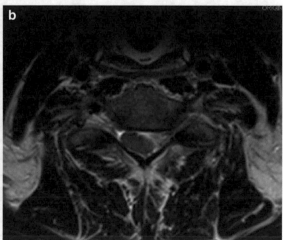

Fig. 2.1 (a) MRI cervical sagittal T2 sequence with fat suppression. Ventral meningioma hyperintense to spinal cord with postero-lateral displacement of the cord.

(b) MRI cervical axial T2 sequence. There is right lateral displacement of the spinal cord by the tumor

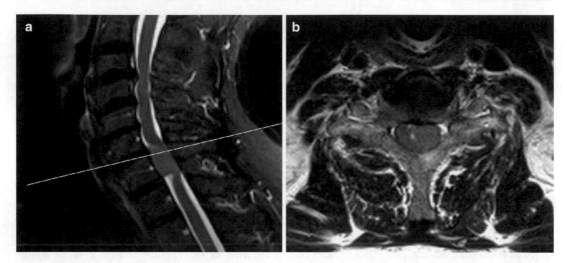

Fig. 2.2 (a) MRI cervical sagittal T2 with additional slices shown. (b) MRI cervical axial T2 with additional slices shown

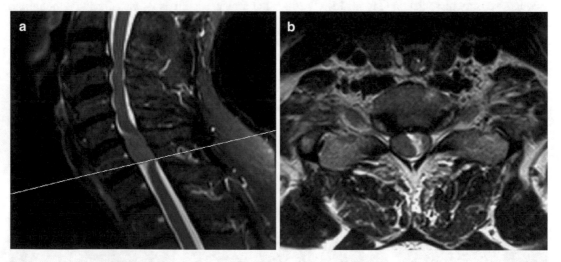

Fig. 2.3 (a) MRI cervical sagittal T2 with additional slices shown. (b) MRI cervical axial T2 with additional slices shown

appear isointense to the spinal cord, whereas they appear mostly hyperintense, but sometimes isointense to fat, on T2-weighted imaging. The contour of the tumor is generally smooth, and it tends to enhance intensely and homogenously with gadolinium. Meningiomas in general have a dural base and, in approximately half of all cases, there is an appreciable dural tail [33]. In a study correlating the dural tail MRI sign with histological analysis of the dura in Simpson Grade 1 resec-

tions, Nakamura and colleagues demonstrated a sensitivity and specificity of 71% and 47%, respectively [14]. Cord signal change is present in approximately half of all cases. Although rare, associated syringomyelia has been reported [34]. Hypo-intensities on both T1- and T2-weighted images correlate with calcifications [32]. Extradural meningiomas exhibit a unique C-shaped half ring sign on axial images and exhibit the same pattern as lymphoma [32].

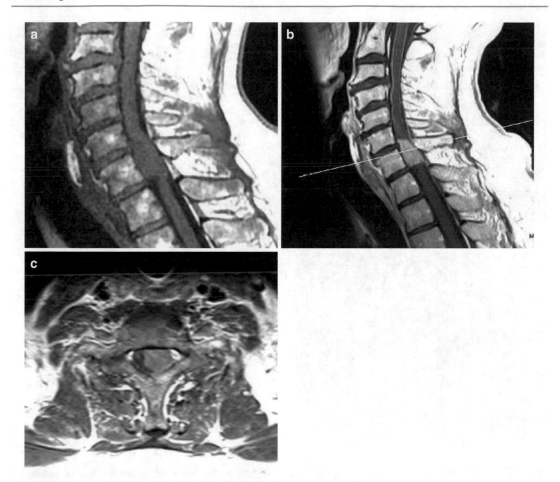

Fig. 2.4 (**a**) MRI cervical sagittal T1-weighted sequence. The tumor is isointense to the spinal cord. (**b**) MRI cervical sagittal T1-weighted sequence with gadolinium. The tumor avidly and homogeneously enhances with contrast.

(**c**) MRI cervical axial T1-weighted sequence with gadolinium. The tumor avidly and homogeneously enhances with contrast and the spinal cord is seen severely displaced to the right

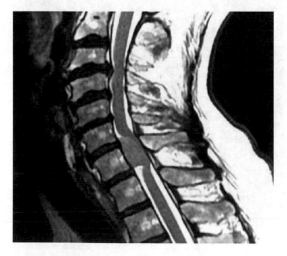

Fig. 2.5 MRI cervical sagittal T2-weighted sequence, without fat suppression. Another view that better shows the relationship of the tumor to the spinal cord

Cerebrospinal Fluid Analysis

In early historical studies, where myelograms were the primary diagnostic modality, CSF samples were also obtained for routine analysis [11, 15]. The majority of patients with spinal meningiomas exhibited elevated levels of protein without any other contributory findings, and, therefore, this practice has been abandoned along with routine myelography.

Operative Management

Gross total resection with radical excision of the dural base, Simpson Grade 1, is the optimal management when surgically feasible and in the

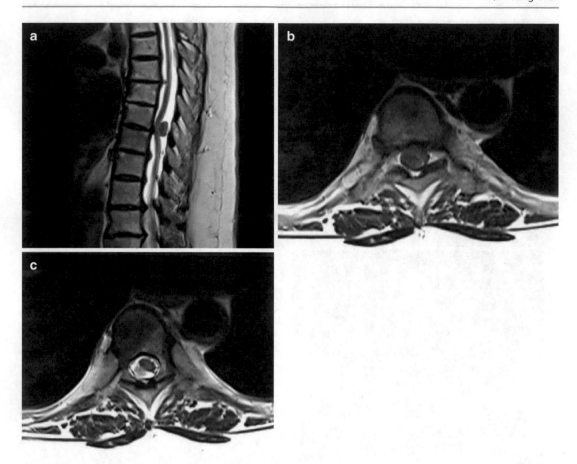

Fig. 2.6 (**a**) MRI thoracic sagittal T2-weighted sequence. The tumor is dorsal and displaces the spinal cord anteriorly. (**b**) MRI thoracic axial T2-weighted sequence. The tumor is dorsal and displaces the spinal cord anteriorly but is difficult to distinguish given the similar intensities. (**c**) MRI thoracic axial T2-weighted sequence. The tumor is dorsal and displaces the spinal cord anteriorly

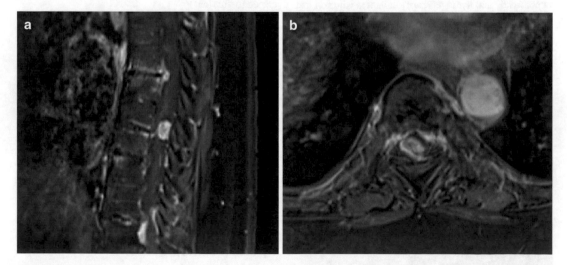

Fig. 2.7 (**a**) MRI thoracic sagittal T1 with gadolinium showing avid and homogeneous tumor enhancement. The tumor is dorsally based with a small dural tail. (**b**) MRI thoracic axial T1 with gadolinium showing vivid and homogeneous tumor enhancement. The tumor is dorsally based with a prominently enhancing dural tail. The spinal cord is displaced anteriorly and to the left side of the canal

absence of major medical comorbidities [14]. Unilateral or bilateral laminectomy can be performed to gain access. Although bilateral laminectomy is the most straightforward technique to access the lesion and provides the widest exposure to the tumor, it can potentially be the most destabilizing surgery [35]. This is especially true in younger patients who have longer postoperative survival and may develop progressive post-laminectomy kyphosis and spinal deformity that require fusion [23]. The rate of iatrogenic instability from laminectomy under 4 levels in the cervical and thoracic spine ranges from 11% to 25% [36, 37].

Open unilateral posterior approaches with hemilaminectomy and medial facetectomy are a less disruptive option [38], with one series [39] reporting overall equivalence of tumor resection extent, peri-operative complications, neurologic outcomes, and recurrence rates in follow-up. As a caveat, they did not achieve better than Simpson Grade 2 resection, and the follow-up was relatively short and incomplete compared to other series in the literature. To build upon the unilateral posterior approach, other authors have utilized expandable tubular retractors for minimally invasive access. This technique was reported to result in faster recovery time, shorter hospitalization, less pain, and fewer post-operative complications [40]. Notably, they achieved Simpson Grade 2 resection in only 67% of their cases and did not report any Simpson Grade 1 resections.

To address the concerns of iatrogenic destabilization or exposure-limited incomplete resection with the aforementioned techniques, some authors advocate the use of laminoplasty. Techniques vary from using sublaminar wire saws to craniotome drills to perform the bilateral laminar cuts. Reconstruction instrumentation ranges from mini-plates typically used for craniotomies to cannulated screws placed through the spinous process into the contralateral pars. Some remove the supraspinous ligament all together, while others reconstruct it [41, 42].

There are no reports of purely anterior approaches for thoracic or lumbar tumors, but there are cases of cervical ventral tumors approached circumferentially, including anterior

corpectomy and cage reconstruction. These cases were highly calcified cervical meningiomas with extensive extraforaminal extension into the anterior neck and were completed in multiple stages with vertebral artery sacrifice [43].

Once sufficient laminectomy is completed, intraoperative ultrasound is used to confirm adequate exposure and localize the lesion. In addition, ultrasound can provide certain clues about the nature of the lesion. Meningiomas are more echogenic, immobile, typically non-cystic, and have a more irregular surface when compared to schwannomas [44].

Laminectomy is typically first performed under loupe magnification and the operative microscope is subsequently brought in for dural opening, tumor resection, and dural closure (Fig. 2.8). The microscope provides superior illumination and magnification (10× and beyond) and its use is the standard of care in modern neurosurgery [45]. Microsurgical techniques are used for dissection of the tumor/neural tissue interface (Fig. 2.9) [9, 12, 46]. The durotomy is generally created in the midline, but a paramedian dural opening tailored toward the side of the tumor is also commonly implemented. The two edges are retracted laterally with dural tack-up sutures sewn to adjacent muscle or clamped off with hemostats to the drape. Sometimes, a much more lateral approach is needed to access ventral lesions and the dural opening can be further enlarged laterally with a T-shaped extension [7]. Sectioning the ipsilateral dentate ligament is a

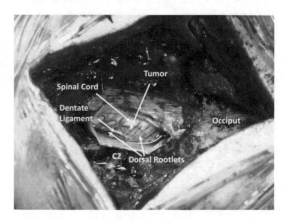

Fig. 2.8 Intraoperative photo of C1 ventral meningioma

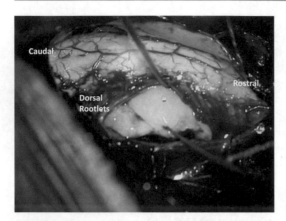

Fig. 2.9 Intraoperative photo of T7 ventral meningioma

critical step that releases the spinal cord and allows it to passively retract away from the tumor, which expands the access corridor and reduces the need for manipulation of the cord itself. Sharp dissection of the tumor away from the spinal cord can then be performed. An ultrasonic aspirator is commonly used to internally debulk the tumor until it is small enough to be collapsed in on itself for en-bloc resection [9, 31, 35, 46–48]. The dural attachment is then either radically excised (Simpson Grade 1) or cauterized with bipolar cautery (Simpson Grade 2) prior to dural reconstruction and closure [49]. Reconstruction strategies for dural defects include the use of local fascia or commercial xenografts grafts such as Durepair (Medtronic) or Bovine Pericardium (Integra) [46, 50]. Fibrin glue sealants such as DuraSeal (Integra) or Tisseel (Baxter) are often injected over the suture lines to ensure a water-tight closure.

Intraoperative neuromonitoring (IONM) with somatosensory evoked potentials (SSEP) and motor-evoked potentials (MEP) are the standard of care for resecting intradural extramedullary spinal tumors to prevent neurologic injury from surgical manipulation [51–53]. In SSEPs, orthodromic stimulation of the median and tibial nerves with electroencephalography recording allows for continuous monitoring of dorsal column integrity [52]. Because SSEPs alone are not sensitive enough for detection of corticospinal tract pathway function, MEP monitoring tech-

niques were also developed and fine-tuned. MEPs induce motor cortex activation by transcutaneous electrical stimulation by scalp electrodes and the resultant recordings at the neuromuscular endplate are measured for circuit integrity [54]. Free-running electromyography (EMG) and direct stimulation-evoked EMG are used to monitor lumbo-sacral nerve root integrity for tumors involving the cauda equina [51, 55].

Histopathology and Cytogenetics

WHO Grade I spinal meningiomas account for greater than 90% of all spinal meningiomas and are benign with no histological evidence of medullary invasion [35, 39, 56]. There are nine histological variants; the most common of which are meningothelial (23–59%), psammomatous (21–66%), and transitional (9–37%) [9, 11, 12, 14, 16, 20, 27, 47, 57]. Grade II lesions are invasive, have 4–19 mitotic figures per 10 high-power field (HPF), and are characterized by either spinal cord invasion or 3 of 5 minor criteria (increased cellularity, high nucleus-to-cytoplasm ratio, large nucleoli, pattern-less or sheet-like growth, and areas of necrosis). These include atypical, clear cell, or chordoid variants [57–59]. Grade III tumors are very rare. They have greater than 20 mitotic figures per 10 HPF, grossly carcinomatous or sarcomatous histological features, and include the anaplastic, papillary, and rhabdoid variants [12, 56–59].

In a karyotyping study of cranial and spinal meningiomas, Ketter et al. [60] were able to correlate the tumor cytogenic profile with histopathologic features with high specificity. Group 0 had a normal diploid chromosomal set. Group 1 had isolated monosomy 22 and correlated with WHO Grade I tumor histopathology. Group 2 were highly hypodiploid, exhibiting loss of additional autosomes, and corresponded to WHO Grade II tumors. Group 3 exhibited deletions in the short arm of chromosome 1 in addition to monosomy 22 and other hypodiploid features, and was associated with WHO Grade III tumors.

Surgical Outcomes

The extent of resection of spinal meningiomas is classified similarly to their cranial counterparts according to Simpson's grading scale, where Grade 1 (SG1) includes radical excision of the involved dural base in addition to gross total resection (GTR) of the tumor. Grade 2 (SG2) resection represents gross total resection and bipolar cautery of the dural base only without radical resection [49]. Given the anatomic constraints of the spinal canal and the typical posterior approach, ventrally-based meningiomas impose a much greater challenge when considering Simpson Grade 1 resection. Excluding a few outlying studies, SG1 is achieved with relatively low rates between 14% and 30% [7, 11, 12, 14, 20, 35]. As a result, a widely accepted practice for treatment of spinal meningiomas is combining Simpson Grade 1 and 2 (S1/2) resections together to represent GTR [11, 14, 23, 35]. The rate of achieving S1/2 GTR is very favorable, as reported in historical series at 82–99%, with most 90% or higher [7–9, 11–14, 20, 27, 35, 46]. Levy's [11] reported rate of 82% GTR represented one of the earliest series and most of their cases pre-dated the modern techniques of microneurosurgery. A notable exception is en-plaque meningioma, which is difficult to achieve S1/2 GTR due to non-encapsulated tumor matrix and aggressive growth that does not respect tissue planes [9, 13, 23]. Not surprisingly, arachnoid/pia scarring in recurrent operations is also associated with a markedly lower success rate for GTR [13, 31].

The overall complication rates of spinal meningioma resection are low. Peri-operative mortality ranges between 0.76% and 3% with no incidences of intraoperative death. These deaths were all secondary to cardiopulmonary complications [7–9, 11–14, 20, 46]. Surgical morbidity is also low with CSF leak and wound complications under 6%. The remaining complications consist of thromboembolic and pulmonary and genitourinary infections that are typical of anesthesia and surgery in general [7, 8, 11–14, 20, 35, 46].

Clinical Outcomes

There are many impressive series in the literature with extensive clinical follow-up. The average duration was 87 months with a range between 23 and 180 months [7–14, 16, 20, 23, 27, 31, 35, 43, 46, 47, 61]. Neurological outcomes, as measured by various validated functional grading scales (Nurick, McCormick, Frankel, Karnofsky, and or Cooper-Epstein), demonstrated improved function in 53% to 95% of the patients. In long-term follow-up with peak neurologic convalescence, these numbers improved to 85% to 95%. With respect to ambulatory rate, the number improved from 65% before surgery to 89% in post-operative follow-up [7, 9, 11–13, 20, 31, 35, 46]. Levy et al. [11] performed further sub-analysis on components of clinical improvement in their series and found that resolution of sensory levels, hyperreflexia, and pain (axial and radicular) occurred in 95%, 66%, and 50% of the cases, respectively. Similarly, in another series, the majority of patients reported significant improvement or resolution of bladder (81%) and bowel symptoms (80%). Eighty-four percent of these patients also reported resolution of their pre-operative sensory symptoms [23]. King [20] reported a 95% improvement or resolution in pre-operative bladder symptoms.

Despite the overall favorable outcomes for spinal meningiomas, a small proportion of patients do not improve or even get worse with surgery, and there are several factors that are associated with these poor outcomes. Setzer et al. [31] reported that invasion of arachnoid/pia by the tumor matrix is an independent predictor of no appreciable neurological improvement and poor long-term outcome. In Levy et al's [11] series, seven patients had a worse neurological outcome post-operatively, including 4 patients who emerged from anesthesia completely paraplegic. Three of these four paraplegic patients had meningiomas that were "rock-hard" with diffuse calcification and adhesion to the spinal cord itself, which required excess manipulation of the spinal cord to dissect. Sandalcioglu et al. [8] corroborated this observation in three of their patients as well. Similarly, Schaller et al. [16] also reported worse outcomes in their subset of patients with psammomatous meningiomas, which are known for their high constitution of concretions/calcifications. Roux et al. [12] noted complete paraplegia post-operatively due to iatrogenic injury to the artery of Adamkiewicz, which was in close proximity to the tumor. Subsequent to that event, they implemented routine use of spinal angiography to evaluate the proximity of the artery to the tumor for pre-operative planning. Due to the delay in diagnosis of spinal meningiomas, many patients are in poor pre-operative neurological condition [15]. Although some authors have reported that older age and poor pre-operative status [11, 31, 35] are associated with worse outcomes, others have reported excellent results even in patients with advanced age [57, 61] and in patients with complete paraplegia who were asymptomatic and independently ambulatory at long term follow-up [8, 20]. Fortunately, with the advent of MRI, time to diagnosis has been shortened significantly and baseline neurologic performance status has been better as a result [13].

It is also important to note that some patients develop delayed iatrogenic spinal instability from the index tumor resection operation [43]. This occurred in younger patients and was reported in 2 of the 40 patients younger than age 50. They were 28 and 38 years of age at the time of index laminectomy for tumor resection, and both patients required fusion surgery for intractable symptomatology and progressive deformity years later [23].

Oncological Outcomes

Sustained clinical success is dependent on oncological cure. Recurrence rates of spinal meningiomas range between 1.3% and 10%. However, in one series, which implemented Kaplan-Meyer statistics accounting for varying follow-up times, Klekamp et al. [13] reported a 21% recurrence rate at 1 year and 40% recurrence rate at 5 years [7–9, 11, 12, 14, 20, 35].

One factor in tumor recurrence is simply length of follow-up. Not surprisingly, the longer the follow-up duration, the more tumor recur-

rences are captured, irrespective of clinical relevance. The Klekamp [13] series of 130 cases with an average 20 month follow-up reported an almost doubled rate of recurrence at 5 years compared to 1 year. Solero et al. [7], with 174 cases in an average follow-up of 15 years, reported a 6% total recurrence rate with 1.3% in the first 5 years. In their study of 68 cases with mean follow-up of 12 years, Nakamura et al. [14] demonstrated a tumor recurrence of 0%, 3.2%, and 8% at 5, 10, and 15 years. As a corollary, patients who are diagnosed and treated at a younger age, and therefore have a necessarily longer follow-up duration, also have recurrence rates as high as 20–35% [23, 28].

Another obvious factor in tumor recurrence is histological grade. Notably, after SG1/2 GTR and a mean follow up duration of 33 months, recurrence rates in WHO I, WHO II, and WHO III were 4.3%, 10.5%, and 30%, respectively [60]. Interestingly, all 23 spinal tumors in this cohort were WHO Grade I. Setzer et al. [31] also segmented their tumor recurrence rate based on histological grading and reported 1.4% for Grade I, 50% for Grade II, and 100% for Grade III with a mean follow up duration of 40 months. There is also a report of 60% recurrence rate in the angiomatous variant of Grade I spinal meningiomas [14].

The third predicting factor is the extent of resection by Simpson Grading [49]. There is no question that SG 3 or worse is associated with a high rate of recurrence as evidenced by the recurrence rates for difficult lesions to resect including en-plaque, epidural/dumbbell, and/or recurrent spinal meningiomas [13, 14, 23, 32]. The point of contention exists between SG 1 and 2 resection among authors. Older historical series report low recurrence rates and thereby suggest that Simpson Grade 2 resection without radical excision of involved dura is sufficient treatment, given the indolent nature and behavior of the majority of these tumors [7, 8, 11, 12, 16, 20, 31]. In fact, Solero et al. [7] reported 8% recurrence for their SG1 and only 5.6% for their SG2 subsets, though the majority of these patients were treated prior to the implementation of the surgical microscope. In their contemporary series, however, Nakamura et al. [14] showed a 0% recurrence rate in their SG1 subgroup, but a 32% recurrence rate in their

SG2 subgroup between 6 and 21 years after surgery. No recurrent tumors in their series had aggressive biologic features and all had a low MIB-1 index of 2%. In addition, they evaluated the dural specimen from their SG1 resections and found infiltrating cells between the inner and outer layers in 35% of specimens, which suggests that late recurrences in Grade I tumors could be explained by residual viable tumor cells within the dura. In another study focusing on an aggressive subgroup of 17 atypical WHO Grade II meningiomas with a mean follow-up of 69 months, the S1/2 GTR resection group had no recurrences [48]. Based on these observations and given the longer average life expectancy of the modern era, the optimal management for spinal meningiomas should be total extirpation including the dural base, or Simpson Grade 1 resection, though we do recognize the obvious challenges in achieving this for meningiomas that have a dural base in the lateral and ventral regions of the canal.

Adjunct Treatments

Recurrent tumors, aggressive tumors (WHO Grade II or III), and patients who are not surgical candidates can undergo radiotherapy, although there is no robust body of literature to support these practices [57]. Roux et al. [12] treated two of their patients who had recurrent tumors with external beam radiation, one of whom underwent the radiotherapy after a second operation. They had no further evidence of progression although length of follow up at the time of publication was insufficient at less than 5 years. Several other studies have reported the use of radiotherapy in treating both recurrent low grade (I) and high grade (II or III) tumors [43, 48, 62]. Although the majority of the literature pertains to radiosurgical treatment of intracranial meningiomas, the advent of frameless stereotactic radiosurgery (Cyberknife) and other new age LINAC systems capable of delivering SRS has opened a new door for modern radiosurgical treatment of spinal meningiomas, and a supporting body of literature is growing [62]. At the current time, radiosurgery should be reserved for treatment of recurrent meningiomas or those that have been resected and proven to be high-grade (II or III) on final pathology. There are select cases where upfront radiosurgery can be considered, such as patients who show minimal to no symptoms and carry elevated risk for open surgery.

Medical adjuvant therapy for spinal meningiomas is lacking. Hydroxyurea showed promise for tumor control, but its efficacy was not consistently reproducible [57, 63, 64]. Anti-angiogenic treatments targeting vascular endothelial growth factor are undergoing clinical trials [57, 63]. The future of medical treatment of spinal meningiomas will likely follow the trend of treatment of other CNS tumors with tailored interventions targeting individual tumor-specific molecular markers.

Conclusion

Spinal meningiomas are rare tumors that mostly affect middle-aged women and are located in the anterolateral thoracic spine. Their diagnosis is often delayed due to slowly progressive symptoms. The optimal treatment of choice is total surgical resection with removal of involved dura, if feasible and safe, though true Simpson Grade 1 resections are rarely achieved. With surgical control of the disease and early diagnosis and intervention, patients generally have an excellent prognosis with full neurological recovery. There is a growing body of literature supporting the use of radiosurgery in the case of recurrent meningiomas, as adjuvant treatment for subtotal or gross total resections of grade 2 and 3 meningiomas, and occasionally as upfront treatment. Given that spinal meningiomas are nearly always uncovered when they have reached clinical significance, surgery will remain the primary modality for the foreseeable future.

References

1. Gowers WR, Horsley V. A case of tumour of the spinal cord. Removal; Recovery. Med Chir Trans. 1888;71(1):377–430.11.
2. Cushing H, Eisenhardt L. Meningiomas: their classification, regional behaviour, life history, and surgical results. Charles C. Thomas: Springfield; 1938. 1 p.

3. Lantos PL, Louis DN, Rosenblum MK, Kleihues P. "Tumors of the Nervous System." Greenfield's Neuropathology, edited by David Graham, Peter Lantos, Arnold Publisher, 2002, pp. 767–980.

4. Horrax G, Poppen JL. Meningiomas and neurofibromas of the spinal cord; certain clinical features and end results. Surg Clin North Am. 1949;29(3):659–65.

5. Hollis PH, Malis LI, Zappula RA. Neurological deterioration after lumbar puncture below complete spinal subarachnoid block. J Neurosurg. (2nd ed, Journal of Neurosurgery Publishing Group). 1986;64(2):253–6.

6. Helseth A, Mørk SJ. Primary intraspinal neoplasms in Norway, 1955 to 1986. A population-based survey of 467 patients. J Neurosurg. 1989;71(6):842–5.

7. Solero CL, Fornari M, Giombini S, Lasio G, Oliveri G, Cimino C, et al. Spinal meningiomas: review of 174 operated cases. Neurosurgery. 1989;25(2):153–60.

8. Sandalcioglu IE, Hunold A, Müller O, Bassiouni H, Stolke D, Asgari S. Spinal meningiomas: critical review of 131 surgically treated patients. Eur Spine J (Springer Berlin Heidelberg). 2008;17(8):1035–41.

9. Gezen F, Kahraman S, Canakci Z, Bedük A. Review of 36 cases of spinal cord meningioma. Spine. 2000;25(6):727–31.

10. Mirimanoff RO, Dosoretz DE, Linggood RM, Ojemann RG, Martuza RL. Meningioma: analysis of recurrence and progression following neurosurgical resection. J Neurosurg. 2nd ed. 1985;62(1):18–24.

11. Levy WJ, Bay J, Dohn D. Spinal cord meningioma. J Neurosurg. 1982;57(6):804–12.

12. Roux FX, Nataf F, Pinaudeau M, Borne G, Devaux B, Meder JF. Intraspinal meningiomas: review of 54 cases with discussion of poor prognosis factors and modern therapeutic management. Surg Neurol. 1996;46(5):458–63; discussion 463–4.

13. Klekamp J, Samii M. Surgical results for spinal meningiomas. Surg Neurol. 1999;52(6):552–62.

14. Nakamura M, Tsuji O, Fujiyoshi K, Hosogane N, Watanabe K, Tsuji T, et al. Long-term surgical outcomes of spinal Meningiomas. Spine. 2012;37(10):E617–23.

15. Pena M, Galasko CS, Barrie JL. Delay in diagnosis of intradural spinal tumors. Spine. 1992;17(9):1110–6.

16. Schaller B. Spinal meningioma: relationship between histological subtypes and surgical outcome? J Neuro-Oncol. 2005;75(2):157–61.

17. Barnholtz-Sloan JS, Kruchko C. Meningiomas: causes and risk factors. Neurosurg Focus. 2007;23(4):E2.

18. Henderson BE, Ross RK, Pike MC, Casagrande JT. Endogenous hormones as a major factor in human cancer. Cancer Res. 1982;42(8):3232–9.

19. Wigertz A, Lönn S, Mathiesen T, Ahlbom A, Hall P, Feychting M. Risk of brain tumors associated with exposure to exogenous female sex hormones. Am J Epidemiol. 2006;164(7):629–36.

20. King AT, Sharr MM, Gullan RW, Bartlett JR. Spinal meningiomas: a 20-year review. Br J Neurosurg. 1998;12(6):521–6.

21. Lloyd SKW, Evans DGR. Neurofibromatosis type 2 (NF2): diagnosis and management. Handb Clin Neurol (Elsevier). 2013;115:957–67.

22. Parry DM, Eldridge R, Kaiser-Kupfer MI, Bouzas EA, Pikus A, Patronas N. Neurofibromatosis 2 (NF2): clinical characteristics of 63 affected individuals and clinical evidence for heterogeneity. Am J Med Genet. 1994;52(4):450–61.

23. Cohen-Gadol AA, Zikel OM, Koch CA, Scheithauer BW, Krauss WE. Spinal meningiomas in patients younger than 50 years of age: a 21-year experience. J Neurosurg. 2003;98(3 Suppl):258–63.

24. Ron E, Modan B, Boice JD, Alfandary E, Stovall M, Chetrit A, et al. Tumors of the brain and nervous-system after radiotherapy in childhood. N Engl J Med. 1988;319(16):1033–9.

25. Hijiya N, Hudson MM, Lensing S, Zacher M, Onciu M, Behm FG, et al. Cumulative incidence of secondary neoplasms as a first event after childhood acute lymphoblastic leukemia. JAMA. 2007;297(11):1207–15.

26. Harrison MJ, Wolfe DE, Lau TS, Mitnick RJ, Sachdev VP. Radiation-induced meningiomas: experience at the Mount Sinai Hospital and review of the literature. J Neurosurg (Journal of Neurosurgery Publishing Group). 1991;75(4):564–74.

27. Albanese V, Platania N. Spinal intradural extramedullary tumors. Personal experience. J Neurosurg Sci. 2002;46(1):18–24.

28. Deen HG, Scheithauer BW, Ebersold MJ. Clinical and pathological study of meningiomas of the first two decades of life. J Neurosurg (Journal of Neurosurgery Publishing Group). 1982;56(3):317–22.

29. Cheng C, Wang J, Zhao S, Tao B, Bai S, Shang A. Intramedullary thoracic meningioma: a rare case report and review of the literature. World Neurosurg (Elsevier Inc). 2019;129:176–80.

30. Constantini S, Lidar Z, Segal D, Corn A. Delay in diagnosis of primary intradural spinal cord tumors. Surg Neurol Int. 2012;3(1):52–8.

31. Setzer M, Vatter H, Marquardt G, Seifert V, Vrionis FD. Management of spinal meningiomas: surgical results and a review of the literature. Neurosurg Focus. (6 ed. American Association of Neurological Surgeons). 2007;23(4):E14.

32. Zhang LH, Yuan HS. Imaging appearances and pathologic characteristics of spinal epidural meningioma. AJNR Am J Neuroradiol. 2018;39(1):199–204.

33. Yeo Y, Park C, Lee JW, Kang Y, Ahn JM, Kang HS, et al. Magnetic resonance imaging spectrum of spinal meningioma. Clin Imaging (Elsevier). 2019;55:100–6.

34. Blaylock RL. Hydrosyringomyelia of the conus medullaris associated with a thoracic meningioma: case report. J Neurosurg (Journal of Neurosurgery Publishing Group). 1981;54(6):833–5.

35. Raco A, Pesce A, Toccaceli G, Domenicucci M, Miscusi M, Delfini R. Factors leading to a poor functional outcome in spinal meningioma surgery: remarks on 173 cases. Neurosurgery. 2017;80(4):602–9.

36. Katsumi Y, Honma T, Nakamura T. Analysis of cervical instability resulting from laminectomies for removal of spinal-cord tumor. Spine. 1989;14(11):1171–6.

37. Papagelopoulos PJ, Peterson HA, Ebersold MJ, Emmanuel PR, Choudhury SN, Quast LM. Spinal column deformity and instability after lumbar or tho-

racolumbar laminectomy for intraspinal tumors in children and young adults. Spine. 1997;22(4):442–51.

38. McGirt MJ, Garcés-Ambrossi GL, Parker SL, Sciubba DM, Bydon A, Wolinksy J-P, et al. Short-term progressive spinal deformity following Laminoplasty versus laminectomy for resection of Intradural spinal tumors. Neurosurgery. 2010;66(5):1005–12.

39. Onken J, Obermüller K, Staub-Bartelt F, Meyer B, Vajkoczy P, Wostrack M. Surgical management of spinal meningiomas: focus on unilateral posterior approach and anterior localization. J Neurosurg Spine. 2018;30(3):308–13.

40. Thavara B, Kidangan G, Rajagopalawarrier B. Analysis of the surgical technique and outcome of the thoracic and lumbar intradural spinal tumor excision using minimally invasive tubular retractor system. Asian J Neurosurg. 2019;14(2):453–8.

41. Wiedemayer H, Sandalcioglu IE, Aalders M, Wiedemayer H, Floerke M, Stolke D. Reconstruction of the laminar roof with Miniplates for a posterior approach in Intraspinal surgery: technical considerations and critical evaluation of follow-up results. Spine. 2004;29(16):E333–42.

42. Park Y-J, Kim S-K, Seo H-Y. Ligament-saving Laminoplasty for Intraspinal tumor excision: a technical note. World Neurosurg (Elsevier Inc). 2019;128:438–43.

43. Lonjon N, Russo V, Barbarisi M, Choi D, Allibone J, Casey A. Spinal cervical Meningiomas: the challenge posed by ventral location. World Neurosurg. 2016;89:464–73.

44. Mimatsu K, Kawakami N, Kato F, Saito H, Sato K. Intraoperative ultrasonography of extramedullary spinal tumours. Neuroradiology. 1992;34(5):440–3.

45. Walker CT, Kakarla UK, Chang SW, Sonntag VKH. History and advances in spinal neurosurgery. J Neurosurg Spine. 2019;31(6):775–85.

46. Gottfried ON, Gluf W, Quiñones-Hinojosa A, Kan P, Schmidt MH. Spinal meningiomas: surgical management and outcome. Neurosurg Focus. 2003;14(6):e2.

47. Riad H, Knafo S, Segnarbieux F, Lonjon N. Spinal meningiomas: surgical outcome and literature review. Neurochirurgie (Elsevier Masson SAS). 2013;59(1):30–4.

48. Noh SH, Kim KH, Shin DA, Park JY, Yi S, Kuh SU, et al. Clinical study treatment outcomes of 17 patients with atypical spinal meningioma, including 4 with metastases: a retrospective observational study. Spine J (Elsevier Inc). 2019;19(2):276–84.

49. Simpson D. The recurrence of intracranial meningiomas after surgical treatment. J Neurol Neurosurg Psychiat (BMJ Publishing Group). 1957;20(1):22–39.

50. Anson JA, Marchand EP. Bovine pericardium for dural grafts: clinical results in 35 patients. Neurosurgery. 1996;39(4):764–8.

51. Kothbauer KF, Deletis V. Intraoperative neurophysiology of the conus medullaris and cauda equina. Childs Nerv Syst. 2010;26(2):247–53.

52. Kothbauer K, Deletis V, Epstein FJ. Intraoperative spinal cord monitoring for intramedullary surgery: an essential adjunct. PNE (Karger Publishers). 1997;26(5):247–54.

53. Ishida W, Casaos J, Chandra A, D'Sa A, Ramhmdani S, Perdomo-Pantoja A, et al. Diagnostic and therapeutic values of intraoperative electrophysiological neuromonitoring during resection of intradural extramedullary spinal tumors: a single-center retrospective cohort and meta-analysis. J Neurosurg Spine. 2019;30(6):839–49.

54. Calancie B, Harris W, Broton JG, Alexeeva N, Green BA. "Threshold-level" multipulse transcranial electrical stimulation of motor cortex for intraoperative monitoring of spinal motor tracts: description of method and comparison to somatosensory evoked potential monitoring. J Neurosurg (Journal of Neurosurgery Publishing Group). 1998 Mar;88(3):457–70.

55. Pang D. Surgical management of complex spinal cord lipomas: how, why, and when to operate. A review. J Neurosurg Pediatr. 2019;23(5):537–56.

56. Kleihues P, Burger PC, Scheithauer BW. The new WHO classification of brain tumours. Brain Pathol. 5 ed. 1993;3(3):255–68.

57. Apra C, Peyre M, Kalamarides M. Current treatment options for meningioma. Expert Rev Neurother. 2018; 18(3):241–49.

58. Louis DN, Perry A, Reifenberger G, Deimling A, Figarella-Branger D, Cavenee WK, et al. The 2016 World Health Organization Classification of Tumors of the Central Nervous System: a summary. Acta Neuropathologica. Springer Berlin Heidelberg; 2016;131(6):803–20.

59. Mawrin C, Perry A. Pathological classification and molecular genetics of meningiomas. J Neuro-Oncol. 2010;99(3):379–91.

60. Ketter R, Henn W, Niedermayer I, Steilen-Gimbel H, König J, Zang KD, et al. Predictive value of progression-associated chromosomal aberrations for the prognosis of meningiomas: a retrospective study of 198 cases. J Neurosurg (Journal of Neurosurgery Publishing Group). 2001;95(4):601–7.

61. Morandi X, Haegelen C, Riffaud L, Amlashi S, Adn M, Brassier G. Results in the operative treatment of elderly patients with spinal meningiomas. Spine. 2004;29(19):2191–4.

62. Sahgal A, Chou D, Ames C, Ma L, Lamborn K, Huang K, et al. Image-guided robotic stereotactic body radiotherapy for benign spinal tumors: The University of California San Francisco preliminary experience. Technol Cancer Res Treat. 2016;6(6):595–603.

63. Sioka C, Kyritsis AP. Chemotherapy, hormonal therapy, and immunotherapy for recurrent meningiomas. J Neuro-Oncol. 2008;92(1):1–6.

64. Newton HB. Hydroxyurea chemotherapy in the treatment of meningiomas. Neurosurg Focus. (6 ed. American Association of Neurological Surgeons). 2007;23(4):E11.

Myxopapillary Ependymoma and Rare Tumors

John Bruckbauer, James Harrop, Kevin Hines, Stephanie Perez, Victor Sabourin, and Anthony Stefanelli

Myxopapillary Ependymoma

Introduction

First described in 1932 by Irish-American neuropathologist James Watson Kernohan [1], myxopapillary ependymomas are rare variants of spinal ependymomas presenting predominantly in adulthood. While they are considered rare tumors, they are actually the most common tumor of the cauda equina region. Often intradural extramedullary, these tumors demonstrate perivascular myxoid pseudorosettes, as well as a distinctive homogeneously enhancing sausage-like appearance on MRI. Given their slow growing, often benign nature, as well as accessible location, they are often good candidates for surgery and complete resection often portends a favorable prognosis.

Demographics and Clinical Presentation

Myxopapillary ependymomas represent 13% of ependymomas in the spinal cord. A rare tumor with an estimated incidence of 0.5–0.8 per

J. Bruckbauer · J. Harrop · K. Hines (✉) · S. Perez ·
V. Sabourin · A. Stefanelli
Department of Neurological Surgery, Thomas
Jefferson University Hospital, Philadelphia, PA, USA
e-mail: kevin.hines@jefferson.edu

100,000 people per year, it actually constitutes the vast majority of all spinal tumors in the cauda equina region. As much as 83% of spinal tumors in this region are identified as myxopapillary ependymoma [2]. They most typically appear in the third or fourth decade. However, there have been variable reported presenting ages, ranging from first decade to eighth decade of life. It has been reported that MPE have a slightly higher predilection for males in both adults and children. Approximately 63% of adults diagnosed with MPE are males and 71% of children diagnosed with MPE are male [3].

Given its similar presentation in most cases to degenerative spine disease, presentation of myxopapillary ependymoma often takes an indolent course. From symptom onset to time of surgery, patient symptom duration may range from several months to years. More commonly average time of symptoms has been reported in the literature as 3–23 months [3–5]. Longer duration of symptoms tended to correlate with larger size tumors at time of diagnosis/treatment [6].

In addition to having a time course very similar to degenerative spine disease, the clinical symptoms and presentation are also very similar. The most frequent presenting symptom in MPE is back pain documented in up to 94% of cases [4]. In addition to this, radicular symptoms such as weakness, numbness, and radicular pain are common symptoms found in more than half of patients reported in prior MPE series. With a lesser rate but still very significant incidence, sacral symptoms, such as urinary/fecal or sexual disturbances were reported in 14–31% presenting cases. Finally, at a variable rate, 9–81% patients reported overall gait dysfunction or increased difficulty with ambulation [3–5, 7, 8]. Given its similarity to lumbar degenerative disease, MPE should remain on the differential for patients with persistent back pain or radicular pain, or symptoms, such as bowel/bladder dysfunction, and when reviewing any advanced spine imaging.

Location

While classic intramedullary spinal ependymomas are located most commonly in the cervical spine, followed by thoracic spine, myxopapillary ependymomas present most frequently at the bottom of the spinal cord [9, 10]. Most commonly, they are considered intradural extramedullary tumors as they are located at the level of the conus medullaris, cauda equina, or filum terminale. In much rarer instances, lesions have been noted in predominantly sacral, cervical, and thoracic distributions (Fig. 3.1) [7]. While these locations are slightly variable, most myxopapillary ependymomas present with a similar constellation of symptoms so location is better determined by advanced imaging.

In a series of 77 MPE by Sonneland et al., the authors noted that 65% of the tumors were restricted to the filum, 30% involved both the filum and the conus medullaris, and 4% were located instead in the cervicothoracic spinal cord [11]. In another series of 107 patients by Abdulaziz et al., it was noted that 50% of MPE arose in the cauda equina/filum region, 31% in the conus medullaris, and 19% originated above the conus medullaris [12]. There have also been reports of MPE originating in the filum that demonstrate locally aggressive behavior with sacral erosion. In addition, there are case reports of myxopapillary ependymal tissue arising from heterotopic ependymal cell clusters in extraspinal locations. These most often present as presacral masses [13, 14]. There have also been reports of extraspinal MPE's presenting as sacrococcygeal masses with no communication with the spinal canal. They may be easily confused for pilonidal cysts on imaging [15, 16]. Finally, it is important to note that while largely considered benign, MPE may result in dissemination to spinal or extraspinal locations. While spinal dissemination has been noted to be relatively low in most studies, a study by Kraetzig et al. noted that distant spinal metastasis was noted in 36.4% of patients upon presentation, most commonly rostrally, including cranial, cervical, and thoracic [17]. Therefore patients with imaging findings concerning for myxopapillary ependymoma should be screened for other sites of disease after presentation.

Macroscopic and Microscopic Pathology

Myxopapillary ependymomas have been described in multiple sources as soft, fleshy tumors. They are often rubbery in consistency and appear vascular with a greyish to reddish-brown color (Fig. 3.2). These fleshy tumors are often fully or at least partially contained in fibrous capsules of filum terminale stroma that may be smooth or nodular [8, 11]. As will be discussed later, this capsule often plays a role in surgical decision making. Given the space they occupy via slow tumorigenesis, myxopapillary ependymomas often become ovoid, or "sausage" shaped

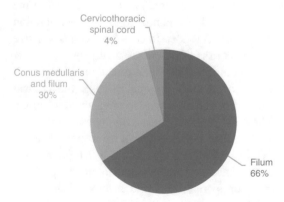

Fig. 3.1 Distribution of spinal location of myxopapillary ependymoma as stated in a study done by Sonneland et al. [11]

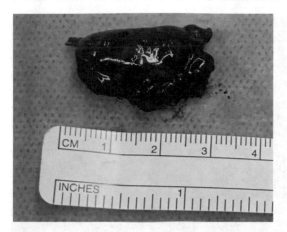

Fig. 3.2 Photograph of en bloc resection of myxopapillary ependymoma. Notice fleshy, vascular appearance of the tumor

as they fill up the lumbosacral spinal canal. While expanding, they may induce dural attenuation or compressive erosion of vertebral bodies [18]. They may be limited to the filum only or extend proximally to incorporate the conus medullaris. In addition, the capsule often forms adhesions or encircles the lumbosacral nerve roots in the vicinity of the tumor.

Microscopically, these tumors are classically described as having pseudopapillary arrangement of tumor cells surrounding hyalinized fibrovascular cores containing myxoid change, also described as pseudorosettes. Mucinous change found in the tumors varies, with most being characterized as mild and moderate mucinous change. Less than 10% of tumors demonstrate marked mucinous change, according to a clinicopathologic study by Sonneland et al. in 1985 [11]. Cytologic appearance of tumors included many cell types, such as flat, cuboidal, and columnar, while cuboidal cells are the classic finding. No mitotic activity is seen in most tumors as well as absent or minimal cytologic atypia. In addition, cellular necrosis was absent in most subjects; however, hemorrhage, hemosiderin deposition, and cystic degeneration were commonly observed in the myxopapillary ependymomas studied [5].

Immunohistochemistry findings of MPE include strong positive findings for GFAP, vimentin, and S-100 protein, while findings are negative for EMA and CK. Immunostaining for EGFR

in the tumor was also strongly positive. Wang et al's clinicopathological study found that most MPE Ki-67 labeling index was 1–6% [11]. Cytogenetically, it has been demonstrated that intramedullary and myxopapillary ependymomas are different genetic subgroups. While both share chromosome 7 gain, other genetic alterations, such as loss of 22q, gain of 15q, gain of 12 did not occur in MPE. Conversely, loss of chromosome 1, 2, and 10 will occur in MPE, but not in intramedullary ependymomas [19].

Imaging Findings

Myxopapillary ependymomas have very distinctive imaging characteristics that should guide physicians' confidence in diagnosis and allow for educated treatment decisions. While MRI is the best modality to evaluate the tumor (Figs. 3.3, 3.4, and 3.5), non-specific findings may occur, leading to findings on plain radiographs or CT. Such findings are more commonly found in cases of larger MPE and include scalloping of vertebral bodies from local erosion of tumor and widened or invaded neural foramina should tumor extend laterally. In addition to this, CT myelogram also demonstrates a sharply demarcated intradural mass associated with distal conus or filum [20].

Characteristically, MPE are found at the conus/cauda equina region and are T1 hypointense to isointense tumors that avidly enhance with administration of gadolinium. While many may be homogeneously enhancing, cystic tumors may be more heterogeneously enhancing [10, 21]. A more unique feature compared to tumors at this location is that T2 sequences demonstrate hyperintensity of the tumor characteristic of the proteinaceous perivascular mucin and may occasionally demonstrate a low intensity rim representative of hemorrhage [22]. This has been helpful in distinguishing the tumor from other potential etiologies in the area. They may or may not demonstrate continuity with the conus that may make resection more challenging. MRI is a very sensitive modality for detection of conus involvement. Finally, hemosiderin/blood prod-

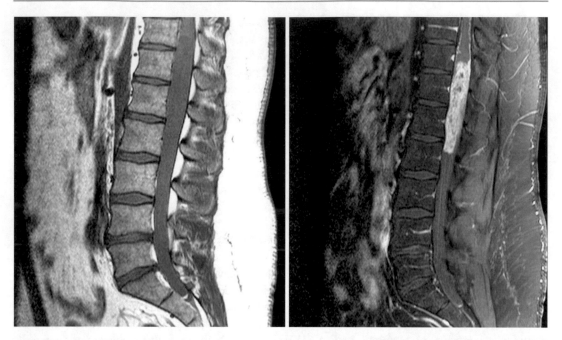

Fig. 3.3 Sagittal MRI T1 pre- and post-contrast sequences depicting a contrast enhancing Myxopapillary ependymoma located at the conus filling the spinal canal

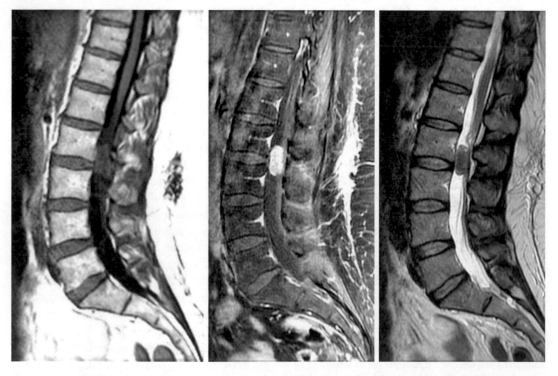

Fig. 3.4 Sagittal MRI T1 pre- and post-contrast as well as T2 sequences depicting a contrast-enhancing Myxopapillary ependymoma of the cauda equina/filum terminale. Note the homogenous enhancement on T1 post-contrast imaging and dorsal displacement of nerve roots. This local compression is often the cause of symptoms leading to presentation of these tumors

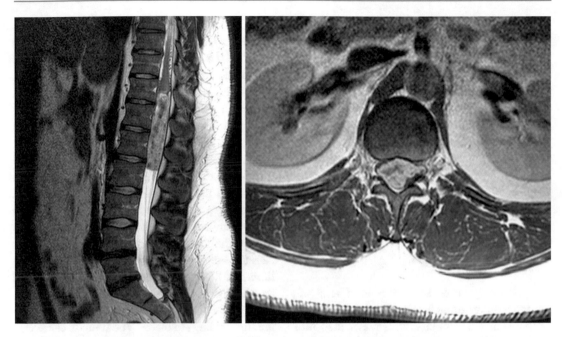

Fig. 3.5 Sagittal and axial MRI T2 depicting a myxopapillary ependymoma at the conus. Note the relative heterogeneous nature of the T2 signal generated by vascularity and mucoid portions of the tumor

ucts may be detectable at the periphery of vascular MPE that have hemorrhaged.

Finally, the tumor appears ovoid or sausage shaped on MRI. While characteristically at the conus/cauda equina, it may demonstrate expansion over many levels, including involvement of lower thoracic cord and the sacrum. The enhancing lesion may protrude through the neural foramina and erode into nearby structures such as vertebral bodies. Occasionally it can be helpful to identify the filum on the MRI and the tumor can sometimes appear to be connected or arising from it.

Natural History

As previously discussed, the natural history of myxopapillary ependymomas is most often a slow, indolent progression. Most commonly diagnosed in third or fourth decade of life, patients notice progressive back/sacral pain and, at times, radicular pain [3]. Less commonly, or in more chronic cases, patients note weakness, ambulatory dysfunction, or bowel/bladder dysfunction. Given the indolent nature and similarity to degenerative lumbar disease, patients often experience

symptoms for months or even years prior to diagnosis and treatment. Over time, symptoms are slowly progressive as the tumor experiences growth. The tumor itself is unlikely to invade or metastasize. They locally expand but often remain encapsulated and localized. However, longer duration of symptoms prior to treatment has been correlated with larger tumor size upon presentation and may leave patients at an increased risk of dissemination or leptomeningeal spread [6]. In addition to longer time to treatment, pediatric patients with MPE have demonstrated more aggressive clinical courses with more frequent recurrence and cerebrospinal dissemination [23].

While often treated prior to progression of symptoms to paraparesis, it has been demonstrated that, if untreated, these tumors have a propensity to progress and cause more severe symptoms, such as paraparesis. In one report, a patient who presented with back pain and bilateral radiculopathy diagnosed with a 3 cm ependymoma refused treatment. Five years later, the patient presented with progressive and severe paraparesis, inability to ambulate, and bladder dysfunction. In that time, the tumor had grown from 3 cm to 20 cm and now involved spinal levels T11 to S1. Despite this, the gross total resection was still achievable because no dissemination or infiltration had occurred in this case [18]. This case, among others, demonstrate that, while the tumor is relatively benign and progression may be slow, lesions treated late have worse outcomes with progression of neurological symptoms. Overall, if treated appropriately, long term survival and progression-free survival are excellent. Studies have demonstrated 5 year survival rates as high as 85–100%, and one retrospective review exhibited an 11 year 94% survival [3].

Treatment/Prognosis

As previously discussed, MPE have relatively benign features often leading to growth and compression of adjacent structures rather than infiltration. This is, in part, due to the capsule surrounding the tumor that may separate pathologic tissue from normal neural tissue. Because MPE are uncommon tumors, there are no definitive therapeutic guidelines for treatment of these tumors. However, because of the characteristics above, it is widely accepted that first line treatment for these tumors is surgical resection with the goal of gross total resection [12].

Surgical Techniques

For typical MPE cases not involving dissemination or sacral invasion, in typical lumbosacral canal distribution, this is achieved through a posterior approach. Patients are typically positioned prone, often times on a Wilson frame. Neuromonitoring is applied and may be useful in differentiating the filum from the nerve roots. Localization is achieved by lateral X-ray and midline subperiosteal dissection over desired levels.

Laminectomies are performed to gain access from the proximal to distal ends of the lesion. At this time, a surgical microscope is brought in the operative field and, often times, the tumor's location may be apparent by visualization through the translucent dura. If desired, ultrasound may also provide clarity on tumor boundaries and relative position of the nerve roots to the tumor before opening dura. The dura is opened midline and

tacked to the muscle laterally. Leaving an arachnoid layer for protection, the surgeon attempts to mobilize the nerve roots laterally to identify the rostral and caudal attachments of the MPE. Since most MPE arise from the filum terminale, this structure is identified rostral to the tumor attachment and may be directly stimulated to confirm that it is not a nerve root attached to the tumor. When visualizing the contents of the dura, the filum's striated membrane is typically a whiter color than the surrounding yellow-tinted cauda equina nerve roots. In addition, a tortuous vessel typically runs along the filum and helps distinguish it from the nerve roots. While preserving tumor capsule, both proximal and distal filum is mobilized past the poles of the tumor in preparation of an en bloc resection. Lateral margins are then mobilized and, if able, freed of all attachments to the surrounding structures. The filum is cauterized and sharply divided and, using the stump near the MPE pole, the tumor is carefully mobilized and rolled out of the resection cavity, while carefully dividing tissue attachments deep and lateral to the tumor. Small cottonoids may be placed to protect the cauda equina roots. After the tumor is mobilized, the other filum pole may be cauterized and sharply divided to deliver the tumor for an en bloc resection. After the tumor is removed, a running stitch is used to primarily close the dura. A Valsalva maneuver is used to test for a watertight closure. After confirming that there is no CSF leak, a xenograft dural substitute may be placed over the dural closure as well as fibrin glue. A subfascial drain is placed and the incision is closed with a watertight fascial closure. The patient may remain flat overnight post-operatively per surgeon preference. Post-operative gadolinium enhanced MRI is obtained to evaluate for residual tumor.

The two main factors that limit en bloc resection are strongly adherent nerve roots to the capsule and an MPE with conus involvement. Both involve tumor invasion into neural elements and a clear dissection plane may not be apparent. The surgeon must make the decision to avoid harming the lumbosacral roots and conus in this scenario, and sacrifice en bloc resection for subtotal resection. By leaving MPE on the neural elements, they may be spared and the patient may undergo radiation post-operatively to preserve their neurological function and enhance their oncologic outcome.

Post-operative Outcomes

Maximal resection of tumor is attempted, as gross total resection may be curative. There have been studies that compare recurrence in patients who achieve subtotal, gross total, and en bloc resection. Given the tumor's propensity to seed the cerebrospinal fluid and recur locally or at distant sites, en bloc resection may lead to better outcomes. It has been reported that progression free survival at 5 years is 100%, 78%, and 49% in en bloc resection, gross total resection with capsular violation, and subtotal resection [12].

Given the low incidence and indolent course of MPE, long-term outcomes have varied. While reported treatment failures vary, multiple sources have correlated GTR with lower treatment failure than STR [4, 11, 12, 17, 20, 23]. In addition, patients undergoing STR may benefit from radiotherapy of residual tumor, as patients receiving adjuvant radiotherapy may have their 10 year PFS increased from <40% to up to 70% [7]. Studies investigating the use of radiotherapy in MPE patients use fractionated treatments with median dosing 40–50 Gy. Even with radiotherapy in addition to STR, control rates are often inferior to GTR [6, 7, 24].

Lastly, although its efficacy has not been fully established in the literature, chemotherapy modalities, such as temozolomide, bevacizumab, etoposide, and carboplatin, have been documented in the treatment of MPE [17, 25]. These therapies are rarely used as first line treatment and may have utility in combating local and distant recurrence, as well as cerebrospinal dissemination. There have not been large enough series in literature to provide recommendations on the use of chemotherapy in MPE patients.

Should tumor location, configuration, and involvement of normal neural structures permit, GTR should be attempted in all of these patients to permit superior outcomes. In addition, MPE is a pathology that may recur locally, have distant spinal metastases, or cranial failure. A larger study carried out by MD Anderson was notable for examining long-term outcomes in 183 patients with MPE. They noted a 10 year survival rate of 92.4%, PFS rate of 61.2%, and reported that of the 31.7% treatment failure rate, 26.8% recurred locally, 9.3% were distant spinal metastasis, and 6.0% were cranial failures [7]. It is interesting to note that although adjuvant radiation appears to be protective in terms of recurrence and PFS in MPE patients, it had not been definitively demonstrated that it improves overall survival [26]. Given the benign nature of the disease, very few patients suffer mortality but instead suffer long term morbidities associated with recurrence such as loss of neurological function, pain, and disability. Besides progression-free survival and overall survival, it is important to investigate the quality of life outcomes in patients undergoing MPE resection, given that presenting symptoms in most patients are, often times, debilitating back or radicular pain. It has been noted that, after the immediate post-operative period, patients who have undergone resection for MPE have decreased Oswestry Disability Index and visual analog scale values, while improving each of the EQ-5D domains in mobility, self-care, usual activities, pain and discomfort, and pain and anxiety [27]. Overall progression-free survival, overall survival, and quality of life seem to be improved by surgical resection of MPE.

Based on this discussion, our recommendations for post-operative management of MPE are based on extent of resection. In patients with GTR confirmed by MRI, we recommend 6-month follow-up MRI, followed by annual MRI to monitor for recurrence. In patients with STR, patients should receive adjuvant radiotherapy, ranging from 45 to 50 Gy in fractions of 1.5–2.0 Gy after resection. Afterward, the patient should receive MRIs to evaluate for recurrence every 6 months for the next several years, at which point patients with stable disease may be monitored with annual MRI.

Differential Diagnosis

MPE only constitutes 13% of all spinal ependymomas. However, it is the etiology for approximately 83% of spinal tumor cases in the conus medullaris and filum terminale regions. As a result, it is strongly favored in the differential diagnosis of this region [2]. While other possibilities are much rarer, the differential diagnosis of intradural extramedullary neoplasms includes schwannoma, meningioma, neurofibroma, and paragangliomas [22, 28, 29]. On imaging, it may be difficult to differentiate between MPE and the other IDEM tumors. Some MRI studies have suggested that a higher ratio T2 hyperintense area of contrast-enhancing tumor may favor an MPE diagnosis over nerve sheath tumors, such as schwannomas; however, pathological studies remain the gold standard of diagnosis. Other differential considerations may include non-neoplastic etiology, such as herniated intervertebral disc, and dermoid cysts [30] mimicking an intradural extramedullary spinal neoplasm. In addition, there are other extradural pathologies that may invade into the dura and should not be confused for IDEM pathology.

Ganglioneuroma

Introduction

Ganglioneuromas (GN) are benign, full-differentiated neuroblastic tumors formed by neural crest cells. They arise from ganglion cells of the sympathetic nervous system, extending from the skull base to the pelvis and adrenal medulla [31]. Pick and Bielschowsky were the first to describe the spinal ganglioneuroma in 1911 [32]. While the spine is an uncommon location for ganglioneuromas, they have been reported in each section of the spine. Extradural and intradural extramedullary varieties are rare. Spinal GN are usually dumbbell-shaped. While typically asymptomatic, ganglioneuroma can cause symptoms due to compression of surrounding tissue. When causing neural compression, they may be resected along with performing a decompression of the spine, such as a laminectomy. Rarely malignant, ganglioneuromas portend a very favorable prognosis when excision is performed. The 10-year survival rate for all ganglioneuromas exceeds 97% [33].

Demographics and Clinical Presentation

Ganglioneuromas are estimated to account for 0.1–0.5% of all central nervous system tumors and 1% of all spinal cord tumors [34, 35]. Often extraspinal, the majority arise within the mediastinum (41.5%), retroperitoneum (37.5%), and neck (8%). However, GN have also been reported in the cervical, lumbar, and sacral regions of the spine [36]. They are more commonly distributed cranially than caudally in the spine. The incidence of ganglioneuromas is estimated to be 1 in 100,000 [33]. About 10% of all ganglioneuromas involve the spinal cord, generally in the paraspinal region, with subsequent intradural invasion [37]. Primary intradural, extramedullary lesions are rare cases. When extraspinal, a ganglioneuroma may present with bowel obstruction, hypertension, virilization, and myasthenia gravis [38]. GN may be asymptomatic and discovered incidentally during imaging. Spinal GN present typically with extremity weakness and paraplegia, as well as sensory loss below the area of tumor [35, 39]. Progressive tetraparesis and neck pain were frequent symptoms in a review of cervical ganglioneuromas [40, 41]. When located in the spine, these tumors more commonly present with signs related to neural element compression. Signs of compression include loss of muscle tone, diminished deep tendon reflexes, clonus, positive Babinski responses, loss of function of the lower extremities, and bowel and bladder disturbances [42]. Smaller lesions often cause non-specific symptoms until lesions become compressive. While ganglioneuromas are most commonly found as solitary lesions, multi-focal lesions may be associated with von Recklinghausen's (NF-1) disease [43]. In the cervical spine, 20% of the ganglioneuromas were associated with the disease [44]. Given the rarity of the tumor, there is little data on gender and demographic predisposition of these tumors. GN are most commonly diagnosed between the ages of 10 and 29 years and 60% occur in children and young adults [33, 40].

Location

GN can arise anywhere within sympathetic nervous system tissue but generally appear in the peripheral nervous system in areas, such as the posterior mediastinum, retroperitoneum, cervical spine, and adrenal gland. Overall, roughly 10% of all GN are in the spine. Cases of GN have been reported in the cervical, thoracic, lumbar, and sacrococcygeal sections of the cord [37]. Most commonly, GN are extradural and also present as intradural extramedullary and intramedullary lesions. The epicenters of the ganglioneuroma of the sympathetic chain arise in the paraspinal space, but extend through the neural foramen intradurally. A review of cervical spine ganglioneuroma cases by Deora et al. found intradural extension occurred in 62.5% of cases. This growth leads to the characteristic dumbbell or hourglass shape. In the cervical spine, 94% of reported GN cases demonstrated this shape. Seventy-five percent of the cervical cases originated above C3. Dumbbell ganglioneuromas can be unilateral or bilateral [44]. In rare cases, GN may develop from the nerve root [43]. Spinal extradural ganglioneuromas can originate from dorsal root ganglions or neural crest remnants. Intramedullary or intradural extramedullary types are extremely rare presentations of GN [34]. Levy et al. described one case of a thoracic GN that was entirely intradural extramedullary [39]. GN infiltrating the conus medullaris have also been reported [45].

Macroscopic and Microscopic Findings

Ganglioneuromas, ganglioneuroblastomas, and neuroblastomas are subgroups of neuroblastic tumors arising from neural crest cells. These subgroups are classified according to cellular and extracellular differentiation [46]. Neuroblastic tumors are classified on a spectrum, with ganglioneuromas being the most mature, while neuroblastomas are the most immature cells. As a general rule, GN have less malignant potential than other neuroblastic tumors because they are composed of more mature, fully differentiated cells [35]. GN are white, well-encapsulated, and firm [43]. Microscopically, GN comprise nerve fibers, Schwann cells, mature ganglion cells, and mucous matrix. Cells with multiple nuclei containing well-defined nucleolus in each nucleus are common. Spinal GN are capable of growing to a large size. The stroma of peripheral GN is composed of connective tissue; however, it is rarely prominent in central GN, where the stroma is usually glial [39]. The absence of immature cells or necrosis is used to rule out malignancy [31]. GN show reactivity with S100 and synaptophysin [35]. In several GN cases, Ki67 index was less than 1% [31, 44]. Reliable and accurate diagnosis before surgery undoubtedly improves disease management, but the nature of ganglioneuromas means they often require histopathological examination to confirm the diagnosis.

Imaging Findings

Characteristically, spinal GN will demonstrate a dumbbell or hourglass shape. Ichikawa et al. described the characteristic features of GN: an oval well-defined mass, and low or intermediate attenuation on CT [47]. Calcification is seen in 40–60% of ganglioneuromas on CT scan. The pattern of calcification in neuroblastomas, a less-mature form of GN, is more amorphous and coarse. This feature can help diagnose ganglioneuromas. Ultrasound is the initial diagnostic modality used in detecting ganglioneuromas. Intraoperative ultrasound has been used to assist with confirming the location of intradural extramedullary lesions [39]. However, the image generally reveals a nonspecific, heterogeneous hypoechoic solid lesion [48]. MR imaging of ganglioneuromas will be hypo-intense, with homogenous low or intermediate signal intensity on T1-weighted images and display heterogeneous hyperintensity on T2-weighted images. Dynamic MR images show gradual increasing enhancement [47]. Curvilinear bands of low signal intensity on T2-weighted images give ganglioneuromas a characteristic "whorled" appearance. Diagnosis by imaging is further complicated by the different proportions of the tumor cell composition, which can cause imaging differences. Specific diagnosis of ganglioneuroma is difficult without histopathological examination.

Natural History

Levy et al. described a case of primary intradural extramedullary ganglioneuroma [39]. The patient presented progressively worsening lower extremity weakness that rapidly progressed to him being unable to walk. Myelography revealed a complete block at T4 due to an intradural extramedullary tumor. Two months after symptoms began, surgical resection was completed via T3-T5 laminectomy to decompress the spine and remove the tumor, which was well-encapsulated. Following the operation, the patient's lower extremity strength improved from preoperative 2/5 to 4/5. No recurrence was reported in this case [39]. In another case reported by Kalyanaraman et al., an intramedullary cervical lesion was identified but not removed 14 years prior [49] . Spinal decompression via laminectomy was completed to alleviate compression, but the tumor was deemed inoperable. The timing and presentation align with the benign, slow growing characteristics of GN. While this lesion was reported as intramedullary, it allows for understanding how these neoplasms can present after a long period of growth.

Treatment/Prognosis

The optimal treatment for ganglioneuroma is surgical resection. Given their benign nature, chemotherapy and radiation have no role in management [33]. The long-term prognosis is generally excellent as long as total excision is performed. The surgical approach typically involves laminectomy or hemilaminectomy of the afflicted area of the spine.

In exceptional cases, lymph node metastasis and recurrence has occurred [33]. Transformation of ganglioneuroma into neuroblastoma and malignant peripheral neural sheath tumors (MPNST) has been reported [33, 50–52]. Therefore, regular radiologic examination is necessary as a follow-up [35]. Resection of spinal cord tumors is a technically demanding procedure, given the proximity of nerve tissue and large vessels. Furthermore, intradural tumors tend to adhere to the dura, posing further challenge to their complete removal. Due to the small chance for recurrence and underlying tumor biology, it is essential to weigh the risks involved with a total resection vs. leaving residual tissue. In a large study of GN in any location, tumors with smaller than 2.0 cm pieces were shown to be less likely to progress than larger residual lesions. Furthermore, cytotoxic therapy was shown to have little effectiveness and secondary surgery was often required [53] . Overall, ganglioneuromas tend to remain silent for a long period of time and long-term survival is likely. Irrespective of location, 10-year survival is 97.7% if total resection is completed [33]. In most cases of spinal ganglioneuroma, surgical resection resulted in significant reversal of their symptoms. Total resection was completed in 6 cases of thoracic GN reviewed by Huang et al. [31]. Sixty percent of cervical GN were subtotally resected in another review [44]. In one case of a 2-year old boy with a ganglioneuroma spanning his entire thoracic spine, his symptoms were reversed within 3 months of decompression. In an extensive review of neuroblastic tumor outcomes by Okamatsu et al., event-free survival was 100% following the resection of mature GN, regardless of location [54]. Other reviews have demonstrated similar excellent recovery and long-term survival [53].

Patients with ganglioneuromas typically present after progressively worsening neurological symptoms over the previous months or years. GN arise from neural crest cells, meaning that the tumor likely appears in childhood or early adulthood. Given the tumors' lack of aggressive growth or metastases, symptoms align with the compression of surrounding nervous tissue. Patients with ganglioneuromas typically have a very good prognosis if resection is successful.

Neurologic function is often improved or restored following resection and subsequent therapy. Patients may present with GN at a young age, so it is imperative that they are assessed and treated before permanent, progressive neurological deficits occur.

Differential Diagnosis

The uncommon locations of spinal ganglioneuromas is due to neural crest cell migration during the embryonic period [55]. Koeller et al. provided a comprehensive review of intradural extramedullary lesions. Differential diagnosis of intradural GN include menigiomas, schwannomas, neurofibroma, and malignant peripheral neural sheath tumors [2]. Other less common diagnoses include myxopapillary ependymoma and paraganglioma, though these tumors typically present in the cauda equina/filum terminale region. GN, meningiomas, and schwannomas are generally T1 hypointense and T2 hyperintense, but they have more specific imaging findings that can be used for diagnosis. Ganglioneuromas have a characteristic T2 weighted MRI of curvilinear bands of low signal intensity, giving the tumor a whorled appearance. In contrast, meningiomas commonly have an intense enhancement with dural tail. Schwannomas have an association with NF2 and heterogenicity that correlates with Antoni B tissues. Neurofibromas have a "can of worms" appearance. Suspected neuroblastic tumor should be evaluated for the presence of necrosis or immature ganglion cells, which are indicative of malignancy [31]. The age at diagnosis is also a factor for the type of tumor, with GN being diagnosed at an average age of 125 months compared to neuroblastoma at 9 months [53]. The presence of one of these characteristic findings in lieu of the previously mentioned GN imaging findings may allow differential diagnosis of another tumor.

It can be difficult to differentiate ganglioneuromas from other neuroblastic tumors using imaging, particularly from other neuroblastic types. Accordingly, ruling out potential malignancies is unlikely until histological analysis can

be completed [35]. Given the heterogeneous composition, GN biopsies are of limited effect in confirming a diagnosis. The numerous potential locations for spinal GN means the misdiagnosis of a more common neoplasm is likely. Ganglioneuroma should be considered when diagnosing any intra- or extraspinal tumor.

Paraganglioma

Introduction

Paragangliomas are rare, slow-growing, and usually benign neuroendocrine neoplasms that arise from cells of the adrenal gland, carotid bodies, middle ear, larynx, and vagus nerve [56, 57]. Spinal intradural paragangliomas were first described by Lerman in 1972, and are an extremely rare presentation of this tumor that generally occur in the filum terminale of the cauda equina, constituting approximately 3.5% of tumors in this region [2, 58]. Spinal paragangliomas occur predominantly in adulthood and often have nonspecific symptoms and similar appearance on imaging to schwannomas and myxopapillary ependymomas, thus requiring immunohistochemical analysis to confirm the diagnosis. Given the low rates of recurrence and metastasis of paragangliomas, complete surgical resection of these tumors yields a favorable prognosis.

Demographics and Clinical Presentation

Paragangliomas are estimated to occur with an incidence of 3 per 1,000,000 people per year. Even rarer in the spine, they have an incidence of 0.07 per 100,000 people per year [59, 60]. Tumors in this region have a slight predilection for males and most commonly occur within the fourth to sixth decades of life, with the average age of diagnosis being 46 years old and ranging from 9 to 75 years [61]. Paraganglioma can occur sporadically or as a result of genetic mutations. In one study of 272 patients by Hamidi et al., 70%

of cases were sporadic. The remaining 30% occurred in connection to a genetic syndrome, such as multiple endocrine neoplasia type 1 (MEN1) (1.15), MEN 2a (2.2%), von Hippel-Lindau disease (VHL) (1.1%), neurofibromatosis type 1 (NF-1) (1.5%), Carney triad (0.4%), and *THMEM127* gene mutations (0.4%). Mutations in the gene that encodes the succinate dehydrogenase enzyme B (SDHB) (15.4%), SDHC (0.7%), and SDHD (2.6%) were correlated. Finally, 5.5% of patients were diagnosed with familial paragangliomas based on family history [62]. Other studies found approximately 40% of patients have paragangliomas from genetic causes [59, 63].

Spinal intradural paragangliomas account for about 3.5% of cauda equina tumors and are most commonly found on the filum terminale [2]. The most commonly reported symptoms are radicular pain and cauda equina syndrome, which can include paraparesis, numbness, and sphincter insufficiency. In a study of 19 patients with spinal paragangliomas, 79% of patients reported lower back pain, 84% reported sciatica, 63% reported motor deficits, 53% reported sensory disturbance, and 26% reported sphincter dysfunction [64]. Increased intracranial pressure and papilledema have also been reported, and increased levels of CSF proteins are a frequent finding [61]. Although pheochromocytomas, which originate in adrenal tissues, are typically the only type of paraganglioma that actively secrete hormones, thoracic paragangliomas have also been found to secrete catecholamines, as well as compress the spinal cord and cause symptoms that are specific to the vertebral level at which it is located [56, 61]. Since the symptoms of intradural paragangliomas are non-specific and similar to those of other types of spinal tumors, they are often misdiagnosed until after resection and tissue diagnosis is achieved.

Location

Paragangliomas occur due to dysfunction of embryonic paraganglia cell migration or non-regression [65]. In the central nervous system, 80–90% of paragangliomas occur in the head and neck regions, including the carotid body, middle ear, larynx, and vagus nerve [65]. Approximately 9% of paragangliomas occur in the spine, the most common location being the filum terminale region of the cauda equina, and they have been reported with extreme rarity in the thoracic and cervical spine [61]. In two studies of 15 patients total with spinal paragangliomas, 1 patient had an extradural lesion at T6–7, and 1 patient had an intradural lesion at C2–3, and the remaining 13 patients had intradural lesions of the lumbar spine [56, 66]. Spinal paragangliomas can occur due to direct invasion of a nearby tumor into the spinal canal, metastatic spread, and, rarely, as a primary localization.

Macroscopic and Microscopic Pathology

Paragangliomas are typically fleshy, friable tumors that appear reddish-brown in color due to high levels of vascularization [67]. They are often oval or sausage shaped and well encapsulated, which contributes to the curative rate of surgical resection. Encapsulated tumors allow for complete surgical resection and very low rates of recurrence, while unencapsulated paragangliomas are more difficult to fully resect and thus have a higher rate of recurrence [2]. Intradural paragangliomas in the cauda equina region are typically fully contained within the dura, but have the potential to transverse the dura and cause destruction of vertebrae [61]. Spinal paragangliomas have been reported on average to be 1–1.2 cm in size, and a size larger than 5-6 cm coupled with a mutation in the SDHB gene is suggestive of malignancy [61].

Post-operative histological examination of paraganglioma is necessary to make the definitive diagnosis due to the ambiguity of its appearance and presenting symptoms. The hallmark microscopic finding in paraganglioma is a "Zellballen" pattern, which denotes a compact and nest-like group of chief cells that is surrounded by supportive connective tissue and a capillary network [56]. Paragangliomas contain neurosecretory granules regardless of origin;

however, only some secrete catecholamines and cause systemic symptoms [59]. Twenty-five percent of intradural paragangliomas contain mature ganglion cell and Schwann cell components [61]. Immunohistochemical analysis of paraganglioma cells has shown expression of synaptophysin (SYN) and chromogranin A (CGA) in chief cells and ganglionic cells, and expression of S100 in sustentacular cells [68]. In a review of 19 spinal paraganglioma cases, Ki-67 was expressed in every tumor in less than 10% of cells [69]. Many of these antibodies are also expressed in ependymomas, therefore a large assay of antibodies should be completed to ensure the correct diagnosis [68]. Due to the rarity of malignant paragangliomas and the nonspecific clinical findings, reliable histological or clinical predictors of malignancy have not been found [70].

Imaging Findings

Imaging, particularly MRI, is instrumental in diagnosis of intradural extramedullary lesions. However, paragangliomas are generally indistin-guishable from schwannomas or ependymomas [61]. The MRI findings for paraganglioma are T1 hypointensity and heterogeneously T2 isointensity/hyperintensity (Fig. 3.6). The tumor is highly vascularized, made evident by flow voids and intense enhancement on MR imaging [71]. One imaging finding useful in identifying a paraganglioma is the cap sign. The cap sign is an area of peripheral T2 hypointensity caused by hemosiderin content [2, 61]. Yang et al's study of 19 spinal paragangliomas identified other characteristic signs that helped differentiate paragangliomas from other spinal tumors. These features include a "salt and pepper" sign on MRI, or speckled appearance due to punctate hemorrhages that appear hyperintense and flow voids that appear hypointense, which appears in richly vascularized tumors [64]. While imaging is the preferred technique to discover lesions like paragangliomas, it is often difficult to definitively diagnose specific lesions as paraganglioma pre-operatively given their rarity. The similarities in presentation of paragangliomas to other spinal cord tumors requires pathological diagnosis after resective surgery.

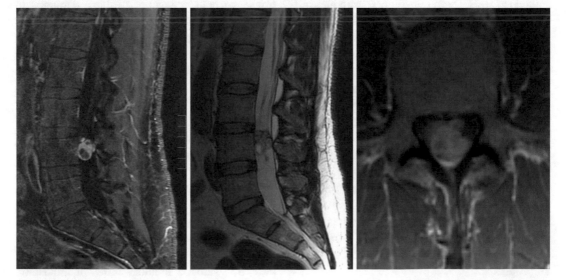

Fig. 3.6 Axial and sagittal post-contrast as well as sagittal T2 sequences depicting a contrast enhancing L4 filum terminale paraganglioma

Natural History

Paragangliomas are typically benign and slow growing, with a median 5-year survival rate of about 65%. Approximately 35% of all paragangliomas are metastatic, with a strong correlation between metastasis and SDHA and SDHB mutations [72]. The origin of spinal intradural paragangliomas is unclear, partly due to the unknown nature of paraganglia cells in the central nervous system and partly due to the rarity of the tumor [56]. Spinal paragangliomas were first described in literature in 1970 and, since then, paragangliomas of the filum terminale have only been reported about 300 times [2]. The tumors are most commonly diagnosed in the fourth to sixth decades of life and can be attributed to genetic mutations such as MEN2, VHL, NF-1, and SHDx up to 40% of the time [57]. The most commonly reported symptoms are sciatic nerve pain, paresthesia, bowel and bladder sphincter dysfunction, and numbness. Paragangliomas are usually encapsulated and thus are good candidates for complete resection with low rates of recurrence.

Honeyman et al. reported a case of intradural extramedullary paraganglioma in a 45-year-old man with a 2-year history of lower back pain and sciatica [73]. His pain transitioned from intermittent to constant over the 2-year period prior to presentation. The pain initially radiated to his right leg, but later began to involve his left leg. Motor power, reflexes, and sensations were all intact in the lower extremities. The patient denied any urinary or fecal issues. MRI revealed a mass at the level of L3 compressing the cauda equina. An en bloc resection was performed and diagnosis of paraganglioma was confirmed via histology. The patient experienced pain relief and no neurological or motor complications from the procedure. At 30 months, there was no recurrence. This case demonstrates the progression of symptoms related to the growth of paraganglioma and subsequent favorable recovery and overall prognosis.

Treatment and Prognosis

Surgical resection is the treatment of choice for paragangliomas. Total resection is advised in order to avoid recurrence, which has been reported in 4% of all cases of both total and subtotal resection. Thus, the vast majority are resected and cured. Paragangliomas are almost always benign, but metastatic potential has been reported in 10–20% of cases [61]. Large tumors (>5-6 cm) are at higher risk for recurrence and metastatic potential. All tumors have the potential for recurrence, making follow-up for at least 10 years strongly recommended [70, 72]. Higher risk patients, such as those presenting at a young age or those who with genetic mutations associated with paragangliomas, should have lifelong surveillance. While surgery is always the recommended treatment for non-metastatic paragangliomas, patients must weigh the risks of surgery for non-functioning or asymptomatic tumors. In the head, neck, and spinal regions, tumors are in close contact with neurovascular structures which increases the risk of surgical complications [72, 74]. If gross total resection is not possible, subtotal resection can be performed to relieve pain and neurological symptoms without causing further damage to neurovascular structures [76]. Radiation therapy is recommended when only subtotal resection is possible; however, the efficacy of radiation and chemotherapy in paraganglioma is undetermined [56, 64]. In one study, it has been suggested that en bloc resection yields a higher progression-free survival rate than subtotal excision with radiation therapy [59, 77]. Overall, the prognosis for paragangliomas is very good. More than 90% of patients with nonmetastatic paragangliomas/pheochromocytomas are alive 5 years after diagnosis [75] In another study of 272 pheochromocytomas and paragangliomas, survival at 5 years was 88.2% and 77.9% at 10-year follow-up for paragangliomas; however, this statistic includes cases of metastatic paraganglioma [70]. Thus, while paragangliomas of the spine can be difficult to diagnose, recovery and long term survival is likely.

Differential Diagnosis

The diagnosis of spinal paragangliomas is difficult, given their low incidence, non-specific symptoms, and radiological findings. Other more common lesions in the intradural extramedullary space, specifically located near the conus, include myxopapillary ependymoma, schwannoma, and meningioma [64]. The clinical presentation of paragangliomas often mimics tumors like ependymoma and schwannoma. Nerve sheath tumors and meningiomas account for almost 80–90% intradural extramedullary lesions. Therefore, paraganglioma is very low on the differential [56, 71]. Diagnosis of paraganglioma in this region is generally not considered prior to surgery. Following resection, IHC is the most commonly used method for definitive identification. A lack of glial fibrillary acidic protein can be used to exclude ependymoma [56]. The presence of GFAP and negative test for chromogranin suggests ependymal origin [67, 69]. Ependymomas are more aggressive and should be kept in mind for any intradural extramedullary lesion. Given the histopathological similarity between ependymomas and paragangliomas, misdiagnosis could potentially result in unnecessary radiotherapy. When the specific imaging and lab findings are present with a cauda equina mass, paraganglioma should be considered in the differential diagnosis [69].

Malignant Peripheral Neural Sheath Tumor

Introduction

Malignant peripheral nerve sheath tumors (MPNST) are a rare subset of soft tissue sarcomas that originate predominately from the Schwann cells of peripheral nerves, both sporadically and in association with neurofibromatosis Type-1 (NF-1). The term MPNST, instituted by the World Health Organization, delineates a category of tumors of similar origins and etiologies which were previously referred to by several different names, including malignant schwannoma, neurofibrosarcoma, malignant neurilemmoma, and neurogenic sarcoma [77]. The rarity, lack of specific immunohistochemical markers, and histological similarity to other soft tissue sarcomas make MPNSTs difficult to diagnose, and they are identified by a combination of MRI, immunohistochemical and histological analysis, physical exam, and evaluation for NF-1. Due to the rapid growth and high likelihood of metastasis, the recommended therapy for MPNST is radical surgical excision with wide margins, often sacrificing surrounding soft tissue and a significant portion of the nerve from which the tumor originates. Despite treatment, these tumors yield a high rate of recurrence and poor prognosis.

Demographics and Clinical Presentation

Malignant peripheral nerve sheath tumors constitute 3–10% of all soft tissue sarcomas, and these rare tumors occur at an incidence of 1 per 100,000 people per year in the general population and 3000–5000 per 100,000 people per year in patients with NF-1 [77, 78]. Spinal intradural MPNSTs are exceedingly rare and, as of 2016, only 23 cases have ever been reported in literature in patients without NF-1 [79]. Patients with NF-1 are at an increased risk of developing this tumor due to genetic predisposition to benign peripheral nerve sheath tumors called neurofibromas, some of which have the potential to become malignant [77, 80]. Approximately 50–60% of MPNSTs occur in patients with NF-1, and 10% are radiation induced [77]. MPNSTs typically develop within the third to sixth decades of life; however, they have been noted to occur 10 years earlier on average in patients with NF-1. They have been reported in patients with NF-1 as young as 7 years old [77, 80]. A study focused specifically on MPNSTs of the spine found the average age of presentation to be 43 years, ranging from 17 to 68 years [81]. This type of tumor shows no predilection for sex or race and occurs with similar incidence in both men and women [77].

Given the rarity and progressive symptom onset of MPNSTs, the time from symptom onset to diagnosis ranges from 1 to 96 months, with a median time of diagnosis of 5.5 months [81]. Common symptoms include pain, weakness, and progressively worsening neurological deficit at the nerve of origin, and duration of symptoms was reported to be longer in patients with NF-1 [77, 80]. In a study of 23 spinal MPNSTs, 74% of patients reported pain, 40% of patients reported lower back pain specifically, 43% reported weakness, 26% reported radiculopathy, and 23% reported paresthesia and/or paraparesis. Other reported symptoms included neck and shoulder pain in patients with cervical spine tumors, and bowel and bladder dysfunction in patients with lumbar and cauda equina tumors [79]. Observation of Tinel's sign (sensation of pins and needles in response to tapping on the mass) is suggestive of a peripheral nerve tumor, and pain, rapid growth, and deteriorating function of the affected nerve indicate likelihood of an MPNST over a benign peripheral nerve tumor, which are typically indolent in course [77].

Location

One of the hallmarks of MPNSTs is that they typically appear along a peripheral nerve, and can be manipulated perpendicularly to the nerve, but not parallel to it, indicating its roots in the myelin sheath of that nerve [77]. According to a study done by Ducatman et al. of 120 MPNSTs, approximately 46% of these

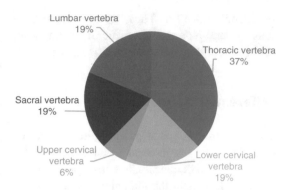

Fig. 3.7 Distribution of spinal location of MPNSTs as stated in a study done by Zhu et al. [78]

tumors occur in the trunk, 34% in the extremities, and 19% in the head and neck [80]. The five most common nerves of origin of these tumors are the sciatic nerve, brachial plexus, spinal nerve roots, vagus nerve, and femoral nerve in order of decreasing likelihood [80]. While spinal MPNSTs are rarer, Zhu et al. found that, of the 16 patients they studied with spinal MPNSTs, 6 were of the thoracic vertebra, 3 of the lower cervical vertebra, 3 of the sacral vertebra, 3 of the lumbar vertebra, and 1 of the upper cervical vertebra (Fig. 3.7) [78].

MPNSTs located in the trunk, especially in the spine, are associated with a poor prognosis and a lower 5-year disease-specific survival rate than tumors located in the head and neck. The reason for worse prognosis is not known, but it is hypothesized that tumors in the spine have higher potential for metastasis to the central nervous system, possibly via CSF dissemination [82]. A study done on the implications of intradural extension in high-grade paraspinal MPNSTs identified 6 patients with tumors that extended into the dura, 5 of which were located in the lumbosacral region and 1 located along the spinal accessory nerve. Sixty-seven percent of patients with intradural extension had metastases to the central nervous system, as opposed to 0% of patients with high-grade paraspinal MPNSTs but no intradural extension [82].

Macroscopic and Microscopic Pathology

MPNSTs appear grossly as globular or fusiform masses with irregular borders and are white and firm, but can be yellow and soft with central necrosis. The tumors are not encapsulated, and tend to demonstrate invasion of the surrounding soft tissue. In later stages, MPNSTs may infiltrate the vertebral bodies and the dura of the spinal cord. Nerve roots are often encased by the mass [77, 78, 80]. Size of the tumor is variable and has been shown to play a role in mortality, with tumors greater than 5 cm in diameter having an almost 2.5× increase in risk of death in all cases [81].

Histological examination of MPNSTs shows spindle-shaped cells arranged in fascicles, giving the appearance of alternating hypocellular and hypercellular areas similar to patterns in schwannomas, with wavy hyperchromatic nuclei [77, 83]. Epithelioid and/or heterologous differentiation of one or two different cell types (and very rarely, more than two) can be found in approximately 15% of MPNSTs. While the most common cell type is rhabdomyoblasts, other possible differentiations include smooth muscle, bone, cartilage, and neuroendocrine cells [83]. The presence of mitotic figures in a peripheral nerve tumor are suggestive of malignancy; however, they can also be present in certain types of benign masses [77]. A grading system of MPNSTs instituted by Ducatman et al. delineates low grade tumors as having mild to moderate hypercellularity, significant nuclear atypia, and 1–6 mitotic figures per 10 high power fields. For high grade tumors, requirements include pronounced hypercellularity and greater than 6 mitotic figures per 10 high power fields. In the same study, 82% of lesions were categorized as high-grade lesions [80].

Another feature of MPNSTs that makes diagnosis difficult is the lack of immunohistochemical markers that are specific to the tumor. The most indicative marker is S-100, a Schwann cell protein, but it can be lost in 10–50% of MPNSTs, so presence or absence of this protein alone is insufficient for diagnosis [77, 83].

S-100 is also a non-specific marker for many soft tissue tumors such as neurofibroma, schwannoma, ganglioneuroma, and synovial sarcoma, so it cannot be used to diagnose MPNST. Other useful markers include neural markers CD56 and PGP 9.5, and recent studies indicate nestin may be a valuable diagnostic finding as well. Immunohistochemical markers specific to differentiated cell types may also be found, such as actin in rhabdomyosarcomatous cells and cytokeratin in epithelial and neuroendocrine cells [83]. The only known predictive genetic marker for development of these tumors is NF-1.

Imaging Findings

Radiologic imaging shows that MPNSTs typically have well defined borders and are irregular, spherical, or lobular in shape. The tumors most often present with a hypo- or isointense T1 signal and hyper- or isointense T2 signal, and show heterogenous enhancement and homogenous enhancement with similar incidence. On CT scans, the tumor presents with isodensity the majority of the time, and no defining characteristics have been reported (Figs. 3.8 and 3.9) [84].

MRI has been found to be an extremely useful tool in distinguishing MPNSTs from other types of malignant soft tissue tumors (MSTTs) [85]. Multiple studies have suggested that benign peripheral nerve tumors have specific characteristics that allow them to be diagnosed with confidence on MRI and additionally that malignancy of soft tissue tumors can be accurately predicted by this modality [85]. One such study consisted of MRI scans of 17 MPNSTs and 18 MSTTs that were blindly reviewed and categorized by radiologists on the basis of location, distribution, nodular morphology, homogeneity, and definition of margins. Analysis of these features showed that intermuscular distribution of the mass, location along the length of a peripheral nerve, nodular morphology, and well-defined margins are all predictive of MPNSTs. Additionally, MPNSTs exhibit T1 and T2 heterogeneity significantly more so than MSTTs [85].

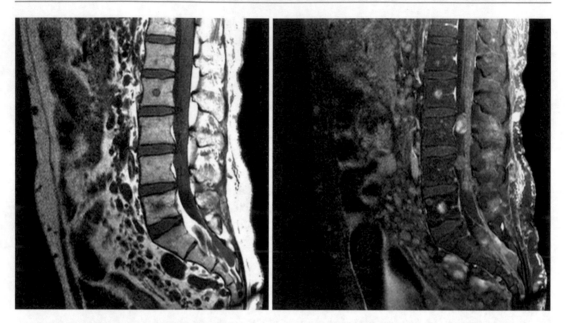

Fig. 3.8 Sagittal MRI T1 pre- and post-contrast sequences depicting a contrast-enhancing L3 MPNST

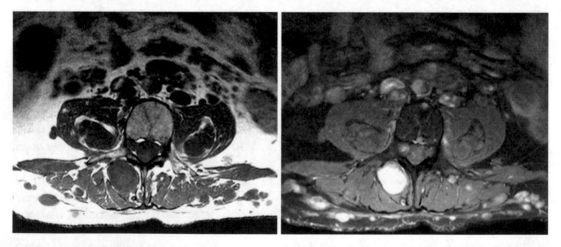

Fig. 3.9 Axial MRI T1 pre- and post-contrast sequences depicting a contrast-enhancing MPNST encroaching upon R neural foramen

MRI and CT scans of the complete neuroaxis may be necessary to evaluate for CSF dissemination and the degree of local invasion of the tumor.

Natural History

The natural history of intradural MPNSTs is typically aggressive, mean time from diagnosis to death reported to be 11.2 months in patients with spinal intradural MPNSTs. Conversely, extradural MPNSTs mean survival was reported as 72 months [82]. The tumors are most commonly diagnosed in the third to sixth decades of life, but are often found earlier in patients with NF-1, who are at a 10% lifetime risk of developing an MPNST [77]. The most commonly reported symptoms are pain and weakness, and other symptoms specific to spinal MPNSTs include bowel and bladder disfunction, paraplegia, and neurologic deficit, all specific to the vertebral level at which the tumor is located [78, 79]. Without treatment, patients develop progressive neurological deficits and poor functional status. MPNSTs yield a high rate of metastasis and recurrence, and in the setting of intradural extension of the tumor, metastasis to the central nervous system is common.

One case study of a 30-year-old woman with NF-1 and a previous history of MPNST, which had been excised with clear margins from her forearm, reports the diagnosis, progression, and treatment of her disease over the course of about 2 years. Two years after the resection of her forearm MPNST, the patient reported an 8 month history of back pain and a 1 week history of paraparesis and was diagnosed with a recurrent MPNST. MRI revealed a mass at T11, destroying the vertebrae and extending into the dura. A vertebrectomy was performed and her spine was stabilized, and this successfully treated her back pain and neurologic deficits. Eight months later, a lung metastasis was discovered and removed, and 14 months after the initial spinal surgery, another MPNST was found at the L5 vertebrae presenting with low back pain and lower extremity weakness. The vertebrectomy procedure was repeated; however, at 22 months from the initial surgery, another lung metastasis was found and treated with resection and chemotherapy, and at 26 months, multiple lung metastases had formed and the patient died [86]. This case highlights the high likelihood of metastasis and recurrence of MPNSTs, as well as the poor prognosis.

Treatment and Prognosis

Due to the high likelihood of metastasis and rapid growth of MPNSTs, the preferred treatment is radical en bloc surgical excision of the tumor with margins of at least 2 cm in every direction [77, 82]. This often includes removal of surrounding muscle and soft tissue and a significant portion of the nerve of origin, leaving the patient with neurologic deficit. Additionally, it can mean removal of adjacent bone, resulting in complete or partial vertebrectomy, sacrectomy, or pelvec-

tomy in the case of spinal MPNSTs [77, 82]. While radical en block surgical incision is preferred, spinal intradural MPNSTs are often not compatible with en bloc resection due to the adherence of the tumor to the dura, the proximity of the spinal cord, surrounding large blood vessels, and the subsequent morbidity associated with removal due to these factors. These tumors are instead removed piecemeal or by curettage, either completely or subtotally to an extent that removes cancerous cells and decompresses affected nerves without increasing morbidity [78, 82]. A study of 14 cases of spinal MPNST by Zhu et al. reported that en bloc resection was only possible for 1 patient, while 11 patients underwent gross total resection via piecemeal removal, and 2 patients underwent subtotal resection [78]. Subtotal resection was performed due to high volume of blood loss and is a clear cause of tumor recurrence, and is likely to complicate additional attempts at resection due to scarring and deformity [78]. Adjuvant chemotherapy and radiation may provide the benefit of prolonging survival and preventing recurrence of the tumor in the same location, notably in tumors of the periphery and in pediatric patients; however, they are not used routinely and more investigation is required to prove the effectiveness of this treatment [77, 78, 82, 86].

Even with aggressive treatment, the recurrence rate of MPNSTs is high and the prognosis is poor. Zhu et al. found the recurrence rate to be 85% after total resection of the tumor, and median survival after the initial resection was 11 months, with a 21.4% 5-year survival rate [78]. Recurrence rate of MPNST of any origin has been measured at 26% after a median interval of 22 months, and metastasis rate at 20% in a study of 54 patients [81]. Patients with spinal intradural MPNST have a mean survival of 11.2 months after diagnosis and 2-year survival rate of 0%. This is in contrast to a 17% 5-year survival rate for extradural spinal MPNST [82]. This is in stark contrast to MPNST patients without involvement of the spine, with a 5-year survival of 46% in over 1800 cases [87].

Certain factors have been found to increase the risk of death in patients with spinal MPNSTs, including location, intradural extension, metastasis, high grade lesions, tumor size, rhabdo-myosarcomatous or neuroendocrine differentiation, subtotal surgical resection, and age at diagnosis [78, 81–83]. Tumors larger than 5 cm in diameter have been reported to increase the risk of death by 2.5× compared to smaller tumors, and gross total resection reduced the risk of death by 92% compared to subtotal resection [81]. In a study of 120 cases of MPNST, 45% of patients with NF-1 experienced at an average of 13 months after initial diagnosis, and 38% patients without NF-1 experienced recurrence at an average of 32 months [80]. MPNST patients with NF-1 and without NF-1were not found to have a significant difference in survival [87].

Differential Diagnosis

Due to the rarity, ambiguous diagnostic features, and non-homogeneity of this tumor, more common types of soft tissue sarcoma should considered as a differential diagnosis unless ruled out by imaging and/or immunohistochemical and histological analysis. In patients with NF-1, benign neurofibromas should be suspected in the absence of pain, irregular shape, and rapid growth, which are typically signs of malignancy. Intradural extramedullary tumors of the thoracic and cervical spine are most often benign and diagnosis of neurofibroma, meningioma, and schwannoma should be considered in the differential [88].

Differential diagnoses based on histology include rhabdomyosarcoma, fibrosarcoma, leiomyosarcoma, synovial sarcoma, osteosarcoma, and chondrosarcoma [80, 83]. MPNST can be distinguished from many of these tumor types because differentiated cells are typically only found in focal locations within the tumor, whereas the characteristic spindle-shaped cells are diffusely spread throughout the tumor. Distinguishing MPNST from rhabdomyosarcoma can be difficult, as rhabdomyosarcomatous cells can sometimes become the most prevalent cell type [83]. MPNSTs with glandular differen-

tiation also bear resemblance to metastatic carcinoma, and the proper identification can be made by determining whether the spindle-shaped cells surrounding the glandular cells are also tumor cells, as in the case of MPNST, or are proliferating fibroblasts, as in the case of metastatic carcinoma [83].

Characteristic features of MPNST, such as T1 and T2 heterogeneity, irregular or spherical shape, well-defined tumor borders, and location along a peripheral nerve can be suggestive of MPNST; however, due to the overlap of features between MPNST and other types of soft tissue sarcoma, such as neurofibroma and schwannoma, a thorough history and physical exam is an important step to contextualize other findings and come to the appropriate diagnosis.

Spinal Lipoma

Introduction

Spinal lipomas are the most commonly diagnosed occult spinal dysraphism amongst pediatric patients, often occurring concomitantly with spina bifida. Spinal lipomas constitute about 1% of all spinal cord tumors, and intradural extramedullary spinal lipomas make up approximately 4% of all occult spinal dysraphisms [89, 90]. These benign masses are composed of adipose and fibrous tissue and generally occur in the lumbosacral spine, but, in rare cases, can also be found in the cervicothoracic region [91]. The tumors are slow growing, and symptoms most commonly arise in the first 5 years of life, the second and third decade, or the fifth decade, most likely due to changes in weight over time. MRI is the first choice for imaging of these lesions and necessary for diagnosis [90]. While spinal lipomas have low mortality rates, they have a 30–40% risk of deterioration if left untreated and can result in significant neurological deficits, and recent studies support complete surgical resection of these tumors in children before they become symptomatic.

Demographics and Clinical Presentation

Symptoms of spinal lipomas are caused by the size of the mass and its compression of the spinal cord as it grows. Patients typically show progressive deterioration as the tumor grows and can cause spinal cord tethering. Symptoms of spinal cord compression include back and leg pain, paresis, bladder and bowel dysfunction, and weakness, and do not typically present acutely, but get worse over time [89, 92]. Lumbosacral lipomas often occur with occult spinal dysraphism and are diagnosed in infants based on skin markers, but can also be diagnosed based on neurological symptoms in children and young adults [92]. Spinal lipomas are considered congenital and commonly present with spina bifida [92]. Intradural lipomas make up just 7% of all spinal lipomas and affect males and females equally [93]. Lipomas that are not associated with an occult spinal dysraphism are completely intradural and have no skin involvement [94]. According to Cogen et al., there are three distinct age groups in which symptoms arise. Twenty-four percent of patients experience symptoms in the first 5 years of life, 54% in the second and third decade, and 16% in the fifth decade [90]. This study notes that the thoracic location of spinal lipomas can be determined based on the corresponding vertebral level of presenting symptoms. For example, bladder and bowel dysfunction is an early finding in lumbosacral lipomas and may present as an isolated finding, but will present only in later stages in combination with other neurological symptoms in cervicothoracic lipomas [90].

Location

Spinal lipomas, including intradural extramedullary, are most commonly found in the lumbosacral region associated with dysraphism. Non-dysraphic lipomas are most common in the thoracic region [94]. Intradural lesions in the cervical and thoracic spine are extremely rare. Intraspinal lipomas are predominantly found in the dorsal spine [90, 91].

Macroscopic/Microscopic Findings

Histopathological examination of spinal lipomas reveal that they are formed of well-vascularized adipose tissue with areas of connective tissue [91]. Neural elements can be found interspersed within the lesion [95]. Şanlı describes the cells in these tumors as "large, polygonal, radiculated and optically empty with delicate cytoplasmic membranes." They contain an unremarkable, eccentric nucleus consistent with mature fat [96]. Analysis of these cells does not show any evidence of malignancy, and some hypothesize these tumors should be classified as hamartomas rather than neoplasms. Macroscopically, these tumors are soft, yellow, and fusiform [96].

Imaging

MRI is required for definitive diagnosis of spinal lipomas, and the lesion appears hyperintense on both T1 and T2 weighted images, and appears hypointense on fat suppressed sequences [90]. Ultrasound can also be used to identify lipomas, and they present as echogenic intraspinal masses adjacent to the spinal cord and are contiguous with subcutaneous fat, which is hypoechoic [89]. CT imaging usually shows a hypodense tumor with a negative Hounsfield number [95]. Plain radiography may show widening of the spinal canal, but findings are not specific for lipoma. Myelography is not usually performed, but may show blockage of contrast at the level of the lesion in the subarachnoid space. Intraoperative ultrasound is useful for determining proper location prior to opening the dura [96].

Natural History

Spinal lipomas are regarded as congenital defects, commonly occurring concomitantly with spina bifida or other neural tube defects. It has been theorized that premature disjunction of ectodermal cells may allow the migration of mesenchymal cells into the neural groove during neural tube formation, resulting in the differentiation and growth of adipose and fibrous tissue along the spinal canal. Lipomas increase in size in correlation with body fat composition, and changes in body fat, such as weight gain and pregnancy, can precipitate symptoms in patients [90]. Most patients are symptomatic for up to 2 years before seeking treatment, and neurological symptoms typically progress for months to years prior to diagnosis of the lipoma [90, 94]. The most common ages for symptoms to present are the first 5 years, the second to third decade, and the fifth decade of life [90].

A case study following an 18-year-old male reported a history of progressively worsening weakness in his legs and lower back pain for a year and half. The patient had no history of spina bifida or other neural tube defects, and X-ray of his spine was clear. Upon further investigation, MRI of the lumbosacral spine showed a hyperintense mass in the spinal canal extending from L1 to L2 and, on fat suppressed scans, the mass appeared hypointense, suggesting a diagnosis of intradural lipoma. The patient underwent a laminectomy and a complete resection of the lipoma, after which the patient experienced a full recovery and resolution of his neurological symptoms [97].

Treatment/Prognosis

A study done by Pang et al. compared the outcomes of different surgical approaches to treating lipomas, including observation only, partial resection, and total resection of the tumor [100]. Historically, partial resection or spinal decompression has been the primary treatment recommendation for spinal lipomas [90, 91, 101]. In the Pang et al.'s review of outcomes, it was demonstrated that total resection conveys a progression-free survival (PFS) of 88.1% at 20 years, while partial resection only yielded a 34.6% PFS at 10.5 years. The risk of symptomatic recurrence is also 5.94 times higher in partial resections over a period of 18 years. These findings contradict earlier studies, many of which state that total resection is accompanied by significant increase in morbidity [90, 91, 100]. Earlier papers also recommend laminectomy and duraplasty to manage symptoms in partial resection. Pang et al. recommend total resection and reconstruction of the neural placode to produce significantly improved long term outcomes for spinal lipomas [96]. In two long term observational studies performed by Kulkarni et al. and Xenos et al., spinal lipomas have a 30–40% risk of deterioration [99, 100]. Thus, Pang also recommends the prophylactic resection of asymptomatic spinal lipomas in children, as these patients had a 98.4% PFS at 16 years [98].

Differential Diagnosis

Only 4% of intraspinal lipomas are intradural extramedullary masses, the rest being lipomyelomeningoceles (84%) and filum terminale fibrolipomas (12%) [95, 97]. It is important to determine, based on imaging, where the masses originate and which layers of the spinal canal they infiltrate in order to accurately classify the lipoma.

Included for comparison of these rare tumors is a summary of common ages of presentation and clinical presentations (Figs. 3.10 and 3.11). To summarize radiographic findings of the various rare intradural extramedullary spinal cord tumors, please see Table 3.1.

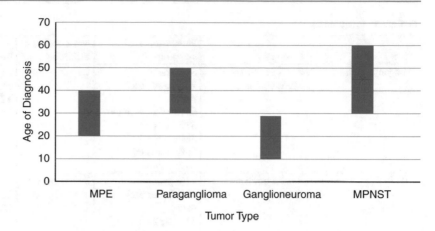

Fig. 3.10 Average age range of diagnosis for each of the four rare tumors

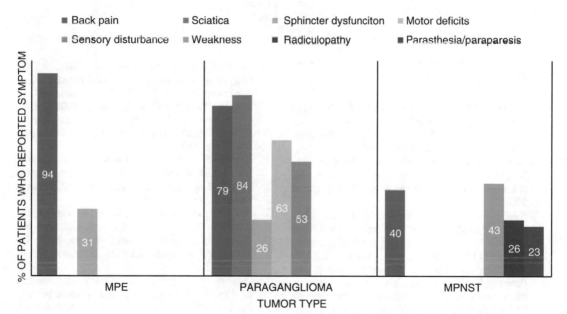

Fig. 3.11 Percentages of patients with MPE, paraganglioma, and MPNST who reported neurological symptoms [5, 64, 79]

Table 3.1 Summary of characteristics of rare intradural extramedullary spinal tumors

Tumor	Frequency	Patient-reported symptoms (%)	Most common location	Imaging
Myxopapillary Ependymoma	Most common tumor of cauda equina	94% back pain 31% sphincter dysfunction 9–81% gait dysfunction	Cauda equina	Sausage shaped T1 hypointense T2 hyperintense
Ganglioneuroma	1% of spinal cord tumors	Lower extremity weakness 33% scoliosis	Cervical spine	T1 hypointense T2 hyperintense and heterogeneous

(continued)

Table 3.1 (continued)

Tumor	Frequency	Patient-reported symptoms (%)	Most common location	Imaging
Paraganglioma	3–4% of tumors of cauda equina	84% sciatica 79% lower back pain 63% motor deficits 53% sensory disturbance 26% sphincter dysfunction	Cauda equina	T1 hypointense, salt and pepper appearance T2 iso or hyperintense Cap sign present
MPNST	3–10% of all soft tissue tumors	74% pain 40% lower back pain 43% weakness 26% radiculopathy 23% paresthesia/paraparesis	Sciatic nerve	T1 iso- or hypointense T2 iso- or hyper intense CT isodense

References

1. Kernohan JW. Primary tumors of the spinal cord and intradural filum terminale. In: Cytology and cellular pathology of the nervous system. New York: P.B. Hoeber, Inc; 1932. p. 993–1025.
2. Koeller KK, Rosenblum RS, Morrison AL. Neoplasms of the spinal cord and filum terminale: radiologic-pathologic correlation. Radiographics. 2000;20(6):1721–49.
3. Bagley CA, Wilson S, Kothbauer KF, Bookland MJ, Epstein F, Jallo GI. Long term outcomes following surgical resection of myxopapillary ependymomas. Neurosurg Rev. 2009;32(3):321–34; discussion 334
4. Al-Habib A, Al-Radi OO, Shannon P, Al-Ahmadi H, Petrenko Y, Fehlings MG. Myxopapillary ependymoma: correlation of clinical and imaging features with surgical resectability in a series with long-term follow-up. Spinal Cord. 2011;49(10):1073–8.
5. Wang H, Zhang S, Rehman SK, Zhang Z, Li W, Makki MS, et al. Clinicopathological features of myxopapillary ependymoma. J Clin Neurosci Off J Neurosurg Soc Australas. 2014;21(4):569–73.
6. Nakamura M, Ishii K, Watanabe K, Tsuji T, Matsumoto M, Toyama Y, et al. Long-term surgical outcomes for myxopapillary ependymomas of the cauda equina. Spine. 2009;34(21):E756–60.
7. Weber DC, Wang Y, Miller R, Villà S, Zaucha R, Pica A, et al. Long-term outcome of patients with spinal myxopapillary ependymoma: treatment results from the MD Anderson Cancer Center and institutions from the Rare Cancer Network. Neuro-Oncol. 2015;17(4):588–95.
8. Balasubramaniam S, Tyagi DK, Desai KI, Dighe MP. Outcome analysis in cases of spinal Conus Cauda Ependymoma. J Clin Diagn Res JCDR. 2016;10(9):PC12–6.
9. Acquaye AA, Vera E, Gilbert MR, Armstrong TS. Clinical presentation and outcomes for adult ependymoma patients. Cancer. 2017;123(3):494–501.
10. Sun B, Wang C, Wang J, Liu A. MRI features of intramedullary spinal cord ependymomas. J Neuroimaging Off J Am Soc Neuroimaging. 2003;13(4):346–51.
11. Sonneland PR, Scheithauer BW, Onofrio BM. Myxopapillary ependymoma. A clinicopathologic and immunocytochemical study of 77 cases. Cancer. 1985;56(4):883–93.
12. Abdulaziz M, Mallory GW, Bydon M, De la Garza Ramos R, Ellis JA, Laack NN, et al. Outcomes following myxopapillary ependymoma resection: the importance of capsule integrity. Neurosurg Focus. 2015;39(2):E8.
13. Gerston KF, Suprun H, Cohen H, Shenhav Z. Presacral myxopapillary ependymoma presenting as an abdominal mass in a child. J Pediatr Surg. 1985;20(3):276–8.
14. Moelleken SM, Seeger LL, Eckardt JJ, Batzdorf U. Myxopapillary ependymoma with extensive sacral destruction: CT and MR findings. J Comput Assist Tomogr. 1992;16(1):164–6.
15. Whittemore DE, Grondahl RE, Wong K. Primary extraneural myxopapillary ependymoma of the broad ligament. Arch Pathol Lab Med. 2005;129(10):1338–42.
16. Helwig EB, Stern JB. Subcutaneous sacrococcygeal myxopapillary ependymoma. A clinicopathologic study of 32 cases. Am J Clin Pathol. 1984;81(2):156–61.
17. Kraetzig T, McLaughlin L, Bilsky MH, Laufer I. Metastases of spinal myxopapillary ependymoma: unique characteristics and clinical management. J Neurosurg Spine. 2018;28(2):201–8.
18. Pusat S, Erbaş YC, Göçmen S, Kocaoğlu M, Erdoğan E. Natural course of Myxopapillary Ependymoma:

unusual case report and review of literature. World Neurosurg. 2019;121:239–42.

19. Hirose Y, Aldape K, Bollen A, James CD, Brat D, Lamborn K, et al. Chromosomal abnormalities subdivide ependymal tumors into clinically relevant groups. Am J Pathol. 2001;158(3):1137–43.

20. Wang AM, Lin JC, Haykal HA, Zamani AA, Rumbaugh CL. Ependymoma of filum terminale: metrizamide-enhanced CT evaluation. Comput Radiol Off J Comput Tomogr Soc. 1986;10(5):239–43.

21. Beall DP, Googe DJ, Emery RL, Thompson DB, Campbell SE, Ly JQ, et al. Extramedullary Intradural spinal tumors: a pictorial review. Curr Probl Diagn Radiol. 2007;36(5):185–1998.

22. Soderlund KA, Smith AB, Rushing EJ, Smirniotopoulos J. Radiologic-pathologic correlation of pediatric and adolescent spinal neoplasms: Part 2, Intradural extramedullary spinal neoplasms. Am J Roentgenol. 2012;198(1):44–51.

23. Feldman WB, Clark AJ, Safaee M, Ames CP, Parsa AT. Tumor control after surgery for spinal myxopapillary ependymomas: distinct outcomes in adults versus children: a systematic review. J Neurosurg Spine. 2013;19(4):471–6.

24. de Jong L, Calenbergh FV, Menten J, van Loon J, De Vleeschouwer S, Plets C, et al. Ependymomas of the filum terminale: the role of surgery and radiotherapy. Surg Neurol Int. 2012;3:76.

25. Fujiwara Y, Manabe H, Izumi B, Shima T, Adachi N. Remarkable efficacy of temozolomide for relapsed spinal myxopapillary ependymoma with multiple recurrence and cerebrospinal dissemination: a case report and literature review. Eur Spine J Off Publ Eur Spine Soc Eur Spinal Deform Soc Eur Sect Cerv Spine Res Soc. 2018;27(Suppl 3):421–5.

26. Akyurek S, Chang EL, Yu T-K, Little D, Allen PK, McCutcheon I, et al. Spinal myxopapillary ependymoma outcomes in patients treated with surgery and radiotherapy at M.D. Anderson Cancer Center. J Neuro-Oncol. 2006;80(2):177–83.

27. Viereck MJ, Ghobrial GM, Beygi S, Harrop JS. Improved patient quality of life following intradural extramedullary spinal tumor resection. J Neurosurg Spine. 2016;25(5):640–5.

28. Chamberlain MC, Tredway TL. Adult primary intradural spinal cord tumors: a review. Curr Neurol Neurosci Rep. 2011;11:320–8.

29. Mathew P, Todd NV. Intradural conus and cauda equina tumours: a retrospective review of presentation, diagnosis, and early outcome. J Neurol Neurosurg Psychiatry. 1993;56(1):69–74.

30. Coppens JR, Sherrill JE. Presumed rupture of a conus medullaris dermoid cyst with cervical intramedullary fat and lipomatous infiltration of the cauda equina. J Neurosurg Spine. 2006;(5):178.

31. Huang Y, Liu L, Li Q, Zhang S. Giant Ganglioneuroma of thoracic spine : a case report and review of literature. J Korean Neurosurg Soc. 2017;60(3):371–4.

32. Pick L, Bielschowsky M. About the system of neuromas and observations on a ganglioneuroma of the brain. J Entire Neurol Psychiatr. 1911;6:391–437.

33. Lopez CB, de la Calle Garcia B, Herrero RS. Intradural Ganglioneuroma mimicking lumbar disc herniation: case report. World Neurosurg. 2018;117:40–5.

34. Kang SH, Lee SM, Ha DH, Lee HJ. Extensive spinal extradural ganglioneuroma of the lumbar spine: mimicking lymphoma. Eur Spine J. 2018 07;27(Suppl 3):520–5.

35. Mounasamy V, Thacker MM, Humble S, Azouz ME, Pitcher JD, Scully SP, et al. Ganglioneuromas of the sacrum-a report of two cases with radiologic-pathologic correlation. Skelet Radiol. 2006;35(2):117–21.

36. Ann Hayes F, Green AA, Rao BN. Clinical manifestations of ganglioneuroma. Cancer. 1989;63(6):1211–4.

37. Pang BC, Tchoyoson Lim CC, Tan KK. Giant spinal ganglioneuroma. J Clin Neurosci. 2005;12(8):967–72.

38. Xu T, Zhu W, Wang P. Cervical ganglioneuroma: a case report and review of the literature. Medicine (Baltimore). 2019;98(15):e15203.

39. Levy DI, Bucci MN, Weatherbee L, Chandler WF. Intradural extramedullary ganglioneuroma: case report and review of the literature. Surg Neurol. 1992;37(3):216–8.

40. Son DW, Song GS, Kim YH, Lee SW. Ventrally located cervical dumbbell ganglioneuroma producing spinal cord compression. Korean J Spine. 2013;10(4):246–8.

41. Tan C, Liu J, Lin Y, Tie X, Cheng P, Qi X, et al. Bilateral and symmetric C1-C2 dumbbell ganglioneuromas associated with neurofibromatosis type 1: a case report. World J Clin Cases. 2019;7(1):109–15.

42. Fagan CJ, Swischuk LE. Dumbbell neuroblastoma of ganglioneuroma of the spinal canal. Am J Roentgenol Radium Therapy, Nucl Med. 1974;120(2):453–60.

43. Hioki A, Miyamoto K, Hirose Y, Kito Y, Fushimi K, Shimizu K. Cervical symmetric dumbbell Ganglioneuromas causing severe paresis. Asian Spine J. 2014;8(1):74–8.

44. Deora H, Kumar A, Das K, Naik B, Dikshit P, Srivastava A, et al. Excision of dumbbell shaped ganglioneuroma of cervical spine using a facet preserving inside out approach – what we know and what we learnt. Interdiscip Neurosurg Adv Techniq Case Manag. 2019;18(100481):1–5.

45. Yılmaz B, Toktaş ZO, Akakın A, Demir MK, Yapıcıer O, Konya D. Lumbar spinal immature Ganglioneuroma with Conus medullaris invasion: case report. Pediatr Neurosurg. 2015;50(6):330–5.

46. He W, Yan Y, Tang W, Cai R, Ren G. Clinical and biological features of neuroblastic tumors: a comparison of neuroblastoma and ganglioneuroblastoma. Oncotarget. 2017;8(23):37730–9.

47. Ichikawa T, Ohtomo K, Araki T, Fujimoto H, Nemoto K, Nanbu A, et al. Ganglioneuroma: computed tomography and magnetic resonance features. Br J Radiol. 1996;69:114–21.
48. Mut DT, Orhan Soylemez UP, Demir M, Tanık C, Ozer A. Diagnostic imaging findings of pelvic retroperitoneal ganglioneuroma in a child: a case report with the emphasis on initial ultrasound findings. Med Ultrason. 2016;18(1):120–2.
49. Kalyanaraman UP, Henderson JP. Intramedullary ganglioneuroma of spinal cord: a clinicopathologic study. Hum Pathol. 1982;13(10):952–5.
50. Moschovi M, Arvanitis D, Hadjigeorgi C, Mikraki V, Tzortzatou-Stathopoulou F. Late malignant transformation of dormant ganglioneuroma? Med Pediatr Oncol. 1997;28(5):377–81.
51. Kulkarni AV, Bilbao JM, Cusimano MD, Muller PJ. Malignant transformation of ganglioneuroma into spinal neuroblastoma in an adult. Case report. J Neurosurg. 1998;88(2):324–7.
52. Drago G, Pasquier B, Pasquier D, Pinel N, Rouault-Plantaz V, Dyon JF, et al. Malignant peripheral nerve sheath tumor arising in a "de novo" ganglioneuroma: a case report and review of the literature. Med Pediatr Oncol. 1997;28(3):216–22.
53. Decarolis B, Simon T, Krug B, Leuschner I, Vokuhl C, Kaatsch P, et al. Treatment and outcome of Ganglioneuroma and Ganglioneuroblastoma intermixed. BMC Cancer. 2016;16(1):542.
54. Okamatsu C, London WB, Naranjo A, Hogarty MD, Gastier-Foster JM, Look AT, et al. Clinicopathological characteristics of Ganglioneuroma and Ganglioneuroblastoma: a report from the CCG and COG. Pediatr Blood Cancer. 2009;53(4):563–9.
55. Takebayashi K, Kohara K, Miura I, Yuzurihara M, Kubota M, Kawamata T. Lumbar Ganglioneuroma from the paravertebral body presenting in continuity between Intradural and extradural spaces. World Neurosurg. 2019;128:289–94.
56. Guohua L, Lu L, Dai Z. Paragangliomas of the spine. Turk Neurosurg. 2017;27(3):401–7. https://doi.org/10.5137/1019-5149.JTN.16276-15.1.
57. Williams M. Paragangliomas of the head and neck: an overview from diagnosis to genetics. Head Neck Pathol. 2017;11(3):278–87. https://doi.org/10.1007/s12105-017-0803-4.
58. Lerman RI, Kaplan ES, Daman L. Ganglioneuroma-paraganglioma of the intradural filum terminale. Case report. J Neurosurg. 1972;36(5):652–8. https://doi.org/10.3171/jns.1972.36.5.0652.
59. Pipola V, Boriani S, Bandiera S, Righi A, Barbanti Bròdano G, Terzi S, Gasbarrini A. Paraganglioma of the spine: a twenty-years clinical experience of a high volume tumor center. J Clin Neurosci. 2019;66:7–11. https://doi.org/10.1016/j.jocn.2019.05.037.
60. Landi A, Tarantino R, Marotta N, Rocco P, Antonelli M, Salvati M, Delfini R. Paraganglioma of the filum terminale: case report. World J Surg Oncol. 2009;7:95. https://doi.org/10.1186/1477-7819-7-95.
61. Louis DN, Ohgaki H, Wiestler OD, Cavenee WK. WHO classification of tumours of the central nervous system (4th ed.) World Health Organization (WHO). Retrieved from https://publications.iarc.fr/Book-And-Report-Series/Who-Iarc-Classification-Of-Tumours/Who-Classification-Of-Tumours-Of-The-Central-Nervous-System-2016
62. Hamidi O, Young WF, Gruber L, Smestad J, Yan Q, Ponce OJ, Bancos I. Outcomes of patients with metastatic phaeochromocytoma and paraganglioma: a systematic review and meta-analysis. Clin Endocrinol. 2017;87(5):440–50. https://doi.org/10.1111/cen.13434.
63. Pang Y, Liu Y, Pacak K, Yang C. Pheochromocytomas and paragangliomas: from genetic diversity to targeted therapies. Cancers. 2019;11(4):436. https://doi.org/10.3390/cancers11040436.
64. Yang C, Li G, Fang J, Wu L, Yang T, Deng X, Xu Y. Clinical characteristics and surgical outcomes of primary spinal paragangliomas. J Neuro-Oncol. 2015;122(3):539–47. https://doi.org/10.1007/s11060-015-1742-0.
65. Murrone D, Romanelli B, Vella G, Ierardi A. Acute onset of paraganglioma of filum terminale: a case report and surgical treatment. Int J Surg Case Rep. 2017;36:126–9. https://doi.org/10.1016/j.ijscr.2017.05.016.
66. Mishra T, Goel NA, Goel AH. Primary paraganglioma of the spine: a clinicopathological study of eight cases. J Craniovertebr Junction Spine. 2014;5(1):20–4.
67. Nagarjun MN, Savardekar AR, Kishore K, Rao S, Pruthi N, Rao MB. Apoplectic presentation of a cauda equina paraganglioma. Surg Neurol Int. 2016;7:37. https://doi.org/10.4103/2152-7806.180093.
68. Midi A, Yener AN, Sav A, Cubuk R. Cauda equina paraganglioma with ependymoma-like histology: a case report. Turk Neurosurg. 2012;22(3):353–9. https://doi.org/10.5137/1019-5149.JTN.3389-10.1.
69. Yang S, Jin YJ, Park SH, Jahng TA, Kim HJ, Chung CK. Paragangliomas in the cauda equina region: Clinicopathoradiologic findings in four cases. J Neuro-Oncol. 2005;72(1):49–55. https://doi.org/10.1007/s11060-004-2159-3.
70. Hamidi O, Young WF, Iñiguez-Ariza NM, Kittah NE, Gruber L, Bancos C, Bancos I. Malignant pheochromocytoma and paraganglioma: 272 patients over 55 years. J Clin Endocrinol Metabol. 2017;102(9):3296–305. https://doi.org/10.1210/jc.2017-00992.
71. Lalloo ST, Mayat AG, Landers AT, Nadvi SS. Clinics in diagnostic imaging (68). Intradural extramedullary spinal paraganglioma. Singap Med J. 2001;42(12):592–5.
72. Nölting U, Pietzsch Z, Eisenhofer G, Pacak K. Current management of pheochromocytoma/paraganglioma: a guide for the practicing clinician in the era of precision medicine. Cancers. 2019;11(10):1505. https://doi.org/10.3390/cancers11101505.

73. Honeyman SI, Warr W, Curran OE, Demetriades AK. Paraganglioma of the lumbar spine: a case report and literature review. Neurochirurgie. 2019;65(6):387–92.

74. Jimenez C. Treatment for patients with malignant pheochromocytomas and paragangliomas: a perspective from the hallmarks of cancer. Front Endocrinol. 2018;9:277. https://doi.org/10.3389/fendo.2018.00277.

75. Hong J, Hur C, Modi HN, Suh S, Chang H. Paraganglioma in the cauda equina. A case report. Acta Orthop Belg. 2012;78(3):418–23.

76. Jia Q, Yin H, Yang J, Wu Z, Yan W, Zhou W, Xiao J. Treatment and outcome of metastatic paraganglioma of the spine. Eur Spine J. 2018;27(4):859–67. https://doi.org/10.1007/s00586-017-5140-5.

77. Perrin RG, Guha A. Malignant peripheral nerve sheath tumors. Neurosurg Clin. 2004;15(2) https://doi.org/10.1016/j.nec.2004.02.004.

78. Zhu B, et al. Malignant peripheral nerve sheath tumours of the spine. clinical manifestations, classification, treatment, and prognostic factors. Eur Spine J. 2012;21(5):897–904.

79. Baharvahdat H, Ganjeifar B, Roshan NM, Baradaran A. Spinal intradural primary malignant peripheral nerve sheat tumor with leptomeningeal seeding: case report and literature review. Turkish Neurol. 2016;28(2):317–22.

80. Ducatman BS, Scheithauer BW, Piepgras DG, Reiman HM, Ilstrup DM. Malignant peripheral nerve sheath tumors. A clinicopathologic study of 120 cases. Cancer. 1986;57(10):2006–21.

81. Baehring J, Betensky R, Batchelor T. Malignant peripheral nerve sheath tumor: the clinical spectrum and outcome of treatment. Neurology. 2003; 61(5):696–8.

82. Gilder HE, Puffer RC, Bydon M, Spinner RJ. The implications of intradural extension in paraspinal malignant peripheral nerve sheath tumors: Effects on central nervous system metastases and overall survival. J Neurosurg Spine SPI. 2018;29(6) https://doi.org/10.3171/2018.5.SPINE18445.

83. Guo A, Liu A, Wei L, Song X. Malignant peripheral nerve sheath tumors: differentiation patters and immunohistochemical features – a mini review and our new findings, J Cancer. 2012;3 https://doi.org/10.7150/jca.4179.

84. Ren X, Wang J, Hu M, Jiang H, Yang J, Jiang Z. Clinical, radiological, and pathological features of 26 intracranial and intraspinal malignant peripheral nerve sheath tumors. J Neurosurg. 2013;119(3):695–708.

85. Van Herendael BH, Heyman SRG, Vanhoenacker FM, De Temmerman G, Bloem JL, Parizel PM, De Schepper AM. The value of magnetic resonance imaging in the differentiation between malignant peripheral nerve-sheath tumors and non-neurogenic malignant soft tissue tumors. Skeletal Radiol. 2006;35(10):745–53.

86. Kett-White R, Martin JL, Jones EW, O'Brien C. Malignant spinal neurofibrosarcoma, vol. 25. Philadelphia: Lippincott Williams & Wilkins; 2000.

87. Kolberg M, Høland M, Agesen TH, Brekke HR, Liestøl K, Hall KS, Mertens F, Picci P, Smeland S, Lothe RA. Survival meta-analyses for >1800 malignant peripheral nerve sheath tumor patients with and without neurofibromatosis type 1. Neuro-Oncol. 2013;15(2):135.

88. Albayrak BS, Gorgulu A, Kose T. A case of intradural malignant peripheral nerve sheath tumor in thoracic spine associated with neurofibromatosis type 1. J Neuro-Oncol. 2006;78(2):187–90.

89. Unsinn KM, Geley T, Freund MC, Gassner I. US of the spinal cord in newborns: spectrum of normal findings, variants, congenital anomalies, and acquired diseases. Radiographics. 2000;20(4):923–38.

90. Cogen A, Michielsen J, Van Schil P, Somville J. An intradural, subpial lipoma. Acta Chir Belg. 2017;117(4):267–9.

91. Klekamp J, Fusco M, Samii M. Thoracic intradural extramedullary lipomas. Report of three cases and review of the literature. Acta Neurochir. 2001;143(8):767–74.

92. Massimi L, Feitosa Chaves TM, Legninda Sop FY, Frassanito P, Tamburrini G, Caldarelli M. Acute presentations of intradural lipomas: case reports and a review of the literature. BMC Neurol. 2019;19:189.

93. Blount JP, Elton S. Spinal lipomas. J Neurosurg. 2001;10(1):e3.

94. Kabir S, Thompson D, Rezajooi K, Casey A. Nondysraphic intradural spinal cord lipoma: case series, literature review and guidelines for management. Acta Neurochir. 2010;152(7):1139–44.

95. Lam W. Cervicothoracic intradural lipoma: features on magnetic resonance imaging. J HK Coll Radiol. 2001;4:281–3.

96. Şanlı A, Türkoğlu E, Kahveci R, Şekerci Z. Intradural lipoma of the cervicothoracic spinal cord with intracranial extension. Childs Nerv Syst. 2010;26(6):847–52.

97. Alam S, Haroon K, Farzana T, Reza MA, Alamgir A, Hossain SS. Intradural spinal lipoma of the Conus: a case report. Bangladesh J Neurosurg. 2019;8(2):112–4.

98. Pang D. Surgical management of complex spinal cord lipomas: how, why, and when to operate. A review. J Neurosurg Pediatr. 2019;23(5):537–56.

99. Kulkarni AV, Pierre-Kahn A, Zerah M. Conservative management of asymptomatic spinal lipomas of the conus. Neurosurgery. 2004;54(4):868–75.

100. Xenos C, Sgouros S, Walsh R, Hockley A. Spinal lipomas in children. Pediatr Neurosurg. 2000;32(6):295–307.

Part II

Intramedullary Tumors

Ependymoma

4

Dominique M. O. Higgins, Mychael Delgardo,
Simon Hanft, and Paul C. McCormick

Introduction

Intramedullary tumors are located within the spinal cord substance and are most commonly of glial origin (Fig. 4.1). Ependymomas are the most common tumor in adults, representing around 60% of all spinal cord tumors [1], followed by astrocytomas at 30% [2]. The goal of this chapter is to describe our operative technique for dealing with ependymomas, both initially and in the recurrent setting. We present multiple cases wherein we demonstrate our fundamental operative approach to this tumor along with surgical nuances. Preoperative goals of surgery, expectations for recovery, and thresholds for adjuvant treatment are discussed to enhance the reader's practical management of these tumors.

D. M. O. Higgins · M. Delgardo
P. C. McCormick (✉)
Department of Neurosurgery, Neurological Institute of New York/Columbia University, New York, NY, USA
e-mail: pcm6@cumc.columbia.edu

S. Hanft
Department of Neurological Surgery,
Rutgers Robert Wood Johnson Medical School,
New Brunswick, NJ, USA

Department of Neurosurgery,
Westchester Medical Center and New York Medical College, Valhalla, NY, USA

Presentation

Spinal ependymomas typically have an indolent presentation at an average age of 40 years, ranging from 8 to 74 years old in recent series [1, 3], with a possible male predominance [4, 5]. Back and neck pain are the most common chief complaint, but patients may also suffer from spasticity, ataxia, and sensory changes [3, 6]. Clinical history often demonstrates gradually progressive radiculopathy or myelopathy occurring over 1–3 years [1, 3, 7]. Sensory symptoms prevail over motor issues given the proximity of the tumor to the spinothalamic tracts and disruption of crossing fibers. Significant motor symptoms are more associated with larger tumors. Some combination of pain and sensory deficits are the presenting features in 85% of patients [8]. Blood and cerebrospinal fluid studies are of limited benefit to aid in diagnosis in most cases, though they may prove crucial in diagnosing nonsurgical intramedullary processes that masquerade as ependymomas. Neuraxis imaging can be employed to determine if metastatic disease is present, though malignant subtypes of this disease are exceedingly rare [3].

Preoperative Consultation

For patients minimally symptomatic (Fig. 4.2), an initial observation period with serial imaging 3–6 months apart may be considered; however,

© Springer Nature Switzerland AG 2021
S. Hanft, P. C. McCormick (eds.), *Tumors of the Spinal Canal*,
https://doi.org/10.1007/978-3-030-55096-7_4

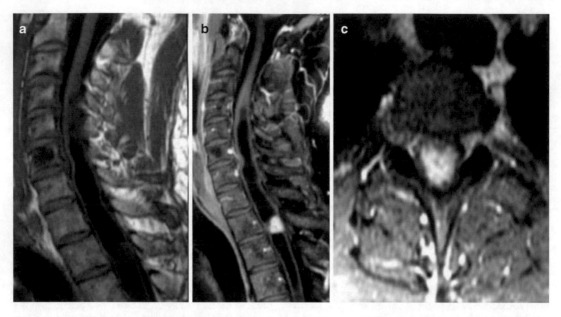

Fig. 4.1 Sagittal MRI pre- (**a**) and post-contrast (**b**) and axial post-contrast (**c**) demonstrating upper thoracic ependymoma with associated large syrinx and avid contrast enhancement

Fig. 4.2 Sagittal (**a**) and axial (**b**) post-contrast MRI demonstrating incidental cervical ependymoma with focal area of enhancement

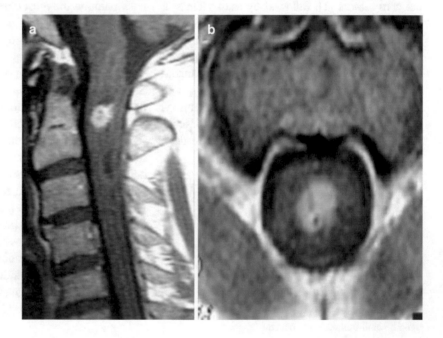

earlier intervention has been shown to improve outcomes, as preoperative functional status is correlated with surgical outcomes (Fig. 4.3) [7]. On the other hand, progressive symptoms inevitably require surgical intervention. Some groups advocate for more aggressive strategies in thoracic ependymomas as the onset of symptoms can be rapid and more difficult to reverse than for their cervical counterparts. Patients must be counseled preoperatively regarding the goals of the surgery and the risks of the intervention. In keeping with the broad goals of any neurosurgical oncologic procedure, a safe maximal resection is the objective. The McCormick Grading Scale is often utilized to assess preoperative clinical/functional status [9]. This scale has

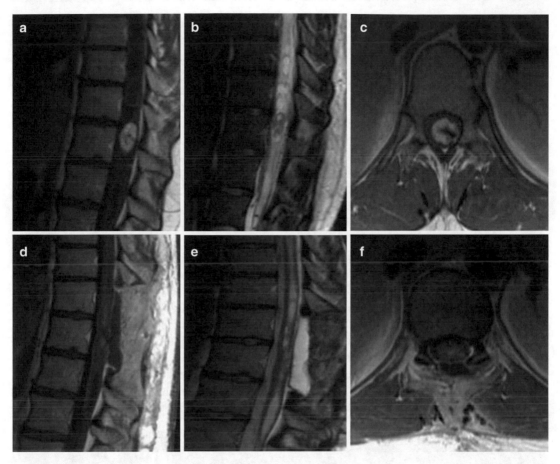

Fig. 4.3 MRI of preoperative (**a–c**) and postoperative (**d–f**) thoracic ependymoma showing complete resection and significant improvement of syrinx

been validated as a predictor of postoperative functional outcome. Complications unique to ependymoma resection begin with dorsal column dysfunction due to the myelotomy – these typically manifest as diminished proprioception and fine touch. The proprioceptive issues often lead to problems with gait. There can also be significant generalized numbness below the level of the myelotomy in isolation or as part of a dysesthetic syndrome. We recommend quoting a fairly high percentage of postoperative sensory dysfunction, roughly in the 30–50% range, on a temporary basis. By 1 month, there should be noticeable improvement in these symptoms in around half of patients, and by 6 months, nearly all of these immediate postoperative morbidities subside, with the likelihood of permanent sensory issues lying somewhere between 5% and 10% [10]. Temporary motor

weakness is an issue for 5–10% of patients with permanent paralysis a rare event. Similar to transient sensory deficits, new motor issues or exacerbation of preoperative motor weakness can take up to 6 months to resolve with most of the improvements coming in the first 1–2 months [11]. Spinal deformity from the laminectomy is uncommon in adults but a major issue in pediatric patients. This can be addressed at a later stage with instrumented fusion [12]. Ideally this can be avoided through consideration of a laminotomy/laminoplasty, especially for long segment ependymomas [13]. In general the aforesaid risks of neurologic deficits are globally elevated in thoracic ependymomas likely due to the tenuous and watershed nature of the blood supply to the thoracic spinal cord [1]. In addition, the caliber of the thoracic cord is smaller than the cervical cord, so patients more commonly present with higher McCormick grades at surgery and therefore have a higher risk of postoperative deficits.

Pathology

Ependymomas are tumors derived from the cerebrospinal fluid-producing ependymal cells that line ventricles and the central canal (Fig. 4.4). Histologically they are marked by the presence of true ependymal rosettes or pseudorosettes (Fig. 4.4a). The 2016 World Health Organization (WHO) classifies four subtypes of ependymal tumors that occur in the spine: myxopapillary ependymoma (WHO I), subependymoma (WHO I), ependymoma (WHO II), and anaplastic ependymoma (WHO III) (Table 4.1). RELA fusion-positive ependymomas, a novel fifth subtype, are almost exclusively intracranial [14]. Myxopapillary ependymomas are discussed in Chap. 3 but are commonly located in the region of the filum. Although they do not have a true capsule, these tumors tend not to invade the sur-

rounding spinal cord. Classic ependymomas can be found anywhere throughout the neuraxis. Intracranial tumors are more commonly found in children, with approximately one third of those occurring in the posterior fossa. In the spine, classic ependymomas are most commonly located in the cervical spine (nearly 50%), followed by thoracic (25%), with the other 25% spanning both cervical and thoracic regions. These tumors are divided into three histologic subtypes: papillary, tanycytic, and clear cell. Papillary ependymomas have fingerlike projections or papillae overlying a single cuboidal cell layer and tumor cells surrounding central fibrovascular foci. Tanycytic ependymomas are the most rare and have fascicles that are irregular and fibrillar in nature due to cells that are elongated. These tumors can be mistaken for astrocytomas due to their projections and subtlety of the pseudorosettes. Clear cell ependymomas demonstrate perinuclear halos, resembling oligodendrogliomas. Prior classification schemes reported a fourth subtype, cellular, but this has since been removed in the new WHO grade classification

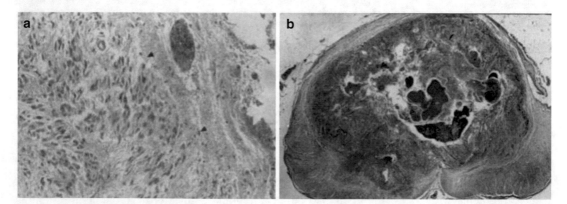

Fig. 4.4 Ependymoma pathology demonstrating typical histology (**a**) and defined margins with intratumoral hemorrhage (**b**)

Table 4.1 Spinal ependymal tumor classification

Type	WHO grade	Location	Prognosis	Management
Myxopapillary ependymoma	I	Lumbar	Good	GTR
Subependymoma	I	Cervical, thoracic, lumbar	Good	GTR
Ependymoma	II	Cervical, thoracic, lumbar	Fair	GTR, STR, adjuvant therapy
Anaplastic Ependymoma	III	Cervical, thoracic, lumbar	Poor	GTR, STR, adjuvant therapy

scheme of 2016 [15]. Anaplastic ependymomas are aggressive tumors that tend to have more local invasion into the normal spine, making gross total resections without neurological compromise a greater challenge. These malignant ependymomas demonstrate frequent mitoses, endothelial proliferation, and infiltration of the surrounding tissue [16]. More recently, molecular sequencing has been utilized to further stratify these tumors. Methylation patterns have demonstrated nine subclasses of ependymal tumors across the three compartments: supratentorial, posterior fossa, and spinal. Tanycytic ependymomas are commonly located in the spine; however, these tumors do not map to a single molecular group. Efforts are ongoing to reconcile histologic, molecular, and clinical findings [4, 14].

Radiographic Features

MRI evaluation should be obtained with and without contrast. Radiographic findings typically demonstrate a T1 isointense or hypointense intramedullary lesion with symmetric expansion of the cord [17, 18]. This symmetric expansion is an important MRI characteristic of these tumors as they arise from ependymal cells of the central canal. Therefore, the growth is centrifugal, from the central canal outward, as opposed to the more eccentric location of astrocytomas and other lesions. Contrast enhancement is avid and often homogeneous except for those tumors containing hemorrhage and cysts. Cystic changes are found in many patients, upwards of 88% of cases in recent studies [2, 17]. These cystic changes can be rostral, caudal (polar cysts), or intratumoral. Most scans demonstrate T2 hyperintensity on MRI consistent with peritumoral edema. A cap sign or hypointense rim of hemosiderin has been noted in a subset of tumors (up to one-third), which is thought to represent recent hemorrhage and potential proclivity for bleeding (Fig. 4.4b).

The process of differentiating ependymomas from astrocytomas and other intramedullary tumors can be challenging (Table 4.2). Beyond symmetric cord expansion seen in ependymo-

Table 4.2 Ependymoma vs astrocytoma: distinguishing radiographic features

Ependymoma	Astrocytoma
Central location with cord expansion	Eccentric location, can appear exophytic
Diffuse homogeneous enhancement	Patchy heterogeneous enhancement
Syringomyelia	Uncommon
Hemorrhage (cap sign)	Uncommon
Polar cysts (rostral-caudal to the mass)	Uncommon
Intratumoral cysts	Slightly less common
Average four vertebral segments	Can extend well beyond four levels

mas, syrinx formation and hydromyelia are more likely to be present in ependymomas than astrocytomas, based on a retrospective review [2]. In fact, syringomyelia is likely to be the main factor in differentiating these tumors [2]. Polar cyst formation (rostral and caudal to the mass), hemorrhage, cap sign, and diffuse enhancement are other distinguishing characteristics (Table 4.2). Though ependymomas can be rather lengthy and involve up to four vertebral levels, longer segment involvement is more common in astrocytomas. Subependymomas are histologically distinct tumors but may also appear similar to ependymomas on MRI (Fig. 4.5). They are more commonly found intracranially, with 50% occurring in the lateral ventricle and 35% in the fourth ventricle in our institutional series and the remaining 17% being found in the spine [19]. Spinal subependymomas are very rare, accounting for less than 2% of intramedullary tumors [20, 21], and tend to be located in the cervical spine [22]. Radiographically, the "bamboo leaf sign" has been proposed as a distinguishing feature, which is a large fusiform expansion of the spinal cord reported in an estimated 76% of cases in the literature [20]. This presentation has been thought to be due to subpial tumor growth [20]. Associated cyst formation has been reported but is uncommon [22]. Surgically, spinal subependymomas behave more like ependymomas than astrocytomas in terms of margins, and gross total resections should be attempted if possible [19].

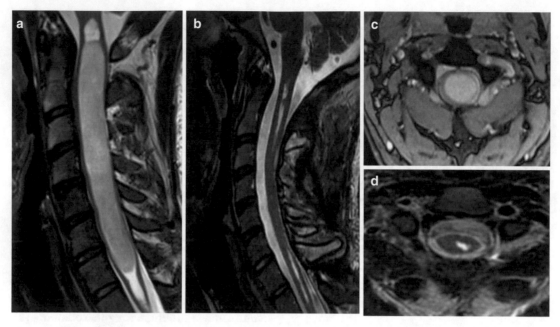

Fig. 4.5 Sagittal (**a**, **b**) and axial (**c**, **d**) MRI of the cervical spine demonstrating large subependymoma with associated syrinx and edema (**a**, **c**) with complete resection and syrinx improvement (**b**, **d**)

Radiographic Mimics

In clinical practice, a neurosurgeon can be faced with an MRI finding of an intramedullary mass that may actually represent a nonneoplastic process. These radiographic mimics of ependymoma need to be recognized and managed appropriately. Performing a biopsy or even attempted resection can be significantly deleterious to the patient. Below we discuss the most common mimic of an ependymoma, which is a demyelinating multiple sclerosis plaque. We also present other such mimics and a general strategy for approaching these nonneoplastic entities (Table 4.3).

Multiple sclerosis can initially present with sensory and motor symptoms. In some cases, these symptoms may prompt a cervical MRI revealing an acutely demyelinating lesion in the cervical spinal cord. If solitary, this plaque can be mistaken for an intramedullary tumor. Though it is rare for MS to present initially with a solitary demyelinating cervical plaque, it is a known phenomenon [23]. The patchy and peripheral enhancement pattern, along with eccentric location in the spinal cord toward the posterior col-

Table 4.3 Is that really an intramedullary tumor? Detecting differences between a tumor and nonneoplastic mimics

Ependymoma/ astrocytoma	Nonneoplastic lesions
Cord expansion	Uncommon
Homogeneous or heterogeneous enhancement	Ring enhancement
Slow symptom onset: Months to years	Rapid symptom onset: Days/ weeks/months
CSF negativity	CSF positivity
Seronegativity	Seropositivity
Focal neurologic findings	Focal and systemic findings
MRI in 2–3 months: Minimal to no change in lesion	MRI in 2–3 months: Dramatic increase or decrease in size/edema/ enhancement

umns, can help to distinguish a plaque from an ependymoma. The cord should also retain its normal caliber. These lesions rarely go beyond two vertebral levels. Perhaps most importantly, the enhancement in an active plaque tends to dissipate after 2–6 weeks, so a repeat MRI showing less enhancement (and perhaps less T2 signal as well) would obviously rule out an ependymoma [24]. In addition, brain MRIs can show more classic periventricular white matter lesions to help rule in MS as the diagnosis. CSF studies, as mentioned above, should be strongly considered in the workup of a solitary enhancing mass in the cervical spinal cord if there is any diagnostic uncertainty.

Beyond MS, there are a litany of rare entities that can confound neurosurgeons in their approach to a perceived intramedullary ependymoma. Dural AV fistulas (causing Foix-Alajouanine syndrome), radiation myelopathy, granulomatous disease (e.g., sarcoid), infection, arterial infarction, arteriovenous malformations, and transverse myelitis are all entities that need to be considered if an atypical intramedullary lesion is identified on MRI.

We recommend caution and a thorough diagnostic workup in such cases. MRI of the brain and remainder of the spine, CSF studies, serum studies, and evaluation by a neurologist and other relevant specialists (e.g., infectious disease) can help to avoid an unnecessary spinal cord biopsy. Repeat MRI with contrast in 2–3 months is a prudent route but can be difficult to advocate on its own if there is significant neurologic decline. This can be especially frustrating for neurosurgeons in the outpatient setting as a complete diagnostic workup can be onerous and slow developing. Some cases might warrant hospital admission for more expeditious evaluation, especially in the setting of more rapid neurologic decline. If a repeat MRI is pursued and ultimately reveals less enhancement or less edema, an ependymoma can confidently be ruled out, as this tumor should not change over such a short period while nonneoplastic lesions can. Table 4.3 presents a useful compendium of radiographic and clinical features that may help to alert the neurosurgeon to a nonneoplastic mimic [7]. When the preoperative workup is exhausted and negative, then an open biopsy must be considered as many of the above entities may not yield a positive result. Figure 4.6 shows a case of a nonneoplastic entity that had some features consistent with ependymoma at first blush (diffuse enhancement, slight cord expansion, somewhat central and symmetric appearance). But the slightly atypical appearance prompted a surveillance MRI in 3 months and additional workup that proved negative. The repeat MRI showed significant resolution of the T2 signal with lack of contrast uptake. A diagnosis was never made as the patient experienced clinical improvement, but a potentially injurious spinal cord biopsy was averted.

Operative Techniques

For cervical ependymomas, patients are positioned prone with head fixation. In our practice, we prefer to utilize three-point fixation with a Mayfield and an electric table. The patient can be placed on a Wilson frame or padded bolsters. Alternatively, Gardner-Wells tongs and an open frame table can be used, especially in the case of a patient with a larger body habitus. Neurophysiologic monitoring of SSEPs and MEPs has become standard practice in the resection of these tumors. Alternatively, D-wave electrodes can be utilized to provide motor monitoring. These electrodes are placed either in the epidural space or along the spinal cord below the myelotomy (subdural) to measure corticospinal tract integrity [25], allowing for reliable, fast real-time feedback signals [26].

During positioning, care must be taken to ensure there is adequate neck flexion. A degree of kyphosis helps keep the tumor in the field of view. Localizing X-rays are obtained to confirm the levels of interest. A midline incision is marked, and local anesthetic with epinephrine is applied. Perioperative antibiotics and high-dose steroids are utilized in our practice. It is not our routine to mandate a baseline MAP level throughout the surgery, though many will use a MAP of 85 mmHg as a goal especially during the tumor resection phase. A standard subperiosteal dissection is carried out. Laminectomies are performed with a combination of Leksell Rongeurs and high-speed drills. For the majority of cases, instrumentation and fusion are not required, but an assessment of cervical sagittal alignment and potential for instability should be done. A laminoplasty may be performed instead for suitable candidates. Great care

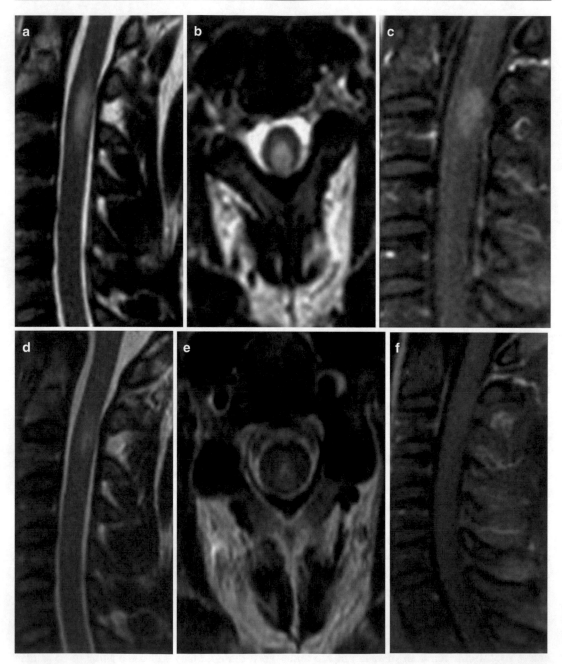

Fig. 4.6 A 42-year-old male with progressive upper extremity numbness and heaviness over 2–3 months. Initial MRI cervical spine with and without contrast (**a–c**) and repeat MRI performed 3 months later (**d–f**). (**a**) Sagittal T2 showing hyperintensity within the spinal cord behind C2-3. (**b**) Axial T2 showing posteriorly situated area of hyperintensity extending to the dorsal cord surface. (**c**) Sagittal T1 post-contrast with diffuse but not avid enhancement throughout the lesion. (**d**) Sagittal T2 with reduced hyperintensity. (**e**) Axial T2 also showing reduced signal. (**f**) Sagittal T1 post-contrast with no more evidence of enhancement

is taken to preserve the facets in an effort to prevent long-term spinal deformity. Transdural ultrasound can be helpful for confirming the level of interest and adequate exposure of the pathology. A midline durotomy is performed using an 11-blade and nerve hook. Care should be taken to preserve the arachnoid layer if possible. 4-0 silk sutures are used to tack up and reflect the dural edges. We do recommend taking an MEP baseline after the durotomy due to the small chance that a change occurred from the laminectomy or dural opening alone – this helps to establish a new baseline, more often improved rather than worsened. Cottonoids can be used to maintain hemostasis. Variable suctions (between 4 and 6 French initially, transitioning to larger 8 and 9 French suctions as the myelotomy is widened and the resection cavity expanded) should be used during the dissection to protect the spinal cord and nerve roots from trauma during aspiration. Once the rostral and caudal poles of the tumor are visible, adequate exposure has been obtained.

Ease of tumor dissection is dependent on natural planes between the tumor and cord parenchyma. Furthermore, size, histology, and the presence of a capsule or syrinx can influence favorability of resection [27]. An irrigating bipolar is used to cauterize the pial surface of the spinal cord along the midline (Fig. 4.7a–d), though some surgeons have moved toward nonstick disposable bipolar forceps. We recommend putting the bipolar on a lower setting for the myelotomy, typically 25. We advocate cauterization over the rostral-caudal extent of the tumor before entering the tumor (7d). The midline between the dorsal columns can be identified by visualizing the dorsal median (or central) septum, though oftentimes it is not clearly apparent due to cord expansion and rotation from the tumor (Fig. 4.7c). As such, identifying exiting vessels from the midline (there can be a confluence of vessels emanating from the septum) and verification by noting the dorsal root entry zones bilaterally have proven to be a reliable marker in our practice (Fig. 4.7b). Some surgeons will utilize dorsal column mapping which involves placement of a grid on the dorsal cord surface or successive stimulation with a bipolar probe. SSEPs are monitored very selectively, and the raphe can be identified between two stimulation peaks of the bilateral posterior tibial nerves. Thus, a physiologic midline is localized and entered into [28]. Pia is then incised with a Beaver Blade (Fig. 4.7e) or sharp microscissors, and the dorsal columns are gently retracted using microdissectors (Fig. 4.7f). If the midline vessels are sizable, they often can be

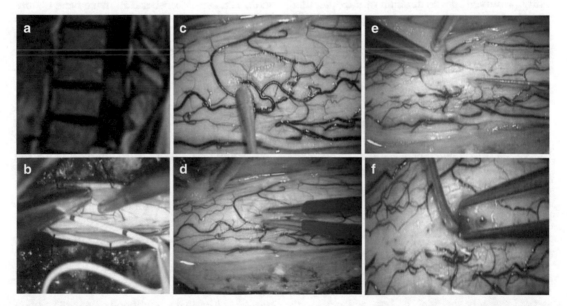

Fig. 4.7 Surgical resection of thoracic ependymoma, midline myelotomy. (**a**) MRI demonstrating contrast enhancing lesion in the lower thoracic spine. (**b**) Subdural D-wave electrode being inserted along spinal cord surface. (**c**) Spinal cord exposed intraoperatively with Penfield marking the position of midline. (**d**) Bipolar cautery used to coagulate midline vessels prior to incision with Beaver Blade (**e**). (**f**) Microdissector and Yasargil bayoneted forceps are used to gently expand the myelotomy

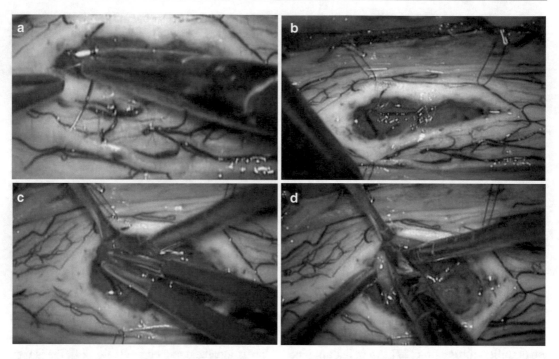

Fig. 4.8 Surgical resection of thoracic ependymoma, tumor exposure. (**a**) 6-0 Prolene pial stitch being carefully placed for retraction after myelotomy. (**b–d**) Bipolar cautery and sharp dissection aiding in defining tumor boundaries

mobilized away from the myelotomy and potentially preserved for the duration of the operation. Smaller vessels are typically cauterized without consequence. The dorsal aspect of the tumor is identified and then exposed (Fig. 4.8). Polar cysts, if present, often identify the rostral-caudal margins of the tumor. SSEPs often diminish after this maneuver, but even significant drops are not reason to abort the operation. They may drop quickly and recover later in the operation or occasionally remain undetectable throughout. Ideally they remain preserved, but their loss does not necessarily mean that there will be sensory dysfunction postoperatively. Regarding MEPs as well as D-waves, the general guidelines regard any drop below 50% in the amplitude as concerning, and therefore the operation should be stopped [29]. A 10% prolongation in latency of MEPs is another recommended guideline for halting surgery (typically latency is not a factor with D-waves). There is a reliable correlation between a drop of 50% in amplitude and long-term postoperative motor deficits. A pause in the resection, irrigation of the cavity with warm saline, and

consideration of MAP elevation with possible additional steroid dose are all maneuvers to consider before aborting the operation [30].

The tumor surface is cauterized and sharply divided (Fig. 4.9). Tumor substance is grasped by forceps for pathologic diagnosis. For larger tumors, we strongly endorse early use of ultrasonic aspiration for internal debulking. For smaller tumors, ideally the tumor can be left intact so as to reduce the risk of seeding the CSF and leading to distant sites of disease in the future. As debulking proceeds, the tumor progressively collapses into the resection cavity, and the planes between the tumor and the normal spinal cord become easier to define. Blunt microdissectors with occasional traction using tumor forceps and suction help to develop these planes. We do emphasize patience with internal debulking as this takes pressure off of the viable spinal cord and reduces the likelihood of causing a pressure or traction-related injury from dissection. The dissection at the margins of the tumor is the key to extent and safety of resection. Emphasis should be placed on excellent microsurgical tech-

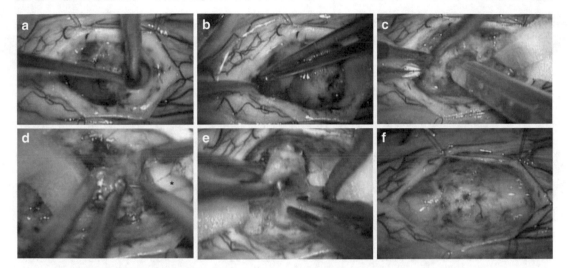

Fig. 4.9 Surgical resection of thoracic ependymoma, tumor resection. (**a**, **b**) Rostral and caudal poles of the tumor are identified with microcottonoids placed to mark the boundaries. (**c**) Ultrasonic aspiration is used to debulk the tumor. (**d**) Ventral tumor boundary (asterisk) is visible as capsule is rolled for further tumor removal. (**e**) Bipolar cautery is used to remove the last remaining tumor attachments. (**f**) Resection cavity following tumor removal

nique under the microscope to gently retract the tumor with slight countertraction on the spinal cord in order to safely develop a plane. It is a balancing act because excessive manipulation and traction on the adjacent spinal cord tissue in an effort to remove the tumor whole can induce neurologic deficits. In some instances, pial stitches with 6-0 Prolene can be helpful to maintain a patent surgical cavity (Fig. 4.8), though excessive traction on the dorsal columns can lead to SSEP loss and possible sensory deficits and may need to be released. Fibrous attachments and feedings vessels should be carefully identified, cauterized, and divided (Fig. 4.8c, d). Minimal bipolar cauterization is used in the cavity as thermal energy may be transduced to the surrounding spinal cord leading to injury. Hemostasis is achieved with injectable thrombin-based gel foam products. As the ventral surface is approached, caution must be used to avoid damage to normal functioning nerve fibers and vessels [13]. As ependymomas receive vascular supply from branches off the anterior spinal artery, these deep reaches of the tumor need to be managed very carefully with tumor left in place if there is significant adhesiveness to ventral spinal cord substance. The ability to safely identify and develop a plane is variable. If a plane is visible, gross total resections can be achieved with minimal risk of recurrence; otherwise, a subtotal resection should be performed (Fig. 4.9).

Following resection, the pia can be approximated by suturing or welding techniques though we do not routinely perform these in our practice [31]. The dura is closed with a running locking 4-0 silk stitch. A Valsalva maneuver may be utilized to confirm a watertight closure. Dural substitutes can be used in addition to aid in a layered closure or as a patch graft if needed. The fascia and layered muscle closure then follow. Subfascial drains are controversial – some use them routinely to evacuate the epidural space of hematoma and to prevent CSF egress beyond the fascia and out through the skin, while others are concerned about CSF fistula formation and have abandoned their use. We typically utilize a dermal layer closure followed by a running 3-0 nylon closure for the skin. Patients remain on bedrest for at least 24 h with progressive mobilization afterward.

For patients with thoracic ependymomas, localization is critical [1]. We prefer to utilize a Jackson frame with padding, and a ProneView or Gardner-Wells tongs. Arm positioning will depend upon surgical levels: upper thoracic with arms down (T4 and above) and lower thoracic with arms above the head and extended less than 90 degrees (below T4). A/P fluoroscopy is utilized preoperatively to mark the incision. Intraoperative localization should be carried out with respect to bony landmarks, such as the pedicle or transverse process and articulation with the ribs. Transdural ultrasound imaging can be particularly helpful in these cases for localization purposes. The operation otherwise proceeds in a similar manner as described above.

Radiation for Spinal Ependymomas

The use of radiotherapy as an adjuvant to resection in spinal cord ependymomas is controversial, with no clear consensus as to its effectiveness in patient outcomes (Table 4.4) [32, 33, 34]. An early retrospective study investigating the role of radiotherapy following resection of spinal ependymomas showed that those who underwent adjuvant radiotherapy had both 59% 5- and 10-year progression-free survival rates, with 62% 10-year overall survival [5]. Lee et al. in their series concluded that radiation therapy had no effect on either progression-free or overall survival [32]. Oh et al. conducted a meta-analysis of

348 patients assessing progression-free survival and overall survival. In this patient population, 77.0% of patients received gross total resections, with 9.5% undergoing subtotal resection alone and 13.5% of patients having subtotal resections with adjuvant radiotherapy [35]. Of the three interventions, however, patients who underwent gross total resection had the most prolonged progression-free survival, and this was the only intervention significantly associated with improvements in overall survival. In patients who underwent subtotal resection alone, the median progression-free survival was 48 months. In contrast, patients who underwent subtotal resection with adjuvant radiotherapy had a median progression-free survival of 96 months. This finding supports the notion that adjuvant radiotherapy could provide some utility in terms of delaying the recurrence of spinal cord ependymomas. A very recent retrospective study by Brown et al. examining outcomes in grade II/III ependymomas similarly found a benefit of radiation for extending progression-free survival in adults but without a significant change in overall survival [36].

Overall, gross total resections are the mainstay of treatment. Grade II ependymomas can be

Table 4.4 Outcomes literature review on published series

Author (Year)	Objective	Patient n	Follow-up (months)	Treatment	Outcomes	Conclusion
Cooper et al. (1989)	Assess intermediate and long-term results of treatment of intramedullary spinal cord tumors via microsurgery	51 (24 ependymomas)	38 (mean) Up to 72 months	Surgery	2 deaths	No deaths or recurrences in patients with ependymomas who underwent gross total resection
Whitaker (1991)	Determine the effect of postoperative radiotherapy on progression-free survival rates of patients with spinal cord ependymoma	58 (40 WHO I, 13 WHO II or greater, 5 indeterminate))	70 (mean) 3–408 months	Biopsy (11), STR (33), GTR (14) Postoperative radiation (43)	5 yr. PFS: 59%, 10 yr. PFS 59%, 5 yr. cause specific survival rate: 69%; 10 yr. cause specific survival rate: 62%	Survival rates in GTR were better than STR, though most GTR patients had low-grade cauda equina tumors

Table 4.4 (continued)

Author (Year)	Objective	Patient n	Follow-up (months)	Treatment	Outcomes	Conclusion
Chang (2002)	To determine prognostic factors and postoperative outcomes in adult spinal ependymomas	31	33 (mean)	STR (8), GTR (23)	5 yr. PFS: 70%; 6 recurrences (2 GTR, 4 STR)	Preoperative functional status and the extent of resection were significantly correlated with improved outcomes. Location and pathology influenced extent of resection
Oh (2013)	Assess the possible correlation between tumor location and disease prognosis	447 (meta-analysis)	62(mean), 1–276 months	STR (24.9%), GTR (75.1%)	PFS shorter in lower spinal regions than those in upper, no difference in overall survival	PFS but not overall survival varied by location
Lee (2013)	Determine predictors for survival for patients who underwent surgical treatment for spinal cord ependymomas	88 (multicenter), age > 18	73 (mean), 2–22 years	Partial removal (1%) STR (15%), GTR (82%), radiation 23% (45–50 Gy, 1.5 or 2 Gy per fraction per day, 10 ependymomas, 3 anaplastic ependymomas)	5 yr. PFS: 87%, 10 yr. PFS 80% Recurrence/progression in 13 patients Not benefit of radiation after STR	Gross total resection, early diagnosis, and surgery improved functional outcome, no clinical benefit from radiation
Wostrack (2018)	Describe the history, prognosis, and management of adult spinal ependymoma patients	158 (multicenter)	19 (mean), 3–127 months	GTR (80%), STR (13%), PR (6%), 10% radiation	5 yr. PFS: 80%, radiation in 15 cases	GTR, WHO grade, and Ki67 index correlated with improved outcomes
Byun (2018)	Analyze outcomes in patients with spinal ependymoma who underwent radiotherapy	25	49 (mean), 9–321 months	Radiation following primarily STR	5 yr. PFS 71%, 5 yr. overall survival 84%	Benefit to radiation in STR patients
Brown (2020)	Determine the effect of adjuvant radiotherapy on survival rates in patients with grade II/III spinal ependymomas	1058 (database query)	n/a	Biopsy/STR (86%) with 93.5% radiation, GTR (14%) with 6.5% radiation;	Grade III vs II, HR 10.3	Radiotherapy improved progression-free survival but did not improve overall survival

safely monitored after gross total resection, but there is controversy regarding adjuvant radiation in cases of residual and recurrence. For grade III ependymomas, even in cases of gross total resection, which are rarely achieved due to local invasion, adjuvant radiation is commonly pursued [37]. Metastatic spinal ependymomas are also considered appropriate targets for adjuvant radiotherapy [33, 34, 38, 39]. As proton therapy and stereotactic radiosurgery (SRS) continue to become more widely utilized, there is the potential for an impact on overall survival to be established with these modalities [40]. Currently there is a very limited role for chemotherapy in recurrent ependymomas, with only one study involving ten patients showing some response to etoposide [41] and another more recent study showing some clinical benefit of Avastin in NF2 patients harboring cystic ependymomas [42].

In our experience, radiation therapy may render a reoperation more challenging in terms of safety and efficacy. There is an increased risk of wound healing failures and other potential complications such as CSF leak and infection. Therefore, it has been our practice to withhold radiation therapy after subtotal resections. An observation period during follow-up allows for an assessment of the biology and regrowth rate of the tumor. If there is early recurrence, which we regard as within a few years, a reoperation is recommended. If we believe that only a subtotal resection is possible, then radiation therapy is considered in lieu of repeat surgery. In general we avoid a rigid paradigm for the management of ependymoma recurrence.

Case Presentations

Case 1: Cervical Ependymoma

Presentation

The patient is a 40-year-old male man generally in excellent health who noted some swallowing issues for about a year and a half prior to presentation. He also reported several months of progressive numbness and tingling, intermittently in both fingers that began to limit functionality. The patient denied any significant change in strength.

Imaging

MRI was obtained showing a large enhancing intramedullary tumor taking up the entire cross-sectional area of the spinal cord between C4 and C6 with expansion of the spinal cord (Fig. 4.10). A significant syrinx was also noted extending rostrally and caudally with associated surrounding edema. Gradient echo sequences (GRE) demonstrated focal areas of hyperintensity, consistent with prior hemorrhage (Fig. 4.10d).

Operation

The patient was taken to the operating room. Standard prone positioning was performed with a Mayfield head clamp fixed to a regular OR table. Neurophysiologic monitoring was set up for intraoperative somatosensory and motor evoked potentials. Steroids and antibiotics were administered. A C3 through C6 laminectomy was performed using a laminoplasty technique, and the bony edges were waxed. The operating microscope was then brought into the wound. The dura was opened in midline and tented laterally with sutures. The spinal cord was quite swollen at this level. Under magnified vision of the operating microscope, irrigating cautery was used to score the posterior median septum, which was then carefully opened with a Beaver Blade. As the myelotomy was extended, the tumor began to expand the spinal cord, and margins became visible. The tumor was approached both rostrally and caudally into the polar cysts, which were drained. The tumor was then internally decompressed with an ultrasonic aspirator. Slight traction on the tumor was then used to develop a plane between the tumor and the surrounding spinal cord fibrous attachments. Feeding vessels were carefully isolated, cauterized, and divided. Using this technique, a radical resection was able to be accomplished with stable somatosensory and motor evoked potential monitoring. At the end, the vast majority of the tumor was removed, though there were certain areas with unclear margins that could not be addressed safely with respect to neurologic function.

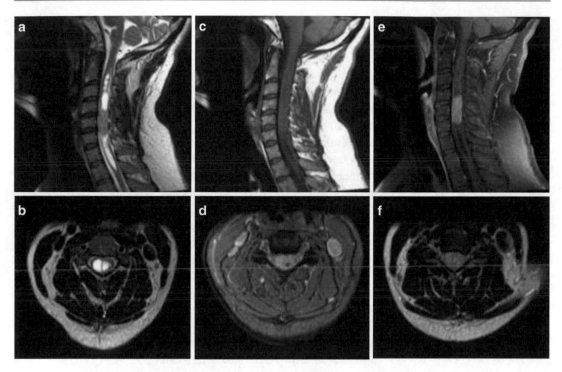

Fig. 4.10 MRI cervical spine of a preoperative ependy-moma. (**a, b**) T2 sagittal (**a**) and axial (**b**) demonstrating cystic changes rostrally and caudally with syrinx. (**c**) Sagittal T1 pre-contrast MRI with isointense tumor with cord expansion and caudal area region of hypointensity. (**d**) Axial gradient echo with area of hypointensity consistent with hemorrhage. (**e, f**) Sagittal and axial T1 post-contrast MRI with homogenous enhancement centrally

Pathology

WHO grade II ependymoma: Hematoxylin and eosin stained sections of the specimen showed a glial neoplasm with perivascular pseudorosettes. The neoplastic cells were round to oval and showed long coarse processes in some areas and cytoplasmic clearing in others. The nuclei were hyperchromatic, irregular, and showed vesicular chromatin. No necrosis or vascular proliferation was recognized. Up to one mitotic figure per ten high-power fields was identified. The Ki67 proliferation index was low (1–2%). The immuno-histochemical profile showed a focally positive subset of GFAP cells and SOX2 positive in a small subset of cells. EBP50 was positive with multiple areas showing dot-like staining. Other common tumor markers such as p53, Olig2, and PDGFRA were negative.

Postoperative Course

The patient did well postoperatively, with intact strength and proprioception. He experienced some asymmetric diminished sensation but was tolerating an oral diet, ambulatory, and voiding. The patient was discharged home on postoperative day 5, after a 2-day period of bed rest. At follow-up he was doing well and independently ambulating with good strength. He reported numbness in his torso and legs with some difficulty feeling bladder and bowel function, but overall he was functionally independent.

Key Technical Observations in Cervical Ependymomas

Adequate exposure is crucial to the safe, effective resection of these tumors. Surgery is performed under high magnification with a limited depth of field, so it is important to have the tumor parallel to the floor. The tumor is at the most dependent point of the surgical field so meticulous epidural hemostasis must be secured before the dura is opened. While polar cysts do not have to be exposed in their entirety, it is important that the midline myelotomy does extend a few millimeters beyond the tumor margin, both for adequate visualization and also to reduce spinal cord retraction. 6-0 Prolene sutures through the spinal cord pia can be clipped laterally to the dura to facilitate exposure and provide gentle consistent retraction of the spinal cord. Intratumoral reduction with an ultrasonic aspirator or laser is useful for substantially larger tumors, but it is often useful to leave the tumor intact and use traction on the tumor to assist in developing tumor margins. The ventral tumor margin is often the most difficult aspect of the resection. Pial sutures do not provide any effective retraction ventrally, and many prominent vessels can complicate removal. Vertical retraction of the tumor can be useful to identity and develop this margin. Finally, skilled surgical assistance is important, especially for dissection of the tumor margins. In essence, this is a "three-hand" operation, one hand for tumor retraction, one hand for suction, and one hand for alternating irrigating bipolar coagulation/sharp division with a micro-knife or scissors.

Case 2: Thoracic Ependymoma

Presentation
The patient is a 51-year-old male with cardiac comorbidities. He presented with asymmetric dysesthesia, complaining of burning sensations down the left leg for almost 2 years prior. The patient pursued conservative management initially but developed back pain with right scapular radiation. He also complained of right lower extremity "heaviness" without weakness, consistent with myelopathy. He denied any upper extremity complaints. On physical examination, marked stiffness and spasticity in the right leg were noted with increased deep tendon reflexes and clonus. No sensory level was noted.

Imaging
MRI of the thoracic spine demonstrated a lesion at approximately T4-T6 with uniform enhancement and cord edema (Fig. 4.11). Scoliosis was also evident on plain films.

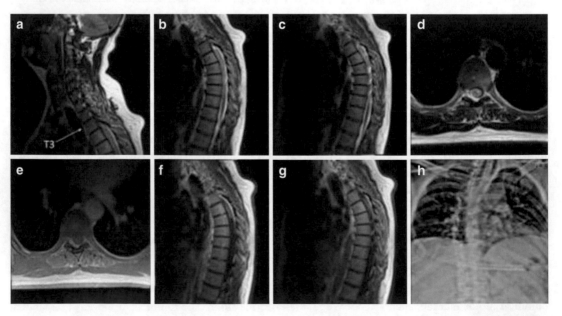

Fig. 4.11 Thoracic MRI of a preoperative thoracic ependymoma. (a–c) Sagittal T2 preoperative with diffuse hyperintensity and cord expansion. (d, e) Axial T2, T1 post-contrast MRI. (f, g) Sagittal T1 post-MRI sagittal demonstrating diffuse enhancement spanning multiple segments. (h) A/P X-ray demonstrating thoracic scoliosis

Operation

The exposure was carried out from T4 to T6 with laminectomies being performed, and care was taken to preserve the facet joints. The bony edges were waxed. SSEPs and MEPs were monitorable during the operation, although there was asymmetry at baseline. The dura was then opened in the midline under the operating microscope and tented laterally with sutures. The operating microscope was then brought into the field. The spinal cord was visibly enlarged. As expected, there was some deviation of the spinal cord because of the patient's scoliosis. The dorsal root entry zones were identified bilaterally. Midline myelotomy was first started by scoring the midline posterior median septum pia with a light cautery under continuous irrigation, which was then opened. The myelotomy was gently deepened at a depth of a millimeter and a half or so where the tumor was identified, eccentric to the right side. The dorsal aspect of the tumor was then slowly identified and noted to be fairly vascular and adherent to the surrounding spinal cord. In most areas there were good planes, but in some, boundaries were difficult to define. Intermittent internal decompression with an ultrasonic aspirator was utilized. Attention was then given to the margins of the tumor where feeding vessels and fibrous attachments were carefully isolated, cauterized, and divided. These scenarios require painstaking effort that takes several hours. The vast majority of the tumor was able to be removed, but there were areas ventrally that would have been too high risk to develop a good plane without harming the spinal cord. There was some diminishment in the SSEPs following the midline myelotomy, but this was stabilized. There was also some variability in the MEPs on one side, but it was not directly related to any surgical maneuver.

Pathology

WHO grade II ependymoma: Hematoxylin and eosin stained sections of the specimen showed a glial neoplasm with prominent perivascular pseudorosettes. The cells had long fibrillar processes and oval elongated nuclei with stippled chromatin. No mitotic figures or areas of necrosis were seen. Hyalinized blood vessels and scattered hemosiderin-laden macrophages were noted. The Ki67 proliferation index was variably increased, with up to 5.6% (56/1000) of tumor cells staining positive. The tumor was positive for GFAP and EBP50.

Key Technical Observations in Thoracic Ependymomas

The core technical aspects for thoracic ependymoma removal are essentially the same as for cervical ependymomas. Adequate exposure, progression of dissection and removal, and techniques are nearly identical. As noted earlier precise localization can be more challenging with thoracic tumors, so it is important to have adequate exposure, ideally prior to dural opening. Intraoperative ultrasound can be particularly useful here to ensure adequate exposure and resection.

Case 3: Recurrent Thoracic Ependymoma

Presentation

The patient described above did well postoperatively. Initial postoperative imaging studies, and again at 1 year, showed a good resection with decreased enhancement. However, 2 years following his initial surgery, he developed worsened spasticity of his right leg and diminished proprioception. He had good motor strength proximally but limited distally. Interval imaging was then obtained to assess for recurrence, which showed some cord expansion with small areas of enhancement rostral and caudal to the prior surgical site. He was observed given the slow progression of symptoms and a recent unrelated surgery. However, at 3 years following surgery, his symptoms had dramatically worsened, and the decision was made to pursue a reoperation.

Imaging

MRI of the thoracic spine demonstrated substantial growth of the tumor and increase in the enhancing portion of the residual ependymoma. The tumor extended from T4 to T6, with slightly

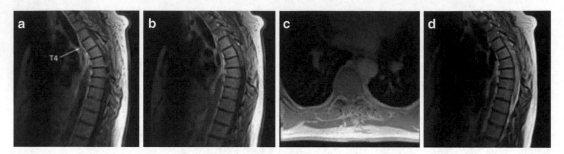

Fig. 4.12 Recurrent thoracic ependymoma. (**a–c**) Sagittal (**a, b**) and axial (**c**) T1 post-contrast MRI images with diffuse enhancement and cord expansion and post-laminectomy changes. (**d**) Sagittal T2 MRI with diffuse T2 signal in the cord

more rostral and caudal extension than prior studies (Fig. 4.12). The residual enhancing portion measured 7.2 cm craniocaudally compared to 4.8 cm the year prior. T2-weighted imaging also demonstrated progression of edema extending from the inferior end plate of C7 to the T9-T10 disc space.

Operation
At the beginning of the procedure, the patient did not have monitorable SSEPs or MEPs on the right leg which corresponded to his preoperative deficit. SSEPs were also not monitorable in the left leg, but MEPs were reliable, and he had stable upper extremity motor and sensory monitoring. A partial laminectomy was carried out that extended up into the T3 level. The dura was identified, and the scar tissue was dissected off the previous dural opening down to the previous level of laminectomy. Ultrasound was used to identify the tumor. Under the operating microscope, the dura was opened rostrally where there was no scar tissue and extended. The cord was substantially enlarged, and recurrent tumor was visible through the very thin posterior elements. Midline was identified, and a midline myelotomy was carefully performed over the rostral-caudal extent of the tumor. The tumor began to bulge out through the myelotomy, and using careful microsurgical techniques, a plane was developed between the outer aspect of the tumor and the inner aspect of the spinal cord. Internal decompression was performed periodically with an ultrasonic aspirator. Ventrally a plane was again difficult to establish, and a more conservative approach was taken in these areas. Evoked poten-

tial monitoring remained stable through the procedure, although only MEP monitoring of the left leg was monitorable.

Pathology
WHO grade II ependymoma: No necrosis or vascular proliferation was identified. The Ki67 proliferation index was up to 3.1%. Reactive gliosis was noted adjacent to the tumor.

Outcomes
At follow-up, the patient predominantly had a right-sided Brown-Sequard with weakness of the right leg, diminished proprioception, and diminished pain and temperature sense on the left side. He had improvement of his strength, particularly in the right leg, and was able to walk independently, but his leg was still spastic. His weakness proximally persisted somewhat, but his quadriceps, hamstrings, and even the ankle improved to some degree. Postoperative imaging showed a near complete resection. There was some enhancement in the rostral area that was planned to be monitored using serial scans with 3-month follow-up appointments.

Key Technical Observations in Reoperations for Ependymomas
Safe exposure can be a challenge here, especially with the previous laminectomy. If possible, it is helpful to expose the polar margins of the previous laminectomy to initially identify midline bone. A small amount of bone removal identifies normal dura at both ends of the prior surgical field, followed by use of both blunt and sharp rostral and/or caudal dissection parallel to the dura.

Such a maneuver is safe and usually allows a clean plane to be developed between the dura and overlying scar tissue. Often the previous myelotomy is not visible, and the midline must be estimated by noting the dorsal root entry zones bilaterally. Often these tumors are under significant pressure and may begin to herniate out of the myelotomy. Early cauterization of the entire rostrocaudal aspect of the tumor prior to any myelotomy prepares you for this possibility and allows rapid completion of myelotomy should this occur. Beyond this, the surgical strategies and techniques are similar to the previously described primary approach. It is important not to be unduly biased by the knowledge of prior subtotal resection, even if you were the initial surgeon. Frequently, margins that were not identified or safely developed at the index surgery may now be more effectively developed at recurrence.

Case 4: Cervical Ependymoma, Indolent

Presentation

The patient is a 57-year-old female who presented with progressive worsening of left arm numbness. This was accompanied by shooting pain down the arm into the hand. She was diagnosed in 2005 with multiple sclerosis per her own report due to the same symptoms. An MRI was done at that time showing a cervical lesion. No additional workup or follow-up was performed, largely because the patient's symptoms improved. Three years prior to her office visit, she underwent a cervical MRI for some right-sided numbness that also improved. We were able to review this MRI and her most recent scan, which showed clear interval progression of the lesion and its associated edema. We did suspect a neoplastic process, either ependymoma or astrocytoma, given its progression and appearance, but it was odd enough to raise the question of a demyelinating MS plaque especially given the patient's history. A lumbar puncture was performed that was negative for oligoclonal bands. MRI imaging of the brain and thoracic cord was negative. We therefore proceeded to surgery given its MRI appearance, growth, and progressive symptoms.

Imaging

MRI showed an intramedullary mass at C5 with ring enhancement and edema above and below. Compared to the 2014 MRI, there was a 2 mm increase in the anteroposterior dimension and an increase in edema (Fig. 4.13).

Operation

The patient was positioned in standard military chin tuck fashion using a Mayfield head clamp. SSEPs and MEPs were utilized in addition to D-waves. These signals were normal at the start of the case. A C5 laminectomy was performed with minimal undercutting of both C4 and C6 lamina. Durotomy was performed with three bilateral tacking sutures to the paraspinal muscles. We then inserted a D-wave electrode underneath the dura along the spinal cord below the planned myelotomy site. The resulting motor monitoring from the D-wave was robust. We identified what appeared to be the dorsal median raphe, though this was a bit challenging as the cord was diffusely swollen. Bipolar cautery was set to 25, and the pial surface was cauterized and cut with microscissors. SSEPs remained stable. We then used fine bayoneted forceps and variable suction to enter into the spinal cord substance. We identified discolored substance that we grasped with tumor forceps and sent for frozen section, which confirmed a neoplastic process. Soon after this we entered into a cyst that released a yellowish fluid consistent with the left lateral cyst on MRI (Fig. 4.13b). We then utilized ultrasonic aspiration with a microtip on a very low setting to gently aspirate the solid portion of the mass. The planes inferior and to the left were difficult to identify, but superior and to the right, there was a more demarcated interface. At its depth we did appear to reach ventral pia, which was alarming, but given SSEP and D-wave preservation, we slowly continued. Our struggle involved the left lateral and inferior portion which ultimately led to a drop in SSEPs in the left arm and MEPs in the left leg first followed by the left arm. The MEP drop reached 60–70%,

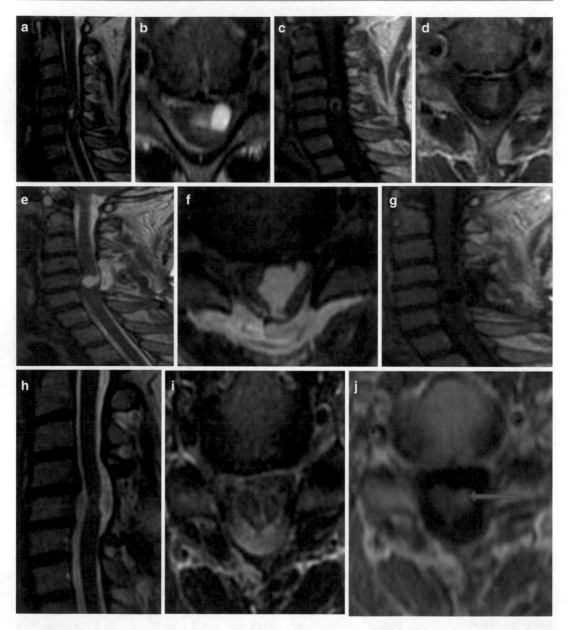

Fig. 4.13 Preoperative MRI with and without contrast. (**a**) Sagittal T2 showing mixed signal in the spinal cord at C5 with a ventral cyst. (**b**) Axial T2 showing a cystic structure mainly to the left and also ventral. (**c**) Sagittal T1 with contrast demonstrating rim enhancement. (**d**) Axial T1 with contrast showing a more homogeneous area of contrast uptake within the central part of the mass but with some rim enhancement out laterally to the left. (**e**) Sagittal T2 postoperative MRI with resection cavity. (**f**) Axial T2 showing dramatic resection cavity up to the ventral pial surface. (**g**) Sagittal T1 post-contrast with no residual enhancement. (**h**) Sagittal T2 MRI 2 years post-resection with some reconstitution of the spinal cord. (**i**) Axial T2 showing collapse of the resection cavity. (**j**) Axial T1 post-contrast showing a small area of left lateral and ventral enhancement (blue arrow)

though the D-waves remained stable. Due to the combined drop of SSEPs and MEPs in the left arm, the resection was halted. There was very little tumor left grossly if any. Irrigation fol-lowed by Surgiflo injection achieved hemostasis. Dural closure was completed with a locking 4-0 silk suture and the fascia with skin closure in standard fashion.

Pathology

Final pathology revealed an ependymoma WHO grade II with a low Ki67 of 2%.

Outcome

The patient did well postoperatively and was discharged to acute rehab on postoperative day 3. She did have new left leg weakness that we graded as 4/5. This improved to near full strength at her 3-week postoperative visit where she was independently ambulatory though using a cane for longer distances. Her left arm numbness was slightly worse after surgery and then back to baseline at the postoperative visit. Her left arm pain was improved. Her immediate postoperative MRI showed no evidence of residual enhancement, though we felt grossly that a small amount of tumor was left behind. There was remarkable volume loss at the level of the resection cavity. MRI done 2 years later showed a small amount of residual enhancement that we have continued to watch. If there is progression, she will proceed to radiation.

Comments

This case demonstrates the incredibly indolent growth profile that some ependymomas possess. This mass appears to have been growing for up to 12 years based on the patient's history and only 2 mm over a 3-year period between MRIs we were able to directly review. This clinical progression is what made us consider a neoplasm as opposed to a demyelinating plaque. Obviously the radiographic features, including eccentricity to the left and ring enhancement, are less typical for an ependymoma. We included this case to show that ependymomas can present in nonca-nonical ways. The postoperative axial T2 image shows a remarkable amount of volume loss – this demonstrates the capacity for these tumors to grow slowly enough that nearly all important traveling fibers are pushed to the periphery. Two years later, the spinal cord shows significant reconstitution on the MRI now that the compressed fiber tracts have had time to re-expand. This annual surveillance will be performed until there is progression of the minimal residual enhancement, in which case she will be referred for radiation therapy.

Regarding surveillance MRIs, there is no absolute timetable, and we resist a doctrinaire approach. In general, for gross total resections, we typically follow the patients with annual MRIs. In patients with near total resections (greater than 90%), especially if there is some elevation to the Ki67 index, we advocate for 6-month surveillance MRIs. If the Ki67 is low in a near total resection case, annual MRI surveillance is reasonable. In some circumstances of subtotal resection, especially if it is less than 80% and the Ki67 is elevated above a threshold of 5%, adjuvant radiation is considered, though we lean toward observing tumor behavior on surveillance imaging. Repeat surgery is often pursued over radiation as the benefits of radiation remain poorly established and can complicate future surgery. One can consider cessation of MRI monitoring after 5–10 years of stability in most patients.

Future Pathways

Outside of important refinements in microsurgical technique, there has been little in the way of technological advancements in the treatment of spinal ependymomas until recently. Doubtless the rarity of these tumors has slowed the search for innovative adjuncts to surgery. Progress has been incremental with regard to nonsurgical treatment as well. Fortunately, techniques that originated in the cranial sphere have shown promise for spinal ependymomas, and that has spurred some appreciable progress in the last few years. As mentioned earlier, the adoption of SRS and proton beam therapy represents some of the newer age methods for delivering targeted radiation to residual and recurrent disease. Corticospinal tract monitoring with D-waves is another fairly new intraoperative tool. Here we briefly highlight some of the recent novel and encouraging developments in the management of these tumors.

With regard to imaging, there have been recent reports of diffusion tensor imaging (DTI) and tractography that can be integrated with intraoperative navigation in the resection of intramedullary tumors [43]. This MRI modality is well-established in preoperative planning for brain tumor removal and can be deployed intraoperatively as part of the neuronavigation system. In similar fashion, DTI can illustrate the descending corticospinal tracts through the spinal cord and their relationship to the tumor, whether they are displaced by the mass (more typical of ependymoma) or coursing through the tumor (indicative of a more invasive entity like astrocytoma). Localization of the tracts and merging with intraoperative navigation can help to avoid the fibers during myelotomy, localize the tumor, and assist with resection. Despite the incorporation of navigation, the strength of DTI with tractography still appears to be in preoperative planning, as the relationship of the tracts to the tumor can help the surgeon more clearly define goals of resection and what areas of the tumor represent higher-risk terrain.

Again taking the lead from the intracranial domain, intraoperative visualization of ependymomas has shown some early promise. 5-aminolevulinic acid (5-ALA), now becoming widespread in the resection of malignant gliomas, has shown the ability in multiple reports to fluoresce spinal ependymomas leading to improvements in resection [44]. A recent study utilized near-infrared indocyanine green video angiography (ICG-VA) to assess the microcirculation of the ventral spinal cord from small anterior spinal artery branches following spinal ependymoma resection. The ICG peak time, if rapid, correlated well to functional recovery, and so ICG-VA showed some predictive potential [45]. ICG has also been used to help identify the posterior spinal artery branches and venous circulation which can then be avoided upon entry into the spinal cord, theoretically reducing morbidity [46].

Genomic studies of spinal ependymomas have collectively been lacking, again due to their relative scarcity. They do appear to be genetically distinct from their intracranial counterparts with a low mutation burden that has yet to lead to any actionable targets for chemotherapy. The genetic drivers of tumor pathogenesis remain poorly understood, thereby limiting the potential for developing and finding ependymoma-specific drugs [47]. Despite this limitation, there is an ongoing clinical trial of marizomib, a proteasome inhibitor, for recurrent spinal ependymomas [48]. The path forward will likely include clinical trials such as this, in which spinal cord ependymomas are grouped with intracranial ependymomas, their more common relative, and even other glial tumors. It is far more likely that a repurposing of currently available drugs as opposed to the selective engineering of new agents will be the way spinal ependymomas are treated in the future.

Conclusion

Spinal ependymomas are rarely encountered tumors though they represent the most common intramedullary tumor in adults. Radiographically they are characterized by expansion of the spinal cord, avid enhancement, central location, syringomyelia, polar cysts, and intratumoral hemorrhage. Histologically, these are generally benign tumors (WHO grades I–II) with a favorable prognosis. Close consideration of the MRI and clinical presentation should allow the neurosurgeon to distinguish a true ependymoma from radiographic mimics. Patient selection and operative timing are critical to optimize outcomes. With meticulous microsurgical technique, safe and effective resections can be achieved. However, more invasive subtypes may preclude gross total resection and eventually warrant a reoperation. Radiation therapy remains an option for recurrence, though the clinical benefit remains uncertain.

References

1. Klekamp J. Spinal ependymomas. Part 1: intramedullary ependymomas. Neurosurg Focus. 2015;39:E6.
2. Kim DH, Kim J-H, Choi SH, Sohn C-H, Yun TJ, Kim CH, Chang K-H. Differentiation between intramedullary spinal ependymoma and astrocytoma: comparative MRI analysis. Clin Radiol. 2014;69:29–35.
3. Celano E, Salehani A, Malcolm JG, Reinertsen E, Hadjipanayis CG. Spinal cord ependymoma: a review of the literature and case series of ten patients. J Neuro-Oncol. 2016;128:377–86.

4. Pajtler KW, Witt H, Sill M, et al. Molecular classification of ependymal tumors across all CNS compartments, histopathological grades, and age groups. Cancer Cell. 2015;27:728–43.

5. Whitaker SJ, Bessell EM, Ashley SE, Bloom HJ, Bell BA, Brada M. Postoperative radiotherapy in the management of spinal cord ependymoma. J Neurosurg. 1991;74:720–8.

6. Tobin MK, Geraghty JR, Engelhard HH, Linninger AA, Mehta AI. Intramedullary spinal cord tumors: a review of current and future treatment strategies. Neurosurg Focus. 2015;39:E14.

7. Schwartz TH, McCormick PC. Intramedullary ependymomas: clinical presentation, surgical treatment strategies and prognosis. J Neuro-Oncol. 2000;47:211–8.

8. Koeller KK, Rosenblum RS, Morrison AL. Neoplasms of the spinal cord and filum terminale: radiologic-pathologic correlation. Radiographics. 2000;20:1721–49.

9. McCormick PC, Torres R, Post KD, Stein BM. Intramedullary ependymoma of the spinal cord. J Neurosurg. 1990;72:523–32.

10. Eroes CA, Zausinger S, Kreth F-W, Goldbrunner R, Tonn J-C. Intramedullary low grade astrocytoma and ependymoma. Surgical results and predicting factors for clinical outcome. Acta Neurochir. 2010;152:611–8.

11. Garcés-Ambrossi GL, McGirt MJ, Mehta VA, Sciubba DM, Witham TF, Bydon A, Wolinksy J-P, Jallo GI, Gokaslan ZL. Factors associated with progression-free survival and long-term neurological outcome after resection of intramedullary spinal cord tumors: analysis of 101 consecutive cases. J Neurosurg Spine. 2009;11:591–9.

12. Nagasawa DT, Smith ZA, Cremer N, Fong C, Lu DC, Yang I. Complications associated with the treatment for spinal ependymomas. Neurosurg Focus. 2011;31:E13.

13. Li T-Y, Chu J-S, Xu Y-L, Yang J, Wang J, Huang Y-H, Kwan A-L, Wang G-H. Surgical strategies and outcomes of spinal ependymomas of different lengths: analysis of 210 patients. J Neurosurg Spine. 2014;21:249–59.

14. Neumann JE, Spohn M, Obrecht D, et al. Molecular characterization of histopathological ependymoma variants. Acta Neuropathol. 2020;139: 305–18.

15. Louis DN, Perry A, Reifenberger G, von Deimling A, Figarella-Branger D, Cavenee WK, Ohgaki H, Wiestler OD, Kleihues P, Ellison DW. The 2016 World Health Organization classification of tumors of the central nervous system: a summary. Acta Neuropathol. 2016;131:803–20.

16. Perry A, Prayson RA. Glial and glioneuronal tumors. Neuropathology. 2012;1:421–88.

17. Kobayashi K, Ando K, Kato F, et al. MRI characteristics of spinal ependymoma in WHO grade II: a review of 59 cases. Spine. 2018;43:E525–30.

18. Yuh EL, Barkovich AJ, Gupta N. Imaging of ependymomas: MRI and CT. Childs Nerv Syst. 2009;25:1203–13.

19. D'Amico RS, Praver M, Zanazzi GJ, et al. Subependymomas are low-grade heterogeneous glial neoplasms defined by subventricular zone lineage markers. World Neurosurg. 2017;107:451–63.

20. Toi H, Ogawa Y, Kinoshita K, Hirai S, Takai H, Hara K, Matsushita N, Matsubara S, Uno M. Bamboo leaf sign as a sensitive magnetic resonance imaging finding in spinal Subependymoma: case report and literature review. Case Rep Neurol Med. 2016;2016: 9108641.

21. Boström A, von Lehe M, Hartmann W, Pietsch T, Feuss M, Boström JP, Schramm J, Simon M. Surgery for spinal cord ependymomas: outcome and prognostic factors. Neurosurgery. 2011;68:302–8. discussion 309

22. Iwasaki M, Hida K, Aoyama T, Houkin K. Thoracolumbar intramedullary subependymoma with multiple cystic formation: a case report and review. Eur Spine J. 2013;22(Suppl 3):S317–20.

23. Lee M, Epstein FJ, Rezai AR, Zagzag D. Nonneoplastic intramedullary spinal cord lesions mimicking tumors. Neurosurgery. 1998;43:788–94; discussion 794–5

24. Watts J, Box GA, Galvin A, Van Tonder F, Trost N, Sutherland T. Magnetic resonance imaging of intramedullary spinal cord lesions: a pictorial review. J Med Imaging Radiat Oncol. 2014;58:569–81.

25. Deletis V, Shils J. Neurophysiology in neurosurgery: a modern intraoperative approach. New York: Elsevier, 2002.

26. Kothbauer KF, Deletis V, Epstein FJ. Motor-evoked potential monitoring for intramedullary spinal cord tumor surgery: correlation of clinical and neurophysiological data in a series of 100 consecutive procedures. Neurosurg Focus. 1998;4:e1.

27. Chang UK, Choe WJ, Chung SK, Chung CK, Kim HJ. Surgical outcome and prognostic factors of spinal intramedullary ependymomas in adults. J Neuro-Oncol. 2002;57:133–9.

28. Sala F, Bricolo A, Faccioli F, Lanteri P, Gerosa M. Surgery for intramedullary spinal cord tumors: the role of intraoperative (neurophysiological) monitoring. Eur Spine J. 2007;16(Suppl 2):S130–9.

29. Costa P, Peretta P, Faccani G. Relevance of intraoperative D wave in spine and spinal cord surgeries. Eur Spine J. 2013;22:840–8.

30. Ghadirpour R, Nasi D, Iaccarino C, Romano A, Motti L, Sabadini R, Valzania F, Servadei F. Intraoperative neurophysiological monitoring for intradural extramedullary spinal tumors: predictive value and relevance of D-wave amplitude on surgical outcome during a 10-year experience. J Neurosurg Spine. 2018;30:259–67.

31. Chacko AG, Daniel RT, Chacko G, Babu KS. Pial and arachnoid welding for restoration of normal cord anatomy after excision of intramedullary spinal cord tumors. J Clin Neurosci. 2007;14:764–9.

32. Lee S-H, Chung CK, Kim CH, Yoon SH, Hyun S-J, Kim K-J, Kim E-S, Eoh W, Kim H-J. Long-term outcomes of surgical resection with or without adjuvant radiation therapy for treatment of spinal ependymoma: a retrospective multicenter study by the Korea Spinal Oncology Research Group. Neuro-Oncology. 2013;15:921–9.

33. Boström A, Kanther N-C, Grote A, Boström J. Management and outcome in adult intramedullary spinal cord tumours: a 20-year single institution experience. BMC Res Notes. 2014;7:908.

34. Lin Y-H, Huang C-I, Wong T-T, Chen M-H, Shiau C-Y, Wang L-W, Ming-Tak Ho D, Yen S-H. Treatment of spinal cord ependymomas by surgery with or without postoperative radiotherapy. J Neuro-Oncol. 2005;71:205–10.

35. Oh MC, Ivan ME, Sun MZ, Kaur G, Safaee M, Kim JM, Sayegh ET, Aranda D, Parsa AT. Adjuvant radiotherapy delays recurrence following subtotal resection of spinal cord ependymomas. Neuro-Oncology. 2013;15:208–15.

36. Brown DA, Goyal A, Takami H, Graffeo CS, Mahajan A, Krauss WE, Bydon M. Radiotherapy in addition to surgical resection may not improve overall survival in WHO grade II spinal ependymomas. Clin Neurol Neurosurg. 2020;189:105632.

37. Rudà R, Reifenberger G, Frappaz D, et al. EANO guidelines for the diagnosis and treatment of ependymal tumors. Neuro-Oncology. 2018;20:445–56.

38. Ryu SM, Lee S-H, Kim E-S, Eoh W. Predicting survival of patients with spinal ependymoma using machine learning algorithms with the SEER database. World Neurosurg. 2018; https://doi.org/10.1016/j.wneu.2018.12.091.

39. Wostrack M, Ringel F, Eicker SO, Jagersberg M, Schaller K, Kerschbaumer J, et al. Spinal ependymoma in adults: a multicenter investigation of surgical outcome and progression-free survival. J Neurosurg Spine. 2018;28:654–62.

40. Amsbaugh MJ, Grosshans DR, McAleer MF, Zhu R, Wages C, Crawford CN, Palmer M, De Gracia B, Woo S, Mahajan A. Proton therapy for spinal ependymomas: planning, acute toxicities, and preliminary outcomes. Int J Radiat Oncol Biol Phys. 2012;83:1419–24.

41. Chamberlain MC. Etoposide for recurrent spinal cord ependymoma. Neurology. 2002;58:1310–1.

42. Morris KA, Afridi SK, Evans DG, Hensiek AE, McCabe MG, Kellett M, et al. The response of spinal cord ependymomas to bevacizumab in patients with neurofibromatosis Type 2. J Neurosurg Spine. 2017;26:474–82.

43. Benjamin CG, Frempong-Boadu A, Hoch M, Bruno M, Shepherd T, Pacione D. Combined use of diffusion tractography and advanced intraoperative imaging for resection of cervical intramedullary spinal cord neoplasms: a case series and technical note. Oper Neurosurg (Hagerstown). 2019;17:525–30.

44. Wainwright JV, Endo T, Cooper JB, Tominaga T, Schmidt MH. The role of 5-aminolevulinic acid in spinal tumor surgery: a review. J Neuro-Oncol. 2019;141:575–84.

45. Arima H, Naito K, Yamagata T, Ohata K, Takami T. Quantitative analysis of near-infrared indocyanine green videoangiography for predicting functional outcomes after spinal intramedullary ependymoma resection. Oper Neurosurg (Hagerstown). 2019;17:531–9.

46. Takami T, Naito K, Yamagata T, Ohata K. Surgical management of spinal intramedullary tumors: radical and safe strategy for benign tumors. Neurol Med Chir (Tokyo). 2015;55:317–27.

47. Zhang M, Iyer R, Azad T, Wang Q, Garzon-Muvdi T, Wang J, et al. Genomic landscape of intramedullary spinal cord gliomas. Sci Rep. 2019;9:18722.

48. Wu J, Armstrong TS, Gilbert MR. Biology and management of ependymomas. Neuro-Oncology. 2016;18:902–13.

Astrocytoma

5

5

Ahmed M. Meleis, M. Benjamin Larkin, and Claudio E. Tatsui

Introduction

Primary spinal cord astrocytomas are uncommon, comprising only 6–8% of all spinal cord tumors [1]. Patients with these types of tumors can have varying presentations, such as back pain, motor deficits, sensory deficits, or bowl and bladder dysfunction. While significant advances in cancer treatment occurred over the last decade, given its low incidence, management of spinal cord astrocytomas has remained largely unchanged. Studies have demonstrated that poor predictors of survival include high-grade morphology, advanced age, and less than a gross total resection (GTR). Surgically, spinal astrocytomas are very challenging because of their infiltrative nature, often affecting several spinal levels, without a distinguishable surgical plane between the tumor and normal spinal cord tissue. High-grade astrocytomas have a near 0% rate of gross total resection because of the challenges previously described. Current standard of care for spinal cord astrocytomas is surgery for confirmation of diagnosis and maximal safe resection followed by radiation therapy in certain cases. The combination of surgery and radiation has demonstrated efficacy primarily for those with lower-grade tumors. Radiation at an optimal dose of at least 45 Gray (Gy) has been shown to improve survival [2]. There are a few reports of utilization of chemotherapy in patients with recurrent and refractory spinal astrocytomas with inconsistent results [3–5].

Background

Spinal cord gliomas are the most common intradural intramedullary neoplasm, accounting for approximately 80% of all spinal cord tumors in all age groups [6, 7]. Among the spinal cord gliomas, astrocytomas comprise 30–40%, and ependymomas comprise 60–70% [6, 8]. There are different subtypes of astrocytomas, including pilocytic astrocytoma (WHO grade I), diffuse astrocytoma (WHO grade II), anaplastic astrocytoma (WHO grade III), and glioblastoma (WHO grade IV). The primary astrocytomas of the spinal cord are generally low grade (WHO grade I and II) 75% of the time, while the remaining are high grade (WHO grade III and IV) [3]. The different WHO grades depend on the various histological appearances and molecular features of the tumor. Typically, higher graded neoplasms (III

A. M. Meleis
Neurological Surgery, University of Texas MD Anderson Cancer Center, Houston, TX, USA

M. B. Larkin
Neurosurgery, Baylor College of Medicine, Houston, TX, USA

C. E. Tatsui (✉)
Neurosurgery, University of Texas MD Anderson Cancer Center, Houston, TX, USA
e-mail: cetatsui@mdanderson.org

© Springer Nature Switzerland AG 2021
S. Hanft, P. C. McCormick (eds.), *Tumors of the Spinal Canal*,
https://doi.org/10.1007/978-3-030-55096-7_5

and IV) demonstrate a more aggressive nature with greater mitotic activity, poorly differentiated features, and infiltration in the neuropil of the spinal cord leading to worse prognosis [9, 10].

The incidence of spinal cord gliomas is estimated to be 0.22 per 100,000 persons per year [8], with 850 to 1700 new cases of primary spinal cord gliomas diagnosed each year in the United States [10]. Peak incidence is in the third to fourth decades, and lesions most commonly occur in the cervical and upper thoracic spine [11, 12].

Patients with neurofibromatosis type 1 are more predisposed to spinal pilocytic astrocytomas, typically presenting as low-grade tumors in children and high-grade tumors in adults [13]. Astrocytomas may involve any region of the spinal cord, with the cervical spine the most commonly affected in children [14]. Patients presenting with spinal astrocytomas usually will have complaints of dysesthesia, paresthesia, motor dysfunction, and non-mechanical back pain. Motor deficits were reported in 30–64% of patients, sensory deficits in 26–43%, and bowel and/or bladder dysfunction in 2–9% [15–18]. In one study, 42% of patients with intramedullary tumors were nonambulatory [16].

Imaging

In general, the best imaging modality is magnetic resonance imaging (MRI) with and without gadolinium [14]. On MRI, astrocytomas usually reveal a hypointense T1-weighted and hyperintense T2-weighted lesion with a heterogeneous pattern of contrast enhancement [6, 7]. The lesion has a diffuse, infiltrative appearance sometimes associated with cysts and/or necrosis [19]. About 60% of astrocytomas are eccentric, as they originate from the glial tissue creating a localized expansion of the spinal cord [20]. Furthermore, the normal tissue of the spinal cord can look displaced to the side relative to the astrocytoma.

On computed tomography (CT), low-grade astrocytomas may be associated with increased interpedicular distance and bone erosion. However, these imaging findings are nonspecific

and can be seen with other intradural tumors and intramedullary lesions such ependymomas [21].

Other types of imaging modalities that have been obtained are diffusion tensor imaging (DTI) and diffusion tensor tractography (DTT) [22]. The information obtained from DTI and DTT have been utilized in surgical planning in patients with spinal cord astrocytomas to try to mitigate the morbidity associated with surgery; however, the results and utility of this advanced imaging are variable. DTI and DTT have been used in assessing the extent of tumor involvement of the spinal cord when looking at images in the axial view [9]. Zhao et al. developed a classification system based on the astrocytoma involvement of the spinal cord. Astrocytomas of the cervical cord were divided into infiltrating type (type I) and displacement type (type II). Type I tumors were further subdivided into simple infiltrating (type IA) and infiltrating with destruction (type IB).

Histology

Spinal astrocytomas are composed of neoplastic astrocytes that demonstrate immunoreactivity for glial fibrillary acidic protein (GFAP) [1]. GFAP immunoreactivity may be lost in some high-grade astrocytomas such as WHO grade IV astrocytomas.

In pilocytic astrocytomas (WHO grade I), the histological phenotype consists of a biphasic neoplasm composed of looser (and cystic) areas with protoplasmic astrocytes and densely cellular areas composed of hairlike (piloid) cells. Eosinophilic granular bodies in the looser cystic areas with Rosenthal fibers are found in the densely cellular areas. Cells with rounded nuclei and perinuclear clearing, known as oligodendroglial-like cells, may be found in some areas as well (Table 5.1).

In diffuse astrocytomas (WHO grade II), the histological phenotype shows relatively low cellularity.

In anaplastic astrocytomas (WHO grade III), the histological phenotype is similar to diffuse astrocytomas.

Table 5.1 World Health Organization grading scale for spinal cord astrocytomas

WHO grade	Histology features
I – Pilocytic astrocytoma	Biphasic neoplasm composed of looser (and cystic) areas with protoplasmic astrocytes and densely cellular areas composed of hairlike (piloid) cells. Eosinophilic granular bodies in the looser cystic areas with Rosenthal fibers found in the densely cellular areas. Cells with rounded nuclei and perinuclear clearing, known as oligodendroglial-like cells, may be found in some areas as well
II – Diffuse astrocytoma	Low cellularity and composed of cells with angulated nuclei and mostly nuclear pleomorphism. The neoplastic astrocytes may have varied appearances such as fibrillary or gemistocytic. Furthermore, there is low mitotic activity without evidence of microvascular proliferation or pseudopalisading necrosis
III – Anaplastic astrocytoma	Similar to diffuse astrocytomas. The main difference is an increased presence of cellularity and mitotic activity. There is no evidence of microvascular proliferation or pseudopalisading necrosis
IV – Glioblastoma	More cellularity and mitotic activity, with microvascular proliferation and/or pseudopalisading necrosis

Based on data from Ref. [52]

In glioblastoma (WHO grade IV), there is even more cellularity and mitotic activity. With this higher-grade astrocytoma, there is a chance of seeing leptomeningeal seeding in the central nervous system (CNS) [23].

Risk Factors and Prognosis

Prognostic factors for patients with spinal astrocytomas include age, histological diagnosis (morphology/WHO grade), and preoperative neurological function [8, 24–27]. Age greater than 60 years old at time of diagnosis, high-grade morphology, and subtotal resection are strong negative predictors of survival [28]. Ebner et al. reported a study of 46 patients with intramedullary spinal cord tumors by demonstrating worse outcomes for patients whose tumors extended beyond three spinal cord segments [29]. Cohen et al. followed 19 consecutive cases of grade III and IV spinal astrocytomas in a younger population (median age 14) and found the median postoperative survival was only 6 months after undergoing a combination of radiation therapy and radical surgical resection [30]. Wong et al. studying risk factors and overall survival for patients with spinal cord astrocytomas found that male gender, the extent of surgical resection, and tumor histology were significant predictors of survival. Interestingly, male patients had double the mean survival versus female patients (24 months versus 12 months), possibly suggesting a level of hormonal or genetic influence [31]. These studies consistently record poor prognostic correlation with higher-grade tumors, with WHO grade IV having a significantly higher rate of mortality. Milano et al. reported a cohort of 664 patients with spinal astrocytomas and that the 5-year overall survival rate was 82% for grade I, 70% for grade II, and declined to 28% and 14% for grades III and IV, respectively [8]. Epstein et al. presented a series of 25 adult patients who underwent gross total resection where the histological grade was the strongest predictor of outcome. Five of six patients with grade IV astrocytoma died within 23 months from surgery, while 17 of 19 patients with low-grade lesions (grade I or II) had a mean survival of 50.2 months [32]. Furthermore, Basheer et al. performed a retrospective study of 89 adult patients with spinal cord astrocytoma (44 grade III and 45 grade IV) and reported that gross total resection, when possible, led to significantly lower mortality when compared to subtotal resection, biopsy, or nonsurgical treatment [25]. Other reviews of high-grade gliomas (grade III and IV) report an 18.7-month post-surgery survival but also quote a low likelihood of gross total resection (approximately 10%) [10]. One must consider though that gross total resection of these lesions is not always possible without severe compromise of a patient's neurologic function. Furthermore, the infiltrative nature of astrocytomas makes gross total resection of these lesions very difficult to attain [33].

Regarding spinal cord glioblastomas (GBM), a literature review found at least 165 primary spinal GBM cases reported since 1938. This disease seems to be more prevalent in young individuals (mean age 26 years), found typically in the thoracic or cervical region and least frequently in the conus medullaris [34]. The average survival for patients with spinal GBM is 14.3 months. Interestingly, age at the time of diagnosis weighs heavily on median overall survival. Patients diagnosed over the age of 50 years had a median overall survival of 2 months, and those diagnosed at less than 50 years of age had a median overall survival of 14 months [35]. Yanamadala et al. reported that patients with spinal GBMs all showed deterioration of functional status within 1 year of diagnosis [36].

Treatment Options

Surgery

The primary goal of any tumor surgery is to obtain tissue for diagnosis. This will help delineate treatment options available for the patient. Safe surgical resection and decompression (such as expansile duraplasty) remain the initial treatment strategy for spinal cord astrocytomas [10, 34, 37–39]. While the literature indicates that aggressive resection generally leads to increased overall survival [38], gross total resection of spinal cord astrocytomas is often not feasible without causing a neurological deficit. This is due to the lack of a tumor–normal spinal cord interface [33]. Karikari et al. looked at their single institution experience of surgical resection of intramedullary tumors, including astrocytomas. They studied whether they could identify a plane of dissection and ability to achieve gross total resection. What these authors found was that a plane was present in 28.6% of astrocytomas and that GTR was achieved in only 14.3% of cases with 47.6% recurrence. This was true only for the

pilocytic astrocytomas. In their review they found that none of the grade II, III, or IV astrocytic tumors had a plane, and gross total resection was not feasible [33].

Minehan et al. report gross total resection being possible in 0% of their grade IV lesions and only 12% of their grade III lesions [40]. In another retrospective review done by Raco et al., of 22 patients with high-grade (grade III or IV) intramedullary astrocytomas, the surgeons were only able to achieve a gross total resection in 2 patients [41]. Babu et al. describe in their experience the morbidity associated with attempted gross total resection of high-grade spinal cord astrocytomas; their results showed that 17 of 46 patients had a worse neurologic function postoperatively as compared to before surgery [39]. Overall, gross total resection should be pursued on certain grounds: if there are good planes of dissection intraoperatively and if there is stable neuromonitoring throughout the case irrespective of tumor grade [33, 42].

Radiation

Conventional external bean radiotherapy remains an effective treatment for various pathologies of the CNS. When treating spinal astrocytomas, it is often used in the postoperative setting, with the typical dose prescription of 45 Gy over 4.5–5 weeks or slightly higher at 50 Gy given in 25 fractions over 5 weeks [2, 43, 44]. A retrospective analysis by Corradini et al. evaluated 16 patients receiving radiotherapy for spinal cord gliomas. In patients who received radiation therapy alone, the mean overall survival was 2.7 months [35]. In contrast, patients who received surgery and then adjuvant radiation therapy had an overall survival of 64 months. Furthermore, a study of 183 patients treated with either surgery alone versus surgery plus radiation found that postoperative radiation therapy was effective at reducing disease progression in low- and moderate-grade (grade I and II) astrocytomas [45]. Overall, the 5-year survival rate for patients with low-grade spinal astrocytomas treated with postoperative radiation is 51–90% [2, 43]. High-grade astrocytomas have a different outlook, however. The outcomes of high-grade astrocytomas (grade III, IV) is very poor, with only 6–8 months of average survival after surgery with our without postoperative radiation [43, 44]. Radiation is not recommended as initial therapy for newly diagnosed spinal cord astrocytoma; however, it can increase overall survival in patients with low-grade (grade I, II) astrocytoma when used after surgery as adjunctive therapy [35].

Chemotherapy

The role of chemotherapeutic agents in the treatment of spinal astrocytomas remains controversial. At the time of writing this chapter, there is no standard chemotherapy used for this patient population. There are those who believe chemotherapeutic agents can be used in patients who have failed conventional treatment of surgery and radiation therapy [3]. Chamberlain et al. describe a multi-institutional retrospective study of 22 adult patients with recurrent grade II and grade III astrocytomas initially treated with surgery and radiation therapy. These patients were then treated with temozolomide after recurrence was observed. The authors note this treatment was effective in providing 2 years of progression-free survival. The probability of survival observed in this cohort was 64% at 6 months, 64% at 12 months, 41% at 18 months, and 27% at 24 months [3]. The combination of procarbazine, lomustine, and vincristine (PCV) has been reported to be used for patients with spinal astrocytomas. One case report describes a case of low-grade spinal cord astrocytoma refractory to radiation, which responded to treatment with PCV with a 23-month progression-free survival [4]. Overall, the collective sentiment towards chemotherapy in patients with spinal astrocytomas is mixed. The gold standard remains surgery and radiation therapy, and chemotherapeutics should be considered if standard treatment fails. Chemotherapy use will continue to remain an area of future research and growth.

Future Direction

Translational research to treat oncologic diseases is one area of tremendous growth that has great potential to find novel ways of treating cancer. Ropper et al. studied the potential ability of a dual-gene therapy in the treatment of high-grade astrocytoma (grade IV) of the spinal cord [37]. Specifically, they investigated the efficacy of dual genc-engineered human neural stem cells in rats injected with human glioblastoma cell lines receiving both 5-fluorocytosine and ganciclovir for 5 days. The authors found that this dual-gene therapy was superior to monotherapy or control group in vitro and in vivo. There was an 83% inhibition of tumor cell proliferation in the dual-gene therapy group compared to 61% in monotherapy with 5-fluorocytosine. Furthermore, postmortem analysis showed incorporation of therapy cells into the tumor. It is our sincere hope that this will translate into clinical progress and that other trials will address this challenging condition.

Patient Evaluation

When evaluating a patient with a primary spinal cord tumor, a thorough history of the patient's complaints is important. The patient can complain of subtle findings, such as a new numbness in an extremity, a clumsiness in a limb, increasing falls, bowl or bladder problems, or back pain that has failed to improve. It is important to elicit duration of symptoms and whether these symptoms are getting worse or have plateaued. Understanding this can help one possibly understand how quickly or slowly the disease is progressing. Furthermore, obtaining a family history is important, as the patient may have a familial or genetic predisposition to spinal tumors (i.e., neurofibromatosis type I). Once the patient history is complete, a thorough neurologic exam is performed. As stated earlier, a patient may have no gross findings, may have subtle findings, or may be more obviously symptomatic. Strength of muscle groups in the upper and lower extremities and sensation in dermatomal distributions are important to document. Patients may have a sensory level that can correlate with the lesion. It is also important to look for long tract signs such as hyperreflexia, Hoffmann sign, clonus, increased muscle tone, Babinski sign, Lhermitte sign, and Romberg sign. All these are important to document as a baseline as well, especially if surveillance of the spinal cord lesion will be pursued as signs of worsening symptoms may only be found objectively and not subjectively.

Reviewing MRI Findings

An MRI with and without gadolinium is the standard imaging modality to evaluate spinal astrocytomas. The imaging characteristics were previously described. Furthermore, in the first patient evaluation, it is important to obtain imaging of the entire CNS to determine if there are any other lesions, leptomeningeal spread, metastatic lesions, and possible other etiologies that can explain the findings in the spinal cord.

Operative Tips

When deciding to perform surgery, it is important to counsel the patient on the inherent risk of neurological decline, specific to the area of spinal cord involvement. Surgery involves a dorsal approach to the tumor. On approach, studying the MRI to see where the tumor comes closest to the dorsal surface of the spinal cord will lead to the safest corridor for entry into the lesion. A midline myelotomy is most often performed, and we find it important to extend the opening of the pia mater to the upper and lower pole of the tumor in order to minimize trauma to spinal cord during resection of the tumor. At this stage, trying to distinguish the tumor from the normal spinal cord can be challenging as the difference may be subtle, and astrocytomas tend to be infiltrative with similar consistency and color of the normal nervous tissue. At this stage obtaining specimen for a frozen section is of paramount importance, as a diagnosis of an infiltrative glioma should limit the surgeon to a more conservative approach. If

there is a clear plane between the tumor and spinal cord, the plane is developed as much as is safely possible. Tumor removal is continued as long as neuromonitoring (discussed below) remains stable and there is a clear distinction between the tumor and the spinal cord. In the event there is a significant change in neuromonitoring or the plane of dissection is lost, the surgeon must decide to change the approach and should consider interrupting the resection to avoid causing irreversible neurological dysfunction. In regard to neuromonitoring, an amplitude decrease of 50% and latency increase of 10% in MEPs typically correlate to new postoperative neurologic deficits [46].

Neuromonitoring

Somatosensory evoked potentials (SSEPs) and motor evoked potentials (MEPs) are important neuromonitoring tools to have during intraoperative resection of intramedullary spinal cord tumors such as astrocytomas [47, 48]. SSEPs monitor the functional status of the somatosensory pathway. Briefly, this is accomplished through the stimulation of a peripheral nerve, usually the median nerve at the wrist and the posterior tibial nerve at the ankle. The stimulation is done at the point of muscle twitch. The electrical potentials generated by this stimulation can then be recorded at various points along the neural pathway, such as Erb's point for upper extremities and popliteal fossa for the lower extremity. These sensory-generated electrical stimulations then enter the spinal cord through dorsal roots at several levels. Monitoring of SSEPs has been shown in previous reports to reduce postoperative spinal cord impairment by warning the surgeon of the potential for spinal cord injury and possibly the need to cease further dissection in order to avoid permanent injury [49]. SSEPs can also be used in the initial planning of the myelotomy incision [50].

Motor evoked potentials (MEPs) can be used to evaluate the functional integrity of the corticospinal tract system from the brain to the spinal cord and target muscle group [51]. This is generally done by a high-intensity stimulus of magnetic or electrical stimulation to the brain via leads placed on the patient's scalp. MEPs offer a better predictor for postoperative neurological outcome than the preoperative motor status of the patient itself. MEPs can be used in conjunction with SSEPs to provide information to the surgeon about the anterior columns and posterior columns of the spinal cord [47]. Direct spinal cord stimulation mapping can also be used to provide the surgeon information on determining the interface between tumor and normal spinal tissue [51]. Furthermore, direct stimulation can give the surgeon information on where a posterior myelotomy can be performed. Initially, the surgeon will visualize the dorsal medullary vein penetrating the medial sulcus. Then, via direct stimulation of the spinal cord, the surgeon can stimulate at midline and 1-mm lateral to where the midline is identified. The region to where there is no stimulation is where a midline myelotomy is performed. If changes in neuromonitoring occurs during resection of astrocytomas, there are certain strategies and maneuvers a surgeon can take to try to evaluate if these changes are reversible or represent real damage to nervous tissue. First, the surgeon should stop the retraction and surgical manipulation of the spinal cord. Warm irrigation should then be placed on the surgical field. One must consider if there is a technical problem with the neuromonitoring leads or machine. Asking the technician to recheck the leads is important. The surgeon should also ask the anesthesiologist if there was a sudden drop in blood pressure, as spinal cord perfusion is important in this instance. If there is not, asking the anesthesiologist to maintain the patient's mean arterial pressures (MAPs) above 85 for the rest of the case will help with spinal cord perfusion. Furthermore, a dose of steroids (typically Decadron 10 mg IV x 1) may be administered to the patient as spinal cord contusion from manipulation can cause a decrease in SSEPs. It is also important to verify with the anesthesiologist if any new anesthetic agent was given to the patient, as these could interfere with neuromonitoring. All these maneuvers can be done in unison to verify if the neuromonitoring signals return back to baseline. The surgeon should then reflect if the most recent surgical manipulation was the cause of the drop. If signals are back at baseline, the surgeon can proceed, taking care to stay in the clear interface of dissection of the tumor with the spinal cord avoiding traumatic manipulation of the spinal cord. If there is no recovery in signals, the surgeon should judge if there is a clear interface between the tumor and the spinal cord; if this interface is not present, probability of neurological decline is certain, and surgery cannot proceed safely at this junction without causing irreversible loss of neurological function. The use of D-waves is discussed in Chapter 4 and has become increasingly adopted in the resection of intramedullary astrocytomas.

Follow-Up and Adjuvant Treatment

In the first postoperative visit, the final pathology results are discussed with the patient. Radiation after surgery for spinal astrocytomas generally commences once the surgeon feels the wound has healed properly and if the patient has adequate improvement in the neurological exam in cases of temporary worsening due to surgical manipulation. A minimum of 2-4 weeks between surgery and commencement of radiation therapy is the general recommendation.

Case Presentations

Case 1 A 53-year-old female presented complaining of several years of recurrent right-sided thoracic radiculopathy, which was largely intermittent. It would be present for a few weeks and then subsided for months. This was not associated with any neurological dysfunction. This was initially diagnosed as neuropathy associated with her diabetes. However, more recently she was having difficulty with proprioception. She had an EMG which was nonspecific and had a left peroneal release without improvement of paresthesias she was experiencing in her left foot. Six months prior to presentation, she experienced episodes of neck and back pain that were not subsiding. This was associated with a burning pain in the mid-thoracic region on the right side running under her right breast. She denied any bowel or bladder dysfunction. She described difficulty with ambulation when trying to walk in a straight line. On neurologic exam she had good motor strength but did have decreased vibratory and proprioceptive sense in both of her lower extremities. She also had significant dysfunction in proprioception of her feet and ankles. Her MRI (Fig. 5.1) showed a

complex mass with cystic components intrinsic to the spinal cord extending from T4 to T6 without gadolinium enhancement. The patient upon counseling was subsequently taken to the operating room for a biopsy, which showed a WHO grade II astrocytoma. Intraoperatively, the plane between the tumor and normal spinal cord became difficult to delineate. The approach was to remove as much safely where the tumor and normal neural tissue were clearly defined, and once that plane of dissection was lost, the deci-

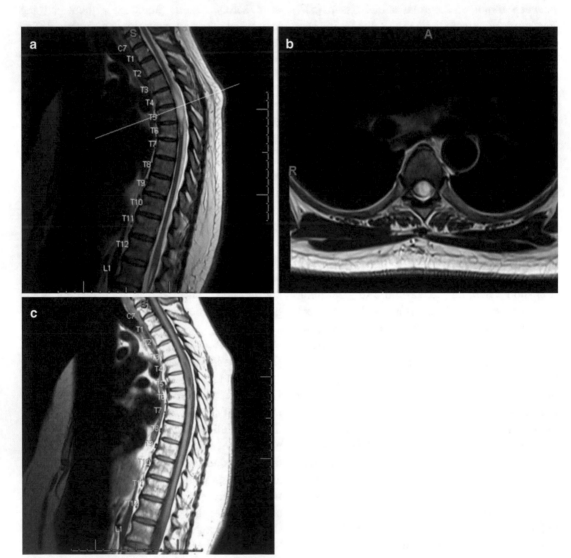

Fig. 5.1 A WHO grade II astrocytoma. (**a**) Sagittal T2 MRI shows a complex mass with cystic components intrinsic to the spinal cord extending from T4 to T6. (**b**) Axial imaging cut through the largest component of the

intramedullary lesion where the lesion is most superficial. (**c**) Sagittal T1 shows areas of iso- to hyperintense areas between the T4 and T6 segments

sion was made to stop before incurring any neu-rologic deficit.

Case 2 A 74-year-old male presented with sev-eral months of progressive lower extremity weak-ness and numbness as well as episodic incontinence of urine and feces. Initially, the symptoms started as numbness in the right heel but then began to extend throughout the right lower extremity into the right buttock. The sen-sory deficit then progressed to right lower extrem-ity weakness, most prominent distally. With his incontinence, initially the episodes were very infrequent, attributing them to his prostatectomy; however, they had become more frequent, and in addition the patient could no longer sense the urge to defecate. The patient then felt new numb-ness from his right chest and back extending down and decreased sensation in his left leg as well. He began using a wheelchair as he felt unsteady and weak in his legs. His neurologic exam was significant for 3/5 motor weakness in his bilateral iliopsoas and 2/5 motor strength in

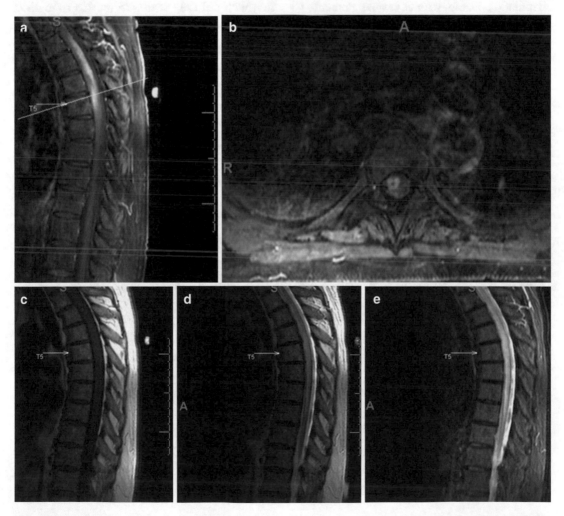

Fig. 5.2 A WHO grade III astrocytoma. (**a**) Sagittal MRI with gadolinium shows a long segment enhancing, expansile lesion of the upper thoracic cord spanning T1 to T8 (**b**) Axial cut with gadolinium shows some enhance-ment centrally and to the right of midline at T5 involving the spinal cord. (**c**) Sagittal T1 shows isointense lesion that expands the cord. (**d**) Sagittal T2 shows a hyperin-tense segment of the cord. (**e**) Sagittal T2 flair once again demonstrates the hyperintense expansile lesion

his quadriceps, hamstrings, dorsiflexion, plantar flexion, and extensor hallucis longus. He had a sensory level at T4, with multiple beats of clonus in his lower extremities. An MRI was obtained (Fig. 5.2) which showed a long segment expansile lesion of the upper thoracic cord spanning T1 to T8 with some enhancement centrally and right of midline at T5 involving the spinal cord. A biopsy was done at the level of enhancement, which showed a WHO grade III astrocytoma. Intraoperatively, there was no clear plane of dissection to attempt to debulk the tumor. Therefore, we stopped the surgery and closed with a referral to radiation oncology for adjuvant treatment.

Case 3 A 46-year-old female presented with a 3-month history of new-onset back pain and bilateral lower extremity weakness. Initially, the symptoms started when she felt tingling and numbness in her legs. This quickly progressed to some abdominal discomfort. The discomfort then was associated with gait difficulty, lower extremity weakness, and upper extremity weakness, especially in the left hand. She said the weakness and numbness made it difficult to ambulate, and she began requiring a cane for ambulation. She denied any bowel or bladder problems. On exam she had increased muscle tone in all four extremities, with diffusely weak 4/5 muscle strength in

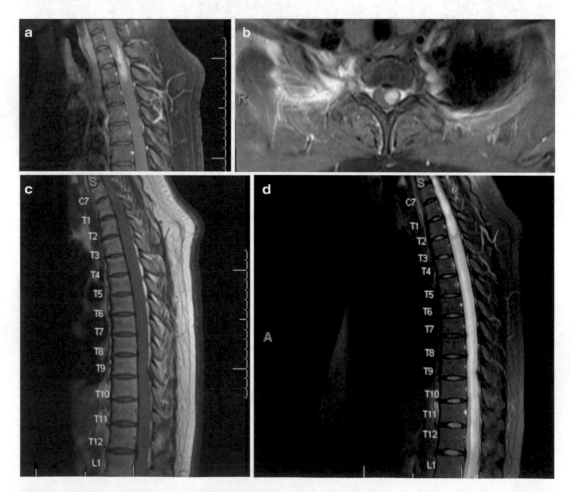

Fig. 5.3 A WHO grade IV astrocytoma/glioblastoma. (**a**) Sagittal T1 with gadolinium shows contrast enhancement between the T1 and T2 space. (**b**) Axial T1 with gadolinium shows contrast enhancement on the anterolateral quadrant of the spinal cord at the level of the left T1–T2 space. (**c**) Sagittal T1 shows enlargement of the entire cervical and thoracic spinal cord. (**d**) Sagittal T2 highlights the diffuse T2 signal changes with enlargement of the entire cervical and thoracic spinal cord

all muscle groups, and had multiple beats of clonus in her left foot. An MRI of the spinal axis (Fig. 5.3) showed diffuse T2 signal changes with enlargement of the entire cervical and thoracic spinal cord and with contrast enhancement of the anterolateral quadrant of the spinal cord at the level of the left T1–T2 space. A biopsy at the level of the enhancing portion at T1–T2 was performed with pathology showing a WHO grade IV astrocytoma/glioblastoma. With the knowledge that this tumor cannot be safely resected in gross total fashion and is infiltrative with T2 signal changes in the cervical and thoracic regions, the decision was made to close and plan for adjuvant therapy.

Conclusion

Primary spinal cord astrocytomas are uncommon, comprising only 6–8% of all spinal cord tumors [1]. There are different subtypes of astrocytomas, including pilocytic astrocytoma (WHO grade I), diffuse astrocytoma (WHO grade II), anaplastic astrocytoma (WHO grade III), and glioblastoma (WHO grade IV). The primary astrocytomas of the spinal cord are generally low grade (WHO grade I and II) 75% of the time [5], while the remaining are high grade (WHO grade III and IV). Typically, higher grade neoplasms (III and IV) demonstrate a more aggressive nature with greater mitotic activity, poorly differentiated features, and a greater potential to infiltrate into the neuropil of the spinal cord, ultimately leading to worse prognosis [9, 10]. On MRI, astrocytomas usually reveal a hypointense T1-weighted and hyperintense T2-weighted lesion with a pattern of contrast enhancement [6, 7]. The lesion has a diffuse, infiltrative appearance and can have intratumoral cysts and/or necrosis [19]. Spinal astrocytomas are composed of neoplastic astrocytes that demonstrate immunoreactivity for glial fibrillary acidic protein (GFAP). Treatment of these lesions remains difficult due to their infiltrative nature in the spinal cord. Patients may present with vague and progressive neurological complaints. It is important to perform a thorough neurologic exam to evaluate for any weakness, sensory level, and/or long tract signs. Surgical resection with the use of intraoperative neuromonitoring remains the first line of treatment to obtain tissue for diagnosis and as much resection as safely possible with care to avoid neurological deficit. Adjuvant radiation therapy has been shown to improve survival. Due to the rarity and overall poor prognosis of spinal cord astrocytomas, large population-based studies are needed to better assess the epidemiology and survival risk factors associated with these tumors in order to better understand the disease [23]. Additionally, further research is necessary for the development of new treatment modalities and combination therapies in hopes of improving patient outcomes.

Disclosures We have no granting organizations or grant numbers, contract numbers, or other sources of financial or material support to disclose.

References

1. Kleihues P. and Cavenee k. (eds). Pathology & Genetics. Tumours of the Nervous System. World Health Organisation Classification of Tumours. IARC Press, Lyon. 2000. No. of pages: 314. ISBN:9283224094.
2. Linstadt DE, Wara WM, Leibel SA, Gutin PH, Wilson CB, Sheline GE. Postoperative radiotherapy of primary spinal cord tumors. Int J Radiat Oncol Biol Phys. 1989;16:1397–403.
3. Chamberlain MC. Temozolomide for recurrent low-grade spinal cord gliomas in adults. Cancer. 2008;113(5):1019–24.
4. Henson JW, Thornton AF, Louis DN. Spinal cord astrocytoma: response to PCV chemotherapy. Neurology. 2000;54:518.
5. Chamberlain MC, Tredway TL. Adult primary intradural spinal cord tumors: a review. Curr Neurol Neurosci Rep. 2011;11:320–8.
6. Parsa AT, Chi JH, Acosta FL, Ames CP, McCormick PC. Intramedullary spinal cord tumors: molecular insights and surgical innovation. Clin Neurosurg. 2005;52:76–84.
7. Lonser RR, Weil RJ, Wanebo JE, DeVroom HL, Oldfield EH. Surgical management of spinal cord hemangioblastomas in patients with von Hippel-Lindau disease. J Neurosurg. 2003;98:106–16.
8. Milano MT, Johnson MD, Sul J, Mohile NA, Korones DN, Okunieff P, et al. Primary spinal cord glioma: a surveillance, epidemiology, and end results database study. J Neuro-Oncol. 2010;98:83–92.

9. Zhao M, Shi B, Chen T, Zhang Y, Geng T, Qiao L, et al. Axial MR diffusion tensor imaging and tractography in clinical diagnosed and pathology confirmed cervical spinal cord astrocytoma. J Neurol Sci. 2017;375:43–51.

10. Raco A, Esposito V, Lenzi J, Piccirilli M, Delfini R, Cantore G. Long-term follow-up of intramedullary spinal cord tumors: a series of 202 cases. Neurosurgery. 2005;56(5):972–81.

11. Osborn AG. Tumor cysts and tumorlike lesions of the spine and spinal cord. In: Osborn AG, eds. Diagnostic neuroradiology. Saint Louis: Mosby; 1994:876–17.

12. Castillo M. Spinal tumors and masses. In: Castillo M, editor. Neuroradiology: the core curriculum. Philadelphia: Lippincott Williams and Wilkins; 2002. p. 387–411.

13. Samartzis D, Gillis CC, Shih P, O'Toole JE, Fessler RG. Intramedullary spinal cord tumors: Part I-epidemiology, pathophysiology, and diagnosis. Global Spine J. 2015;5:425–35.

14. Townsend N, Handler M, Fleitz J, Foreman N. Intramedullary spinal cord astrocytomas in children. Pediatr Blood Cancer. 2004;43:629–32.

15. Sandler HM, Papadopoulos SM, Thornton AF Jr, Ross DA. Spinal cord astrocytomas: results of therapy. Neurosurgery. 1992;30(4):490–3.

16. Grem JL, Burgess J, Trump DL. Clinical features and natural history of intramedullary spinal cord metastasis. Cancer. 1985;56(9):2305–14.

17. Villegas AE, Guthrie TH. Intramedullary spinal cord metastasis in breast cancer: clinical features, diagnosis, and therapeutic consideration. Breast J. 2004;10:532–5.

18. Hoshimaru M, Koyama T, Hashimoto N, Kikuchi H. Results of microsurgical treatment for intramedullary spinal cord ependymomas: analysis of 36 cases. Neurosurgery. 1999;44:264–9.

19. Constantini S, Houten J, Miller DC, Freed D, Ozek MM, Rorke LB, et al. Intramedullary spinal cord tumors in children under the age of 3 years. J Neurosurg. 1996;85:1036–43.

20. Koeller KK, Rosenblum RS, Morrison AL. Neoplasms of the spinal cord and filum terminale: radiologic-pathologic correlation. Radiographics. 2000;20:1721–49.

21. Epstein F, Epstein N. Surgical treatment of spinal cord astrocytomas of childhood. A series of 19 patients. J Neurosurg. 1982;57(5):685–9.

22. Ducreux D, Lepeintre JF, Fillard P, Loureiro C, Tadié M, Lasjaunias P. MR diffusion tensor imaging and fiber tracking in 5 spinal cord astrocytomas. Am J Neuroradiol. 2006;27:214–6.

23. Ogunlade J, Wiginton JG 4th, Elia C, Odell T, Rao SC. Primary spinal Astrocytomas: a literature review. Cureus. 2019;11(7):e5247.

24. Tseng J-H, Tseng M-Y. Survival analysis of 459 adult patients with primary spinal cancer in England and Wales: a population-based study. Surg Neurol. 2007;67(1):53–8.

25. Basheer A, Rammo R, Kalkanis S, Felicella MM, Chedid M. Multifocal Intradural Extramedullary Pilocytic Astrocytomas of the spinal cord: a case report and review of the literature. Neurosurgery. 2016;80(2):E178–84.

26. Minehan KJ, Shaw EG, Scheithauer BW, Davis DL, Onofrio BM. Spinal cord astrocytoma: pathological and treatment considerations. J Neurosurg. 1995;83(4):590–5.

27. Adams H, Avendaño J, Raza SM, Gokaslan ZL, Jallo GI, Quiñones-Hinojosa A. Prognostic factors and survival in primary malignant astrocytomas of the spinal cord: a population-based analysis from 1973 to 2007. Spine (Phila Pa 1976). 2012;37(12):E727–35.

28. Tobin MK, Geraghty JR, Engelhard HH, Linninger AA, Mehta AI. Intramedullary spinal cord tumors: a review of current and future treatment strategies. Neurosurg Focus. 2015;39(2):E14.

29. Ebner FH, Roser F, Falk M, Hermann S, Honegger J, Tatagiba M. Management of intramedullary spinal cord lesions: interdependence of the longitudinal extension of the lesion and the functional outcome. Eur Spine J. 2010;19(4):665–9.

30. Cohen AR, Wisoff JH, Allen JC, Epstein F. Malignant astrocytomas of the spinal cord. J Neurosurg. 1989;70(1):50–4.

31. Wong AP, Dahdaleh NS, Fessler RG, Melkonian SC, Lin Y, Smith ZA, et al. Risk factors and long-term survival in adult patients with primary malignant spinal cord astrocytomas. J Neuro-Oncol. 2013;115(3):493–503.

32. Epstein FJ, Farmer J-P, Freed D. Adult intramedullary astrocytomas of the spinal cord. J Neurosurg. 1992;77(3):355–9.

33. Karikari IO, Nimjee SM, Hodges TR, Cutrell E, Hughes BD, Powers CJ, et al. Impact of tumor histology on resectability and neurological outcome in primary intramedullary spinal cord tumors: a single-center experience with 102 patients. Neurosurgery. 2015;76(Suppl 1):S4–13.

34. Shen C-X, Wu J-F, Zhao W, Cai Z-W, Cai R-Z, Chen C-M. Primary spinal glioblastoma multiforme: a case report and review of the literature. Medicine (Baltimore). 2017;96(16):e6634.

35. Corradini S, Hadi I, Hankel V, Ertl L, Ganswindt U, Belka C, et al. Radiotherapy of spinal cord gliomas. Strahlentherapie und Onkol. 2016;192(3):139–45.

36. Yanamadala V, Koffie RM, Shankar GM, Kumar JI, Buchlak QD, Puthenpura V, et al. Spinal cord glioblastoma: 25years of experience from a single institution. J Clin Neurosci. 2016;27:138–41.

37. Ropper AE, Zeng X, Haragopal H, Anderson JE, Aljuboori Z, Han I, et al. Targeted treatment of experimental spinal cord glioma with dual gene-engineered human neural stem cells. Neurosurgery. 2015;79(3):481–91.

38. McGirt MJ, Goldstein IM, Chaichana KL, Tobias ME, Kothbauer KF, Jallo GI. Extent of surgical resection of malignant Astrocytomas of the spinal

cord: outcome analysis of 35 patients. Neurosurgery. 2008;63(1):55–61.

39. Houten JK, Cooper PR. Spinal cord Astrocytomas: presentation, management and outcome. J Neuro-Oncol. 2000;47(3):219–24.

40. Minehan KJ, Brown PD, Scheithauer BW, Krauss WE, Wright MP. Prognosis and treatment of spinal cord astrocytoma. Int J Radiat Oncol Biol Phys. 2009;73(3):727–33.

41. Raco A, Piccirilli M, Landi A, Lenzi J, Delfini R, Cantore G. High-grade intramedullary astrocytomas: 30 years' experience at the neurosurgery Department of the University of Rome "Sapienza". J Neurosurg Spine SPI. 2010;12(2):144–53.

42. Garcés-Ambrossi GL, McGirt MJ, Mehta VA, Sciubba DM, Witham TF, Bydon A, et al. Factors associated with progression-free survival and long-term neurological outcome after resection of intramedullary spinal cord tumors: analysis of 101 consecutive cases. J Neurosurg Spine. 2009;11(5):591–9.

43. Shirato H, Kamada T, Hida K, Koyanagi I, Iwasaki Y, Miyasaka K, et al. The role of radiotherapy in the management of spinal cord glioma. Int J Radiat Oncol Biol Phys. 1995;33:323–8.

44. Merchant TE, Nguyen D, Thompson SJ, Reardon DA, Kun LE, Sanford RA. High-grade pediatric spinal cord tumors. Pediatr Neurosurg. 1999;30(1):1–5.

45. Abdel-Wahab M, Etuk B, Palermo J, Shirato H, Kresl J, Yapıcıer O, et al. Spinal cord gliomas: a multi-institutional retrospective analysis. Int J Radiat Oncol Biol Phys. 2006;64(4):1060–71.

46. Nuwer MR. Spinal cord monitoring. Muscle Nerve. 1999;22(12):1620–30.

47. Morota N, Deletis V, Constantini S, Kofler M, Cohen H, Epstein FJ. The role of motor evoked potentials during surgery for intramedullary spinal cord tumors. Neurosurgery. 1997;41:1327–36.

48. Kothbauer K, Deletis V, Epstein FJ. Intraoperative spinal cord monitoring for intramedullary surgery: an essential adjunct. Pediatr Neurosurg. 1997;26:247–54.

49. Nuwer MR. Spinal cord monitoring with somatosensory techniques. J Clin Neurophysiol. 1998;15(3):183–93.

50. Quinones-Hinojosa A, Gulati M, Lyon R, Gupta N, Yingling C, Cooper PR, et al. Spinal cord mapping as an adjunct for resection of intramedullary tumors: surgical technique with case illustrations. Neurosurgery. 2002;51:1199–207.

51. Quinones-Hinojosa A, Lyon R, Ames CP, Parsa AT. Neuromonitoring during surgery for metastatic tumors to the spine: intraoperative interpretation and management strategies. Neurosurg Clin N Am. 2004;15:537–47.

52. Koh J-S, Chang U-K, Haddiz T. Intramedullary tumors. In: Kim DH, Chang U-K, Kim S-H, Bilsky M, editors. Tumors of the spine. Philadelphia: Saunders Elsevier; 2008. p. 93–114.

Hemangioblastoma

6

Ryan G. Eaton and Russell R. Lonser

Epidemiology and Etiology

Spinal cord hemangioblastomas are the third most common intramedullary spinal cord tumor. They represent 3–8% of all spinal cord tumors and have an incidence of 0.01 to 0.02 per 100,000 persons [1–5]. The spinal cord is the second most common location for central nervous system (CNS) hemangioblastoma (25–40%), arising only slightly less often than hemangioblastomas of the cerebellum [6, 7]. While approximately 25–33% of spinal cord tumors are found in associated with von Hippel-Lindau disease (VHL) patients, 66–75% are arise sporadically.

VHL

VHL is a heritable multisystem cancer syndrome associated with a germline mutation in the *VHL tumor suppressor gene* located on the short arm of chromosome 3 [8]. The overall incidence of VHL is estimated at 1 per 45,500 live births with a point prevalence of 1 per 85,000 people [9]. VHL is inherited in an autosomal dominant manner and is highly penetrant (over 90% penetrance over the age of 65 years). Spinal hemangioblasto-

mas are found in over 50% VHL patients and are diagnosed at a mean age of 33 (range, 12–66 years) with a male to female ratio ranging from 1.6:1 to 5.5:1 [7, 10, 11].

Sporadic

The etiology of sporadic spinal cord hemangioblastomas is unknown (see below). Sporadic spinal cord hemangioblastomas are often diagnosed later in life than VHL-associated hemangioblastomas. Mean age of diagnosis of spinal cord hemangioblastomas is 41 years (range, 24–70 years) with a male to female ratio similar to that of VHL-associated hemangioblastomas [12, 13]. Sporadic lesions are less likely to be located in the lower spinal segments and are not multifocal [12].

Genetic Characteristics

VHL

The *VHL gene* is a tumor suppressor gene located on chromosome 3p25–26. The *VHL gene* consists of three exons and encodes for the VHL protein (pVHL). pVHL is involved in ubiquitin-mediated proteolysis of hypoxia-inducing factor (HIF)-1 and HIF-2 which mediate the release of pro-angiogenic factors such as

R. G. Eaton (✉) · R. R. Lonser
Department of Neurological Surgery,
The Ohio State University Wexner Medical Center,
Columbus, OH, USA
e-mail: ryan.eaton@osumc.edu

© Springer Nature Switzerland AG 2021
S. Hanft, P. C. McCormick (eds.), *Tumors of the Spinal Canal*,
https://doi.org/10.1007/978-3-030-55096-7_6

Fig. 6.1 Interaction of VHL protein with other proteins to form VCB-CUL2 complex Glut-1 = glucose transporter 1 and subsequent cell singling under conditions of normoxia and hypoxia. (From Lonser et al. [10])

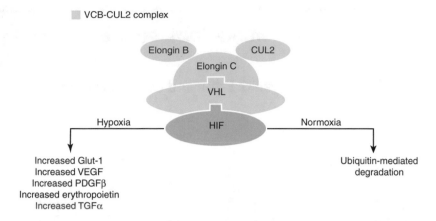

erythropoietin, platelet-derived growth factor, vascular endothelial growth factor, and transforming growth factor (Fig. 6.1) [14]. Based on the Knudson "two-hit" model of gene inactivation, the *VHL gene* requires mutations of both alleles for loss of function. VHL patients have a "first hit" germline mutation and a second somatic mutation/inactivation required for tumor formation [15]. The two most common germline mutations are missense (51.1%) and microdeletions mutations (19.7%) [16]. Missense mutated proteins retain some intrinsic functional capacity to degrade HIF, but the mutated pVHL is an unstable complex that is quickly degraded in a chaperonin binding-mediated sequence [17]. With aging, the chaperonin protein-mediated degradation occurs less robustly allowing for extended life span of the mutated protein [18], which may underlie the decrease in new tumor burden with age in VHL.

Sporadic

The genetic mechanism underlying sporadic hemangioblastoma formation is still unclear. Most sporadic hemangioblastomas do not have germline or somatic alterations of the *VHL gene* [19, 20]. The occurrence of biallelic inactivation of *VHL gene* in sporadic hemangioblastomas using next-generation sequencing was found to be less than 50%. These findings indicate that biallelic inactivation that initiates hemangioblastoma formation in VHL may not be necessary for tumorigenesis in sporadic hemangioblastomas [19, 21]. Two hypotheses that may explain sporadic tumorigenesis are aberrant epigenetic regu-

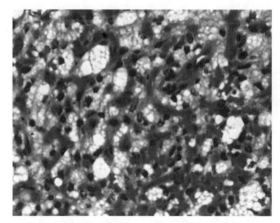

Fig. 6.2 Hematoxylin and eosin staining from a resected hemangioblastoma showing the lipid-laden stromal cells encased by numerous vessels. (From Lonser et al. [29])

lation of the *VHL gene* leading to tumor formation and/or genetic alterations in tumor-suppressing genes that regulate hypoxic-sensing pathways that support tumor formation. At the microscopic level, hemangioblastomas (VHL-associated and sporadic) appear as lipid-laden stromal cells within a dense vascular matrix (Fig. 6.2).

Clinical Features

Tumor Location

Spinal hemangioblastomas most frequently arise in the cervical spinal cord (19–39%) followed by thoracic (19–28%) and least frequently lumbar (2–7%) (Fig. 6.3). The vast majority (over 95%) of spinal cord hemangioblastomas are located posterior to the dentate ligament. Sixty-six percent of hemangioblastomas are located in the dorsal root entry zone. Approximately 50% of hemangioblastomas have both intra- and extramedullary components with 30% being entirely intramedullary and 20%

being primarily extramedullary (cases where 50% of the tumor was located extramedullary). Cyst formation occurs at an even frequency between cervical, thoracic, and lumbar lesions [22].

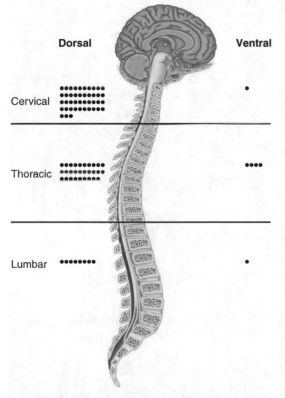

Fig. 6.3 Hemangioblastoma distribution by location in spinal cord based on 86 spinal cord hemangioblastomas resected in patients with von Hippel-Lindau disease. (From Lonser et al. [22])

Signs and Symptoms

Symptom formation is most frequently caused by a combination of mass effect from the hemangioblastoma and an associated peritumoral cyst (syringomyelia). Over 90% of symptomatic spinal cord hemangioblastomas are associated with a syrinx [23]. Consistent with their anatomic location, the most common symptom associated with spinal cord hemangioblastomas is sensory changes (symptom frequency of over 80% of affected individuals). Other common signs and symptoms are weakness (65%), gait ataxia (65%), and hyperreflexia (52%). Pain was a presenting symptom in 20% [24]. Symptom formation is associated with tumor size, growth rate, and/or presence of associated syringomyelia [25].

Diagnostic Imaging

Magnetic Resonance Imaging (MR Imaging)

Contrast-enhanced MR imaging is the most accurate method for visualization and serial monitoring of hemangioblastoma (Figs. 6.4, 6.5,

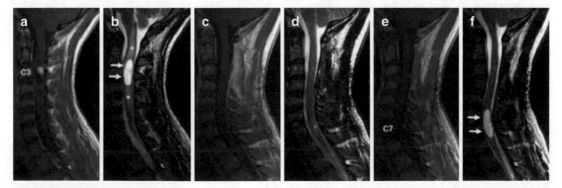

Fig. 6.4 Cervical spine MR images demonstrating the effect of tumor resection. Preoperative contrast-enhanced image (**a**) and T2-weighted image (**b**) of hemangioblastoma at C3 with associated syrinx (arrows) and cord edema (asterisks). Postoperative image at 7 months post resection (**c**) showing resolution of syrinx and edema (**d**). At 20 months, the development of another hemangioblastoma at C7 is seen (**e, f**) as well as associated syrinx development (arrows). (From Mehta et al. [13])

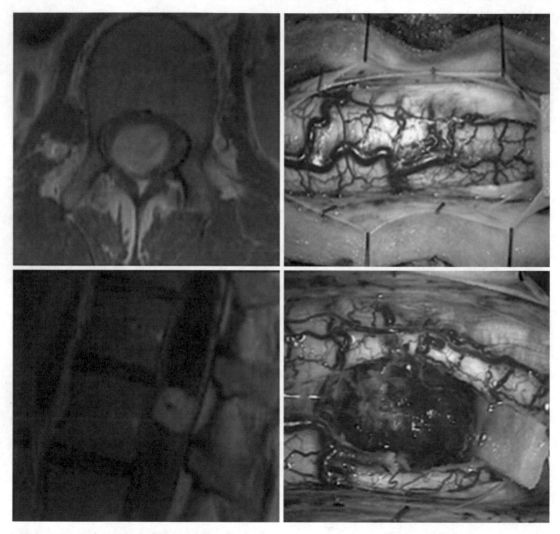

Fig. 6.5 Contrast-enhanced T1-weighted MR image of hyperintense nodule in axial section (Top left) and sagittal section (Bottom left)). Intraoperatively, a collection of large draining veins are appreciated dorsal to the tumor (Top right) with the lesion eventually isolated from the surrounding medullary tissue after careful dissection (Bottom right)

and 6.6). While post-contrast MR imaging will typically reveal a homogenous enhancing tumor, the non-enhanced regions of the hemangioblastomas can be dependent on tumor size. Generally, hemangioblastomas less than 10 mm in diameter appear isointense on pre-contrast T1-weighted imaging and hyperintense on T2-weighted imaging. Larger tumors (greater than 10 mm) are usually hypointense on pre-contrast T1-weighted images and heterogeneous on T2-weighted images and can enhance homogeneously or heterogeneously [26]. Given the highly vascular nature of hemangioblastomas, these tumors will often show intratumor and perimedullary vascular flow voids on MR images [27]. MR imaging features of hemangioblastoma often differentiate them from other intramedullary tumors. T2-weighted MR sequences are useful for defining the extent of peritumoral edema and syringomyelia [28].

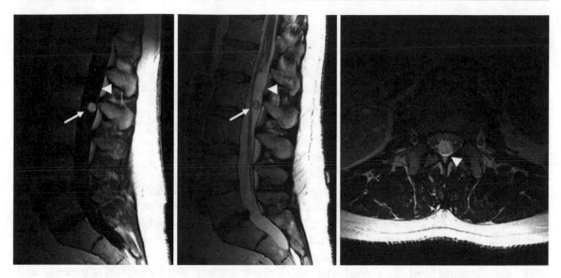

Fig. 6.6 Sagittal T1-weighted post-contrast MR (left) and T2-weighed image (center) of L2 hemangioblastoma (white arrow) with associated cystic mass (white arrow-head). Axial T2-weighted image (right) shows the cystic mass displacing the cauda equina [48]. (From Mehta et al. [48])

Arteriography

Hemangioblastomas are defined by a central tumor blush with prominent feeding arteries and dilated draining veins on arteriography. Angiography is usually not necessary for diagnostic purposes. However, in rare situations there may be utility in defining the vascular supply of very large lesions during preoperative planning.

Natural History

Pattern of Progression

Hemangioblastomas follow a variable growth pattern and can demonstrate a linear, exponential, or saltatory pattern with saltatory being the most common. VHL patients with known hemangioblastomas were observed over a 32-month follow-up period, and it was observed that 44% of hemangioblastomas grew. Of the hemangioblastomas with associated cysts in these patients, 67% demonstrated growth of the cyst during this follow-up period [25]. When observed for over

5 years, approximately half of all CNS hemangioblastomas in VHL will grow, while the others will remain stable in size [7]. This growth was observed to occur over a mean of 13 months followed by a subsequent quiescent period that lasted a mean of 25 months [23]. With patients followed over a sufficient time period, this saltatory pattern characterized by the presence of multiple growth and quiescent periods was the most frequently seen pattern of progression [25].

Over a 10-year period, CNS hemangioblastomas associated with VHL will undergo an average of 1.85 quiescent periods before becoming symptomatic [23]. It has also been observed that the rate of cyst growth usually exceeds the rate of tumor growth in symptomatic tumors [25]. Many lesions that will eventually require treatment are often not present on initial MR imaging done to evaluate other tumors. This highlights the sporadic genesis and growth of these tumors and the importance of serial neuroimaging. Growth pattern is also dependent on anatomic location with hemangioblastomas of the spinal cord growing significantly slower (0.3 mm³/year) than cranial lesions [7].

Syringomyelia

Peritumoral cysts (syringomyelia) are the most frequent cause of symptoms and neurologic dysfunction in patients with spinal hemangioblastomas. Syringomyelia forms when plasma ultrafiltrate extravasates from the permeable thin walled tumor vessels, which leads to elevated pressure within the tumor interstitial spaces. The increased hydrostatic pressure drives the plasma ultrafiltrate into the surrounding tissue causing the edema. When the rate of fluid extravasation from the tumor exceeds resorptive capacity of the peritumoral tissue, a peritumoral cyst forms. As the cyst continues to grow, the rate of resorption from the expanded cell wall will eventually approximate the rate of fluid extravasation, and cyst growth will cease increasing in size. In most cases, the cyst is larger than the associated tumor with the probability of cyst formation increasing with increasing tumor size [25]. Because the cyst formation is a direct consequence of the permeable vessels of the hemangioblastoma, surgical resection will result in cyst resolution and shunting or cyst fenestration is unnecessary [24, 29]. Natural history studies have shown cyst formation to occur in almost 33% of VHL-associated spinal cord hemangioblastomas and are associated with 80–90% of symptomatic spinal cord hemangioblastomas [7, 25].

Management

Decision-Making

For symptomatic sporadic or VHL-associated hemangioblastomas, en bloc surgical resection is the standard of care. Currently, given the characteristic radiographic appearance of hemangioblastomas, asymptomatic lesions in patients without a personal or family history of VHL generally may be safely monitored with serial imaging and clinical follow-up. However, in some sporadic cases, surgeons may opt for resection for tissue diagnosis. VHL patients with asymptomatic tumors should not be resected but monitored for symptom development. Long-term

VHL natural history studies show that tumor size, location, and growth rate were associated with symptom formation [23, 25]. Serial imaging at 1–2 year intervals is recommended in these situations or sooner with the onset of signs/symptoms [30].

Pregnancy

Case reports have suggested that pregnancy may accelerate CNS hemangioblastoma growth and/or peritumoral cyst progression. However, a prospective study of female VHL patients during child bearing years showed that the rate of development of new tumor/cyst, rate of tumor growth, and rate of cyst growth did not differ between those that became pregnant and those that did not [31]. For lesions that do become symptomatic requiring surgery during pregnancy, resection can be achieved depending on gestational age and maternal comorbidities. A study on spinal cord hemangioblastoma outcomes in pregnancy found that paresthesia suspected to be related to the lesion could be successfully managed symptomatically to avoid tumor resection during pregnancy [32]. While prospective mothers with VHL can undergo non-contrasted MR imaging during pregnancy, contrast-enhanced MR imaging is contraindicated during pregnancy.

Surgical Technique

Patients undergo endotracheal intubation. Perioperative antibiotics and corticosteroids are given (solumedrol trauma protocol). Somatosensory and motor evoked potentials monitoring is typically not employed. The posterior approach is the most common operative trajectory for hemangioblastomas given the majority are located posterior to the dentate ligament. Patients are positioned prone and supported by gel rolls from shoulder to the anterior iliac crest with adequate padding of contact areas to prevent ischemic injury. For lesions rostral to T6 level, the head is placed in three-point pin fixation, and for caudal lesions the head is placed on a padded head frame. The incision is planned using fluoroscopy or plain film localization [33].

The surgical field is prepared and draped in a sterile fashion. The predetermined incision site is infiltrated with 0.25% Marcaine (1:200,000 epinephrine). A skin incision is made, and dissection is carried anteriorly through the subcutaneous fat layer with dissection in periosteal plane to reflect the paraspinal muscles to visualize the spinal column. Laminectomies are made 1 to 2 cm rostral and caudal to the tumor to facilitate adequate visualization. The medial portions of the facets are preserved. Once the dura is exposed, intraoperative ultrasound is used to confirm the adequacy of the bony opening. The operative microscope is brought into the field, and a midline dural incision is made taking care to preserve the underlying arachnoid layer. The dura is reflected laterally and retained using 40 silk sutures fixed to the adjacent paraspinal muscle (Fig. 6.7). Superficial feeding arteries/arterioles (Fig. 6.8) are bipolar cauterized and sharply sectioned. The hemangioblastoma is generally located at or immediately adjacent to the posterior nerve root involving the entry zone. If the dorsal root fascicles involve and obscure the tumor, they are mobilized and divided. It is may necessary to dissect through and/or around sensory nerve fibers to reach the margins of the tumor [33].

Because the majority of hemangioblastomas are pial based, careful opening of the pia mater is made to maintain the dissection plane between the spinal cord and tumor capsule. A diamond knife is used to incise at the tumor-pial interface. This is followed by circumferential microsurgical dissection at the tumor-spinal cord interface. If the tumor is completely intramedullary, it can be accessed directly via a midline (or dorsal root zone) myelotomy. A circumferential plane is developed by interrupting the vessels entering and leaving the tumor. The vessels are coagulated using irrigated bipolar microforceps and transected with microscissors. This devascularizes the tumor and provides mobility needed to release the intramedullary component from the spinal cord tissue. The use of cottonoids is important at this stage to define the tumor margin, to protect surrounding medullary tissue, and to maintain the resection cavity. The dissection is continued rostrally and caudally. Care is taken throughout the circumferential dissection to maintain the associated cyst (if present) to facilitate dissection. Importantly, the cyst wall is composed of nonneoplastic glial tissue and is not resected [34].

Once the tumor is adequately released, the poles of the tumor must be reflected during which it is important to avoid excessive tenting of the spinal cord. Bleeding from the tumor surface is best controlled with Gelfoam. The dissection should proceed anteriorly with fine bipolar forceps and microscissors eventually severing the deep attachment of the tumor. The dura is then closed in a watertight manner. This is followed by a tight fascial closure, and the operation is completed with subcutaneous and cutaneous closure.

Surgical Outcomes

Outcomes for surgical resection of spinal cord hemangioblastomas are favorable, and complete resection is curative with a recurrence of less than 1% [13]. A long-term analysis by Mehta and colleagues of 108 VHL patients that underwent spinal cord hemangioblastoma resection found that 85% of patients were stable or improved immediately postoperatively with 96% functionally stable or improved at 6 months post resection. Of the 218 spinal cord hemangioblastomas resected in the study, over 99% achieved gross total resections and syrinx (when present) resolution or inactivation after resection of tumors occurred in all cases [13]. With regard to sporadic hemangioblastomas, a meta-analysis found 89% of patients were improved (65%) or stable (24%) at long-term follow up [12]. Overall, large cohort studies have suggested surgical outcomes for individuals with VHL-associated lesions are worse than those with sporadic hemangioblastomas [2, 12].

Complications

Mehta and colleagues (108 VHL patients that underwent resection of 218 spinal cord heman-

Fig. 6.7 Illustration of microsurgical resection of spinal cord hemangioblastoma. Vessels along the margin of the tumor are coagulated and divided (**a**, **b**) after which the pia is carefully incised (**c**, **d**). The tumor is then dissected circumferencially with a cottonid eventually being used to reflect the caudal pole for deep resection (**e**, **f**). (From Mehta et al. [13])

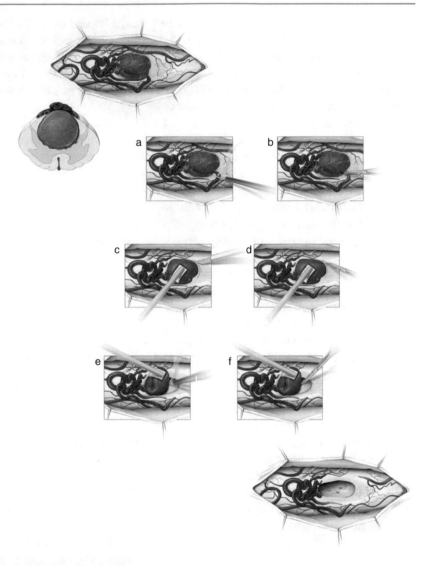

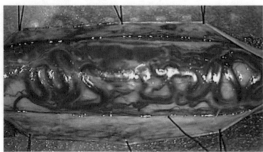

Fig. 6.8 Intraoperative photograph of intramedullary hemangioblastoma with enlarged draining veins surrounding the lesion

gioblastomas) found that cerebrospinal fluid leak (CSF) was the most common complication (3%). Half of these patients were successfully managed with CSF diversion, while the other half required surgical repair. Superficial wound infections occurred in three patients (1%), and all were successfully managed with oral antibiotics. Wound site hematomas occurred in three patients with two located extradural (1%) and one intradural (0.5%) all of which required reexploration. There was one case of aseptic meningitis (0.5%) resolved after 1 week without treatment [13].

Other Management Strategies

Radiosurgery

Stereotactic radiosurgery (SRS) may have benefit in patients with residual or unresectable hemangioblastomas [35, 36]. Hemangioblastomas with associated peritumoral cysts do not respond well to SRS, which can exacerbate cyst progression by increasing tumor/tumor vessel permeability [36]. A study of SRS performed on 46 patients with spinal cord hemangioblastomas demonstrated favorable short-term outcomes with local control rates of greater than 90% at 5-year followup with no adverse radiation events or complications [37]. SRS long-term control rates are less favorable. In a long-term prospective study, hemangioblastomas treated with SRS progressed (after 7 years) at similar rates to the natural history of untreated hemangioblastomas. Control rates continued to decline over time revealing limited long-term control potential [35].

Chemotherapy

Previously, the medical management for hemangioblastoma was with antiangiogenic drugs. The earliest studied drug was SU5416 (Semaxanib), a potent inhibitor of the tyrosine kinase receptor for VEGF. Case reports demonstrated clinical response to SU5416 therapy in two of six VHL patients due to a reduction in edema, but the treatment had no effect on tumor progression/size [38]. Recently, reports on pazopanib have shown benefit in individuals with multiple CNS hemangioblastomas [39, 40]. Another antiangiogenic drug, thalidomide, achieved stabilization of progressive, multifocal spinal cord hemangioblastomas [41]. Proteostasis modulators have also shown promise in preclinical models. They act by retaining the pVHL function by limiting proteasomal degradation via histone deacetylate inhabitation and have shown promise at preserving pVHL function [17].

Large clinical trials are required to assess the true efficacy of all these antineoplastic agents. Moreover, the challenge with evaluating the therapeutic effect of chemotherapy and radiotherapy is the saltatory growth pattern of hemangioblastomas, a process that can confound the definition of "local control" as it has been described that untreated tumors will undergo extended intervals of stability. Surgical resection remains the mainstay for hemangioblastomas of the spinal cord amenable to resection.

Angiographic Embolization

Few authors have recommended endovascular embolization to reduce surgical bleeding and possibly facilitate total removal, though we have not found it useful [42, 43]. The blood supply to hemangioblastomas is predominantly through small feeding vessels in addition to any dominant vessel that would be amenable to embolization. Therefore, the embolization only partially reduces intraoperative blood loss and carries a risk of post-embolization hemorrhage, infarction, and mortality [44]. Using careful microsurgical technique will obviate the need for preoperative embolization.

Genetic Advances in Hemangioblastoma

Genetic research on sporadic hemangioblastoma over the past decade has sought to reconcile the lower frequency of mutation in VHL gene compared to VHL-associated hemangioblastoma. One theory is that previous bulk sequencing methods were unable to fully characterize VHL inactivation in this population, and next-generation sequencing may more accurately approximate VHL gene changes. In a 2017 study, VHL gene alterations were low when analyzed by direct sequence (4 of 21 sporadic). However, targeted deep sequencing identified alterations in nine more samples. Along the same lines, a 2014 study found that VHL inactivating events were present in 25/32 (78%) of sporadic CNS hemangioblastomas by deep-coverage DNA sequencing far exceeding the 10–44% mutation rate of sporadic hemangioblastomas previous reported [19,

45]. The same study found biallelic VHL inactivation to occur in 64% of VHL-associated versus
52% of sporadic hemangioblastomas with all
VHL-related hemangioblastomas harboring a
mutation or deletions of the VHL gene [20].
When methylation-specific PCR and bisulfite
sequencing were used to evaluate the epigenetic
regulation of the VHL gene, it was observed that
VHL promoter hypermethylation was unique to
sporadic hemangioblastomas (7 of 21 samples)
with bisulfite sequences.

The alternative explanation is in a subset of
sporadic hemangioblastomas, there is a causative
gene unrelated to the VHL gene, and the neoplasm is caused by alterations in other hypoxic-
sensing pathways. In one study, two-thirds of
sporadic hemangioblastomas without chromosome 3 LOH showed LOH at chromosome 6 or
10 when screened for copy number abnormalities
with comparative genomic hybridization.
Phosphatase and tension homolog (PTEN) is a
well-known tumor suppressor gene located on 10
and has been suggested as a possible culprit given
its co-deletion with VHL in renal epithelial cells
and can lead to precancerous cysts by the same
pathogenetic pathway to hemangioblastoma [46].
ARID1B is another potentially causative gene
that was found to be mutated or epigenetically
suppressed in 20% of sporadic hemangioblastomas [19, 20].

Finally, it is important to recognize that
patients with a single CNS hemangioblastoma
may still harbor a VHL-specific germline mutation with no extra-neural manifestations of VHL
[47]. A large cohort study showed a putative VHL
mutation in 7 of 188 individuals with sporadic
tumors. In three of these patients with the classic
frameshift mutation in B1, two of these went on
to develop non-CNS manifestations of VHL [21].

Conclusions

Spinal cord hemangioblastomas are primary
benign tumors that occur sporadically or in association with VHL. The vast majority of hemangioblastomas are located posterior to the dentate
ligament (66% are found in the dorsal root entry

zone) and found most frequently in the cervical
and thoracic spinal cord. The most common presenting symptoms are pain and/or sensory
changes. Hemangioblastomas progress in a saltatory pattern typified by quiescent and growth
periods and are best characterized on T1-weighted
post-contrast magnetic resonance. Surgical resection is the treatment of choice and is typically
curative with resolution of peritumoral edema/
syringomyelia (when present).

References

1. Tredway TL. Minimally invasive approaches for the
   treatment of intramedullary spinal tumors. Neurosurg
   Clin N Am. 2014;25(2):327–36.
2. Conway JE, Chou D, Clatterbuck RE, Brem H, Long
   DM, Rigamonti D. Hemangioblastomas of the central
   nervous system in von Hippel-Lindau syndrome and
   sporadic disease. Neurosurgery. 2001;48(1):55–62;
   discussion 62-53
3. Browne   TR,   Adams   RD,   Roberson
   GH. Hemangioblastoma of the spinal cord. Review
   and report of five cases. Arch Neurol. 1976;33(6):
   435–41.
4. Westwick HJ, Giguere JF, Shamji MF. Incidence
   and prognosis of spinal hemangioblastoma: a surveillance epidemiology and end results study.
   Neuroepidemiology. 2016;46(1):14–23.
5. Siller S, Szelenyi A, Herlitz L, Tonn JC, Zausinger
   S. Spinal cord hemangioblastomas: significance of
   intraoperative neurophysiological monitoring for
   resection and long-term outcome. J Neurosurg Spine.
   2017;26(4):483–93.
6. Takai K, Taniguchi M, Takahashi H, Usui M, Saito
   N. Comparative analysis of spinal hemangioblastomas in sporadic disease and Von Hippel-Lindau syndrome. Neurol Med Chir (Tokyo). 2010;50(7):560–7.
7. Lonser RR, Butman JA, Huntoon K, et al. Prospective
   natural history study of central nervous system
   hemangioblastomas in von Hippel-Lindau disease. J
   Neurosurg. 2014;120(5):1055–62.
8. Latif F, Tory K, Gnarra J, et al. Identification of the
   von Hippel-Lindau disease tumor suppressor gene.
   Science. 1993;260(5112):1317–20.
9. Maddock IR, Moran A, Maher ER, et al. A genetic
   register for von Hippel-Lindau disease. J Med Genet.
   1996;33(2):120–7.
10. Lonser RR, Glenn GM, Walther M, et al. von Hippel-
    Lindau disease. Lancet. 2003;361(9374):2059–67.
11. Yousef A, Rutkowski MJ, Yalcin CE, Eren OC,
    Caliskan I, Tihan T. Sporadic and Von-Hippel Lindau
    disease-associated spinal hemangioblastomas: institu-
    tional experience on their similarities and differences.
    J Neuro-Oncol. 2019;143(3):547–52.

12. Sun HI, Ozduman K, Usseli MI, Ozgen S, Pamir MN. Sporadic spinal hemangioblastomas can be effectively treated by microsurgery alone. World Neurosurg. 2014;82(5):836–47.
13. Mehta GU, Asthagiri AR, Bakhtian KD, Auh S, Oldfield EH, Lonser RR. Functional outcome after resection of spinal cord hemangioblastomas associated with von Hippel-Lindau disease. J Neurosurg Spine. 2010;12(3):233–42.
14. Wind JJ, Lonser RR. Management of von Hippel-Lindau disease-associated CNS lesions. Expert Rev Neurother. 2011;11(10):1433–41.
15. Chittiboina P, Lonser RR. Von Hippel-Lindau disease. Handb Clin Neurol. 2015;132:139–56.
16. Zbar B, Kishida T, Chen F, et al. Germline mutations in the Von Hippel-Lindau disease (VHL) gene in families from North America, Europe, and Japan. Hum Mutat. 1996;8(4):348–57.
17. Yang C, Huntoon K, Ksendzovsky A, Zhuang Z, Lonser RR. Proteostasis modulators prolong missense VHL protein activity and halt tumor progression. Cell Rep. 2013;3(1):52–9.
18. Kourtis N, Tavernarakis N. Cellular stress response pathways and ageing: intricate molecular relationships. EMBO J. 2011;30(13):2520–31.
19. Shankar GM, Taylor-Weiner A, Lelic N, et al. Sporadic hemangioblastomas are characterized by cryptic VHL inactivation. Acta Neuropathol Commun. 2014;2:167.
20. Takayanagi S, Mukasa A, Tanaka S, et al. Differences in genetic and epigenetic alterations between von Hippel-Lindau disease-related and sporadic hemangioblastomas of the central nervous system. Neuro-Oncology. 2017;19(9):1228–36.
21. Woodward ER, Wall K, Forsyth J, Macdonald F, Maher ER. VHL mutation analysis in patients with isolated central nervous system haemangioblastoma. Brain. 2007;130(Pt 3):836–42.
22. Lonser RR, Weil RJ, Wanebo JE, DeVroom HL, Oldfield EH. Surgical management of spinal cord hemangioblastomas in patients with von Hippel-Lindau disease. J Neurosurg. 2003;98(1):106–16.
23. Ammerman JM, Lonser RR, Dambrosia J, Butman JA, Oldfield EH. Long-term natural history of hemangioblastomas in patients with von Hippel-Lindau disease: implications for treatment. J Neurosurg. 2006;105(2):248–55.
24. Butman JA, Linehan WM, Lonser RR. Neurologic manifestations of von Hippel-Lindau disease. JAMA. 2008;300(11):1334–42.
25. Wanebo JE, Lonser RR, Glenn GM, Oldfield EH. The natural history of hemangioblastomas of the central nervous system in patients with von Hippel-Lindau disease. J Neurosurg. 2003;98(1):82–94.
26. Chu BC, Terae S, Hida K, Furukawa M, Abe S, Miyasaka K. MR findings in spinal hemangioblastoma: correlation with symptoms and with angiographic and surgical findings. AJNR Am J Neuroradiol. 2001;22(1):206–17.
27. dos Santos MP, Zhang J, Ghinda D, et al. Imaging diagnosis and the role of endovascular embolization treatment for vascular intraspinal tumors. Neurosurg Focus. 2015;39(2):E16.
28. Lonser RR. Surgical management of sporadic spinal cord hemangioblastomas. World Neurosurg. 2014;82(5):632–3.
29. Lonser RR, Vortmeyer AO, Butman JA, et al. Edema is a precursor to central nervous system peritumoral cyst formation. Ann Neurol. 2005;58(3):392–9.
30. Van Velthoven V, Reinacher PC, Klisch J, Neumann HP, Glasker S. Treatment of intramedullary hemangioblastomas, with special attention to von Hippel-Lindau disease. Neurosurgery. 2003;53(6):1306–13; discussion 1313-1304
31. Ye DY, Bakhtian KD, Asthagiri AR, Lonser RR. Effect of pregnancy on hemangioblastoma development and progression in von Hippel-Lindau disease. J Neurosurg. 2012;117(5):818–24.
32. Ma XJ, Zhang GB, Guo TX, et al. Management and outcomes of pregnant patients with central nervous system hemangioblastoma. J Clin Neurosci. 2018;57:126–30.
33. Mandigo CE, Ogden AT, Angevine PD, McCormick PC. Operative management of spinal hemangioblastoma. Neurosurgery. 2009;65(6):1166–77.
34. Lonser RR, Oldfield EH. Microsurgical resection of spinal cord hemangioblastomas. Neurosurgery. 2005;57(4 Suppl):372–6; discussion 372–6
35. Asthagiri AR, Mehta GU, Zach L, et al. Prospective evaluation of radiosurgery for hemangioblastomas in von Hippel-Lindau disease. Neuro-Oncology. 2010;12(1):80–6.
36. Pan J, Jabarkheel R, Huang Y, Ho A, Chang SD. Stereotactic radiosurgery for central nervous system hemangioblastoma: systematic review and meta-analysis. J Neuro-Oncol. 2018;137(1):11–22.
37. Pan J, Ho AL, D'Astous M, et al. Image-guided stereotactic radiosurgery for treatment of spinal hemangioblastoma. Neurosurg Focus. 2017;42(1):E12.
38. Madhusudan S, Deplanque G, Braybrooke JP, et al. Antiangiogenic therapy for von Hippel-Lindau disease. JAMA. 2004;291:943–4.
39. Migliorini D, Haller S, Merkler D, et al. Recurrent multiple CNS hemangioblastomas with VHL disease treated with pazopanib: a case report and literature review. CNS Oncol. 2015;4(6):387–92.
40. Riklin C, Seystahl K, Hofer S, Happold C, Winterhalder R, Weller M. Antiangiogenic treatment for multiple CNS hemangioblastomas. Onkologie. 2012;35(7–8):443–5.
41. Sardi I, Sanzo M, Giordano F, et al. Monotherapy with thalidomide for treatment of spinal cord hemangioblastomas in a patient with von Hippel-Lindau disease. Pediatr Blood Cancer. 2009;53(3):464–7.
42. Lee DK, Choe WJ, Chung CK, Kim HJ. Spinal cord hemangioblastoma: surgical strategy and clinical outcome. J Neuro-Oncol. 2003;61(1):27–34.
43. Saliou G, Giammattei L, Ozanne A, Messerer M. Role of preoperative embolization of intramedullary hemangioblastoma. Neurochirurgie. 2017;63(5):372–5.

44. Cornelius JF, Saint-Maurice JP, Bresson D, George B, Houdart E. Hemorrhage after particle embolization of hemangioblastomas: comparison of outcomes in spinal and cerebellar lesions. J Neurosurg. 2007;106(6):994–8.

45. Kim WY, Kaelin WG. Role of VHL gene mutation in human cancer. J Clin Oncol. 2004;22(24):4991–5004.

46. Sato Y, Yoshizato T, Shiraishi Y, et al. Integrated molecular analysis of clear-cell renal cell carcinoma. Nat Genet. 2013;45(8):860–7.

47. Muscarella LA, la Torre A, Faienza A, et al. Molecular dissection of the VHL gene in solitary capillary hemangioblastoma of the central nervous system. J Neuropathol Exp Neurol. 2014;73(1):50–8.

48. Mehta GU, Montgomery BK, Maggio DM, Chittiboina P, Oldfield EH, Lonser RR. Functional outcome after resection of Von Hippel-Lindau disease-associated cauda Equina Hemangioblastomas: an observational cohort study. Oper Neurosurg (Hagerstown). 2017;13(4):435–40.

Metastases

Mohammad Hassan A. Noureldine, Nir Shimony,
and George I. Jallo

Introduction

A rare manifestation of systemic malignancy, intramedullary spinal cord metastases (ISCMs) are increasingly reported in the literature as the debate on the best strategy to manage this pathology has been fueled by studies supporting surgical treatment, chemotherapy, radiotherapy, radiosurgery, or various combinations of these modalities [1–5]. In addition to increased awareness and improved detection on contemporary imaging studies, prolonged survival of patients with various types of primary malignancies may have contributed to higher numbers of ISCMs being diagnosed. At this stage of systemic spread, the goals of management are individualized to each patient but generally include preserving neurological function, extending survival, and improving quality of life in terminally ill patients.

The role of surgical resection is still unclear, owing to the scarcity of studies on this topic as well as the neurosurgeon's hesitancy to pursue a procedure with a relatively high risk-to-benefit ratio. With progressive neurological decline and impending paraparesis or quadriplegia, it is recommended to pursue surgical intervention in spite of the high risk in order to improve the neurological status or at least halt the progression of neurological decline [6]. The aim of this chapter is to explore the surgical parameters and decision-making in patients with ISCMs as well as describe the technical nuances of ISCM resection.

M. H. A. Noureldine
Department of Neurosurgery, Johns Hopkins University School of Medicine/Johns Hopkins All Children's Hospital, Saint Petersburg, FL, USA

N. Shimony
Institute of Neuroscience, Geisinger Medical Center, Geisinger Commonwealth School of Medicine, Danville, PA, USA

Johns Hopkins University School of Medicine, Institute for Brain Protection Sciences, Johns Hopkins All Children's Hospital, Saint Petersburg, FL, USA

G. I. Jallo (✉)
Institute for Brain Protections Sciences, Johns Hopkins All Children's Hospital, Saint Petersburg, FL, USA
e-mail: gjallo1@jhmi.edu

Epidemiology

The rarity of ISCMs is observed in epidemiologic data and remains consistent across various categories. For all cancer patients, autopsy studies suggest an ISCM incidence of 0.9–2.1% [7, 8]. Among all CNS and spinal metastases, the incidence of ISCMs increases to 8.5% and 3.5%, respectively [7, 9, 10]. It is also estimated that ISCMs comprise 0.6% of all spinal cord tumors [10] and 1–3% of all intramedullary tumors [11]. Moreover, ISCMs accounted for 3.4–6% of myelopathies in patients with different cancers [9, 12–14]. Across multiple studies, 34–77% of

© Springer Nature Switzerland AG 2021
S. Hanft, P. C. McCormick (eds.), *Tumors of the Spinal Canal*,
https://doi.org/10.1007/978-3-030-55096-7_7

ISCMs involved the thoracic segment, whereas 26–41% and 14–38% involved the cervical and lumbar/conus medullaris segments, respectively [2, 15–19].

Origin, Spread, and Natural History

Among the largest ISCMs series, the most common origin of the primary tumor is by far lung cancer, followed by breast cancer [16, 17, 19]. Melanoma, renal cell carcinoma, colorectal cancer, prostate cancer, and tumors of central nervous system (CNS) origin usually follow with no clear and consistent ranking in many other studies [2, 5, 15–23]. Other primary tumors reported in the literature include lymphoma, sarcoma, ovarian cancer, endometrial carcinoma, esophageal cancer, gastric cancer, thyroid carcinoma, choroid plexus carcinoma, epithelioid hemangioepithelioma, carcinoid tumor, bladder carcinoma, liver cancer, cervical cancer, esthesioneuroblastoma, and sinonasal carcinoma [2, 4, 6, 16, 17, 19–21, 23, 24]. Multiple theories have been proposed regarding the mechanism of dissemination. Hematogenous spread of the primary tumor and arterial embolization into the spinal cord matter are the most plausible theory [25–27], although retrograde dissemination through Batson's venous plexus that surrounds the spinal cord, antidromic cellular migration through the nerve roots, direct crossing from the penetrating vessels of Virchow-Robin spaces into the spinal cord, and infiltrating the cerebrospinal fluid (CSF) through intraspinal perineural sheaths are also potential metastatic mechanisms [13, 28]. If left untreated, the natural history of ISCMs leads to rapid buildup of local pressure, cord swelling, and ischemia and potential occurrence of ISCMs at other sites, all of which are associated with permanent neurological injury [14, 29, 30].

Diagnostic Approach

Clinical Assessment

In patients with established malignancy, the occurrence of metastasis is always a possibility, even in treated patients who are thought to be in complete remission. Therefore, the importance of active surveillance in cancer patients, including a full clinical and neurological examination on every follow-up visit, cannot be overstated [31]. Localizing the pathology to the spinal cord as opposed to the brain or peripheral nervous system can be suspected on neurological examination alone in many patients with ISCMs. Subtle or profound clues of myelopathy and bilateral signs and symptoms point to lesions in the spinal cord. Depending on the size, growth rate, and location of the ISCM mass as well as any compression of neurovascular structures, patients may present with back/neck pain, extremity pain, motor deficits, sensory deficits, sphincter and sexual dysfunction, and/or even spinal cord syndromes such as Brown-Sequard [12, 32]. Back/neck pain is usually constant in intensity and worsened with lying down, possibly due to dural distension and irritation [33], and pain that wakes up the patient during the night is a red flag. Spasticity, weakness, and clumsiness may occur with intradural nerve root compression, and paresthesia/dysesthesia may start distally and unilaterally and then progress to become proximal and bilateral [33]. Cord expansion may lead to tethering of the dorsal/ventral nerve roots and dentate ligament, and lumbosacral lesions may lead to radiculopathy. Involvement of spinal tracts leads to specific deficits: compression of dorsal columns is associated with proprioceptive and gait deficits, spinothalamic tract with loss of pain and temperature sensation, corticospinal tract with upper motor neuron signs and deficits, etc. Severe disability and paraplegia are common (12.5–42.6%) in patients with ISCMs [16, 17] and can progress quite rapidly, within an average of 22.85 days as reported in a recent study [17].

Many patients with ISCMs have metastases in other critical organs [6, 16, 17], with anticipated short life expectancy. It is, therefore, not reasonable to attempt extreme surgical measures to remove the ISCMs that will potentially reduce the quality of life, while knowing that these patients will die from their systemic disease soon after surgery. Assessing the overall disease burden and performance status of the patient will help in the decision-making process. Objective scoring systems, such as the Karnofsky Performance Scale (KPS), Recursive Partitioning Analysis Index (RPAI), and Modified McCormick Score (MMCS), are regarded as successful prognosticators [6, 16, 34, 35]. Patients with poor prognoses are not candidates for major or high-risk surgical interventions; less invasive or palliative procedures directed toward improving the quality of life are better suited in these patients.

Radiologic Characteristics

Radiologic evaluation of a cancer patient with suspicion of ISCMs on clinical examination warrants full body imaging to delineate the overall burden of the disease. Multiple modalities are used to detect lesions at various stages of growth and in different body organs. For example, whole-body positron emission tomography (PET) screens for metastatic deposits by detecting elevated metabolic activity; it is especially helpful in exposing bone marrow involvement with no apparent bony destruction. Computed tomography (CT), however, is the imaging study of choice to evaluate lytic versus blastic lesions and spot tumor calcifications. Spinal instability is best identified on dynamic X-ray imaging. Detailed discussion of these modalities is beyond the scope of this chapter.

Owing to its powerful tissue characterization, magnetic resonance imaging (MRI) is the most useful imaging modality and the current gold standard for evaluation of ISCMs. Typically, ISCM manifests as a solitary lesion involving 2–3 vertebral segments, most commonly in the thoracic and cervical regions. Administering intravenous contrast further enhances the sensitivity of MRI and allows for better delineation of the ISCMs from the normal spinal cord tissue, which reveals homogenous and intense enhancement of the metastatic lesion [2, 36, 37]. ISCMs usually have a hypointense central area on T1-weighted and are hyperintense on T2-weighted imaging. Peritumoral cyst formation is rarely associated with ISCMs, unlike primary spinal

cord tumors [37]. Extensive edema and spinal cord expansion out of proportion to relatively small lesion are common findings, probably due to the accelerated growth of most metastatic lesions. Other than the known history of cancer, however, there are no specific characteristics that may help in differentiating ISCMs from other primary intramedullary spinal cord lesions such as hemangioblastoma, transverse myelitis, demyelinating diseases, and sarcoidosis, among others.

Mimics of Intramedullary Lesions

Several lesions may radiographically mimic intramedullary spinal cord tumors, including ISCMs. Such mimics fall into three main categories: vascular (dural arteriovenous fistula, cavernous malformation, infarction), inflammatory (paraneoplastic myelopathy, transverse myelitis, demyelination, abscess), and traumatic (spinal cord contusion) [38] (Figs. 7.1 and 7.2).

In cancer patients with advanced disease and those who are undergoing radiation therapy, however, two specific entities are of special concern:

1. Paraneoplastic myelopathy occurs in cancer patients, by definition, but is quite rare, and its pathophysiology is poorly understood [39]. Lymphoma, breast, ovarian, thymic, and lung malignancies, especially SCLC, have been associated with paraneoplastic syndromes [40]. MRI findings are variable and range from normal spinal cord signal to T2 hyperintensity, typically extending over >3 spinal segments with symmetric gray matter or tract specific abnormalities. Contrast enhancement is seen in 2/3 of cases and is usually symmetric [41].
2. Postradiation myelopathy is the most feared complication of radiation therapy in cancer patients with cervico-thoraco-abdominal metastases. Histopathologic studies are limited to advanced disease on autopsies in humans, where radiation injury may manifest as malacia, demyelination, and/or white matter necrosis [42]. MRI is the gold standard to

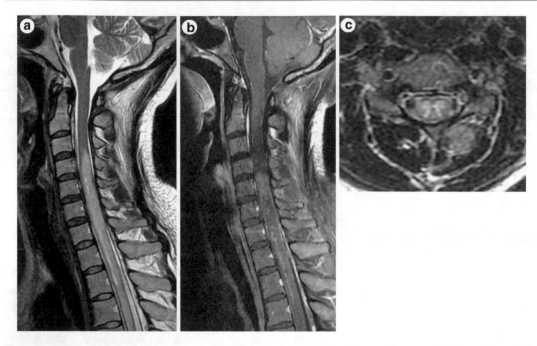

Fig. 7.1 Acute spinal cord infarction. A 34-year-old patient with type 1 diabetes mellitus presented with acute onset of myelopathy and paraplegia. (**a, c**) Sagittal and axial T2-weighted sequences show holocord abnormal increased signal and cord swelling extending from C4 inferiorly. (**b**) Post-contrast T1-weighted sagittal image demonstrates linear enhancement along the anterior aspect of the lower cervical and thoracic cord, which may represent vascular enhancement within the ventral median fissure. No enhancing mass is seen. (Reprinted from Hazenfield et al. [50]. With permission from Elsevier)

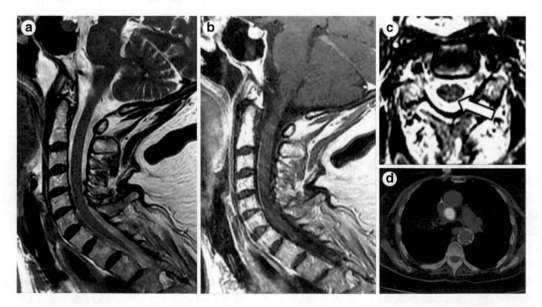

Fig. 7.2 Paraneoplastic syndrome. A 77-year-old woman with symptoms of progressive generalized muscle weakness, poor coordination, bowel/bladder control problems, and uncontrolled movement of her hands. Workup showed motor and sensory axonal demyelinating neuropathy and positive anti-Hu (ANA-1) antibodies. Biopsy of a pretracheal lymph node revealed small cell carcinoma. (**a, b**) No definite cord abnormality is seen on sagittal T2- and post-gadolinium T1-weighted images. (**c**) However, on T2 axial images subtle abnormal increased signal is noted in the bilateral posterior tracts (arrow). (**d**) PET-CT shows prominent FDG uptake in a pretracheal node. PET-CT, positron emission tomography-computed tomography; FDG, fluorodeoxyglucose. (Reprinted from Hazenfield et al. [50]. With permission from Elsevier)

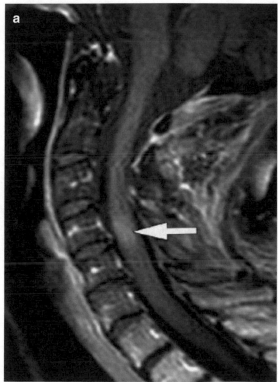 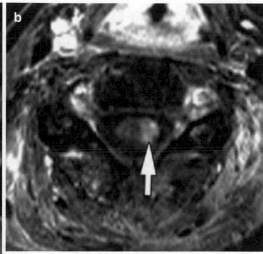

Fig. 7.3 Acute radiation myelopathy. Sagittal fat-saturated, post-contrast, T1-weighted image (**a**) and axial post contrast, T1-weighted image (**b**). Patchy enhancement within the left side of the cervical spinal cord at the C4–C5 level (arrow) in a patient who received radiation to the neck. (Reprinted from Fenton [51]. With permission from Elsevier)

detect radiation injury-related lesions, which range from low-to-moderate T1- and high T2-weighted signals representing spinal cord edema to variable, patchy or ring-like, contrast enhancement and atrophy later in the disease process (Fig. 7.3).

Perhaps the most important nuance in the context of systemic malignancy treated with radiation therapy is to be able to recognize paraneoplastic and/or postradiation myelopathy as these lesions may be mistaken for ISCMs, and surgical exploration is absolutely contraindicated in this scenario.

Surgical Resection

Decision-Making

The role of surgery in cases of ISCMs remains ambiguous, which may be attributed to several factors. First, small-cell lung cancer (SCLC) is the most common lesion in large ISCMs series in the literature [11, 12, 29, 36], in which early detection of the lesion and radiation therapy were associated with survival benefit. Although many other cancer types were reported in these series as well, the considerably high number of SCLC would statistically skew the data in favor of non-surgical interventions, given that surgery has little to no role in the management of this tumor subtype [36, 43]. Second, ISCMs patients with advanced systemic disease and poor prognosis on preoperative evaluation are less likely to attain a measurable benefit from surgical resection of the ISCMs due to the anticipated short survival, and they are more likely to develop perioperative complications. Third, studies that attempt to answer this specific question about the role of surgery are scarce and observational in nature. Yet, those studies that accounted for patient-related factors concluded that surgery is indeed effective in selected patients with progressive neurological decline [6, 20].

Gross total resection (GTR) of the ISCMs is possible but largely depends on the tumor histology and extent of invasion. For example, series reporting lung cancer, breast cancer, and melanoma [5] reported higher rates of GTR compared to series reporting sarcoma and poorly differentiated carcinoma [10]. Patients with solitary ISCMs will most likely benefit from surgical resection as described in small reports [5, 20, 44–46], where patients had better quality of life or prolonged survival. In small series of non-SCLC [47] and renal cell carcinoma [48] patients with ISCMs who were treated with chemoradiation and radiation therapy (except for one patient who underwent surgery), respectively, neurological function stabilized but did not improve in any patient, and the median survival was around 10 months, although two patients underwent surgery to stop neurological deterioration. Leptomeningeal disease, often seen in patients with advanced breast cancer, portends very poor prognosis due to direct parenchymal invasion. Survival is significantly decreased in these patients [44]. Surgery, however, may have a role in breast cancer patients with ISCMs but no parenchymal invasion or leptomeningeal disease [6].

In summary, patients who will benefit the most from surgical resection of their ISCMs are those with (1) good preoperative overall performance status, (2) solitary ISCMs, (3) fast-growing lesions with rapid neurological decline, (4) lesions with favorable histological types, and/or (5) lesions not responding to radiation therapy. Transient postoperative neurological deterioration may occur and should not deter the surgeon from undertaking the operation since gradual recovery is expected shortly afterward.

Radiation therapy, in the form of conventional external beam radiotherapy (EBRT), spinal radiotherapy, and stereotactic spinal radiosurgery, is a less invasive alternative treatment modality in patients who are not eligible for surgical resection and has also been used as primary treatment in many series. However, the discussion of the role of radiation therapy in the management of ISCMs is beyond the scope of this chapter and discussed in Chap. 9.

Case Example

A 70-year-old male patient with a known history of SCLC presented with acute and rapid neurological deterioration that progressed to functional quadriplegia and loss of bladder control over 1 week prior to presentation. Imaging studies revealed a heterogeneously enhancing intramedullary spinal cord lesion extending between C4 and T1 and associated with significant rostrocaudal cord edema (Fig. 7.4). Note the resulting severe cervical canal stenosis and cord compression imposed by edema in the context of degenerative disc disease. Although suspicion of ISCM from SCLC recurrence was high, the decision was made to perform urgent surgical decompression and simultaneously confirm the diagnosis by obtaining tissue from the lesion. Maximal safe resection (80–90% of the lesions) was attained under intraoperative neuromonitoring (IONM), and the patient was able to walk and use his hands again by postoperative day 5.

Technique Tenets and Nuances

The primary goal of surgery is maximal safe resection. In patients with more than one ISCM, a thorough clinical and radiological evaluation will help the surgeon decide on which lesion(s) are causing the neurological decline, and the removal of which will be most beneficial to the patient. Before proceeding with surgery, the surgeon should discuss the surgical plan, anticipated benefits and risks, and all nonsurgical alternatives with the patient.

After intubation and securing all necessary neurophysiologic electrodes for IONM in place, the patient is flipped to a prone position, and all bony prominences are padded. For lesions in the cervical cord, a clamp with pins is used to fix the head and neck in a semi-flexed position; a Wilson frame with no head fixation is used for thoracic or lumbar lesions. The anesthetic team should be knowledgeable about all controllable factors that may affect the IONM: choice of the anesthetic

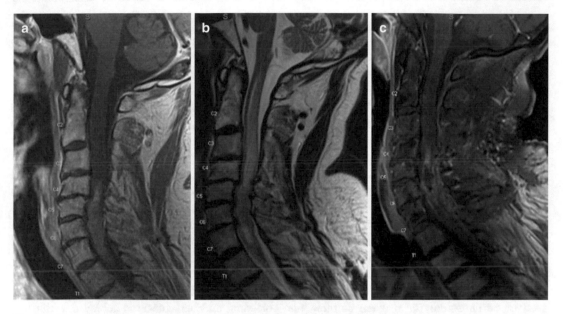

Fig. 7.4 Sagittal preoperative contrast-enhanced T1- (**a**), preoperative T2-, and (**b**) postoperative contrast-enhanced T1-weighted (**c**) images of an ISCM from a biopsy-confirmed, metastatic SCLC

agent, maintaining a mean arterial pressure between 80 and 90 mmHg, etc.

The skin is marked just above the lesion using image-guided localization. A midline skin incision is performed, followed by subcutaneous and subperiosteal muscular dissection to expose the posterior spinal elements; the facet joint capsules should be preserved to avoid potential development of instability and postoperative kyphosis. Laminoplasty is preferred over laminectomy if no stenosis is present at the surgical level, which proceeds with bilateral laminotomies using BoneScalpel or small Kerrison punches. After transecting the interspinous ligaments and dissecting the ligamentum flavum off the laminae on top, the posterior elements are removed en bloc and preserved for reattachment at the end of the surgery through the laminoplasty technique. In cases where there is concern for significant post-procedural cord edema or local mass effect, the posterior elements may not be reinstalled. Bleeding from the epidural venous plexus is managed with a low-voltage bipolar.

Before opening the dura, the rostrocaudal extent of the lesion is estimated using intraoperative ultrasound; this will confirm the adequacy of bony exposure as well as determine the size of durotomy. The durotomy should span the full length of the lesion, reducing the need to retract the spinal cord during resection. Then, a D-wave electrode is inserted epidurally; in case the epidural reading is not adequate or consistent, the surgeon may relocate the D-wave electrode subdurally, just on top of the spinal cord. A scalpel and tenotomy scissors are used to perform a midline dural incision while trying to preserve the underlying arachnoid membrane. To further expose the dural window and prevent blood products from entering the intradural space, several tenting sutures are applied bilaterally. The arachnoid membrane is then cut with a micro-scalpel or an arachnoid knife to expose the spinal cord, the surface of which may or may not be distorted by the ISCM lesion. Often, a focal surface discoloration or bulge and/or cord rotation or hypervascularity is noted near the ISCM site. If no hints as to the exact location of the lesion can be seen at the surface, the intraoperative ultrasound is used to guide the myelotomy site. Important anatomical landmarks such as the dorsal median, dorsal intermediate, and dorsolateral sulci are then identified by following the surface veins, which dive deep into these sulci. If no cord rotation is present, myelotomy is performed through the dorsal median sulcus; otherwise, the dorsal intermediate or dorsolateral sulcus is chosen depending on which one offers the shortest route and easier maneuverability around the lesion with minimal spinal cord retraction. A very low-voltage bipolar is used to coagulate the small bleeding veins. Lesions are typically encountered after only few millimeters of dissection through the cord tissue. Depending on the histological type of the ISCM, a dissection plane may or may not be identified. For example, it is easier to find a plane for metastatic lesions from breast and non-SCLC as opposed to those from a sarcoma, SCLC, and poorly differentiated carcinoma; the latter is usually associated with poorly demarcated and invasive patterns within the cord tissue. Extreme care should be taken not to damage the normal spinal cord or corticospinal tracts when defining the tumor interface. Unlike dissecting and removing metastatic lesions from the intracranial compartment, the plane of dissection is not as easily defined or discernable for ISCM lesions. In many cases, it is preferable to work from in an inside-out fashion to preserve the normal spinal cord tissue. After taking a biopsy for histopathologic examination, the tumor is debulked starting at the center using suction or an ultrasonic aspirator; the goal is to minimize cord retraction as much as possible. The lesion margins are removed at the end of resection using microsuction. Coagulation with a bipolar should be minimized and avoided if possible while working inside the cord tissue as thermal injury may lead to irreversible damage. Plated bayonets can be used for dynamic retraction while avoiding extended periods of working in the same surgical zone. Somatosensory evoked potentials (SSEPs) are usually lost after the midline myelotomy and are not usually used as a reliable source. On the other hand, any changes in D-wave and/or motor evoked potentials (MEPs) should be taken seriously, and the surgeon should proceed with the resection according to the information obtained from MEPs and D-wave signals. The D-waves are a much more reliable source. Studies have shown a 50% reduction in peak-to-peak amplitude of D-wave signals is considered a major alarming criterion [49]. In the context of normal D-wave signals or a signal drop of less than 50%, MEP signal deficits are usually

ignored, though transient postoperative deficits may still occur. Techniques that may be used to facilitate the return of signals include releasing any traction on the cord, irrigation with warm saline, introduction of a papaverine-soaked cotton into the surgical cavity, and increasing the mean arterial pressure [49]. In fact, changes in these signals are the main determinant of the extent of resection. After all, the goal of surgery is to improve or at least preserve the current level of neurological functioning in these patients, and the surgeon should not pursue GTR while causing irreversible neurological injury. This is in contrast to intracranial lesions, where gross total resection is standard of care and much more easily achieved.

The surgical field is then surveyed for any bleeding and hemostasis is achieved within the dural compartment. The dura is then closed using running Nurolon or polyproline sutures, with or without a dural patch to expand the thecal space if needed, and an overlying layer of fibrin glue or dural sealant is used to decrease the risk of postoperative CSF leakage. The D-wave electrode is removed after dural closure, and laminoplasty is prepared, fixed with plates and screws, and reattached to the exposed bony edges within the surgical field. Finally, the musculocutaneous flap is closed layer by layer in a watertight fashion.

Conclusion

Management of ISCMs in patients with systemic malignancy is complex since the literature is scarce and studies are small and observational in nature. Surgery may be the best initial option in a selected group of patients, and decision-making should be judicious as the surgical sequelae can be unforgiving. Future clinical trials that compare the benefits and risks of surgery alone versus radiation therapy alone versus surgery plus radiation therapy are dearly needed to solve the dilemma of managing ISCMs. And as advances in immunotherapy continue to prolong patient survival, we as a field need to be prepared for an increase of ISCMs. It is our hope that in the coming years, we will more thoroughly define our collective approach to this daunting disease.

References

1. Saeed H, Patel R, Thakkar J, Hamoodi L, Chen L, Villano JL. Multimodality therapy improves survival in intramedullary spinal cord metastasis of lung primary. Hematol Oncol Stem Cell Ther. 2017;10(3):143–50.
2. Payer S, Mende K, Westphal M, Eicker S. Intramedullary spinal cord metastases: an increasingly common diagnosis. Neurosurg Focus. 2015;39(2):E15–E.
3. Miura S, Kaira K, Kaira R, Akamatsu II, Ono A, Shukuya T, et al. The efficacy of amrubicin on central nervous system metastases originating from small-cell lung cancer: a case series of eight patients. Investig New Drugs. 2015;33(3):755–60.
4. Veeravagu A, Lieberson R, Mener A, Chen Y, Soltys S, Gibbs I, et al. CyberKnife stereotactic radiosurgery for the treatment of intramedullary spinal cord metastases. J Clin Neurosci. 2012;19(9):1273–7.
5. Wilson D, Fusco D, Uschold T, Spetzler R, Chang S. Survival and functional outcome after surgical resection of intramedullary spinal cord metastases. World Neurosurg. 2012;77(2):370–4.
6. Strickland B, McCutcheon I, Chakrabarti I, Rhines L, Weinberg J. The surgical treatment of metastatic spine tumors within the intramedullary compartment. J Neurosurg Spine. 2018;28(1):79–87.
7. Costigan D, Winkelman M. Intramedullary spinal cord metastasis. A clinicopathological study of 13 cases. J Neurosurg. 1985;62(2):227–33.
8. Chason J, Walker FB, Landers JW. Metastatic carcinoma in the central nervous system and dorsal root ganglia. A prospective autopsy study. Cancer. 1963;16(6):781–7.
9. Hashizume Y, Hirano A. Intramedullary spinal cord metastasis. Pathologic findings in five autopsy cases. Acta Neuropathol. 1983;61(3–4):214–8.
10. Gasser T, Pospiech J, Stolke D, Schwechheimer K. Spinal intramedullary metastases. Report of two cases and review of the literature. Neurosurg Rev. 2001;24(2–3):88–92.
11. Connolly JE, Winfree CJ, McCormick PC, Cruz M, Stein BM. Intramedullary spinal cord metastasis: report of three cases and review of the literature. Surg Neurol. 1996;46(4):329–37; discussion 37–8
12. Schiff D, O'Neill B. Intramedullary spinal cord metastases: clinical features and treatment outcome. Neurology. 1996;47(4):906–12.
13. Edelson R, Deck M, Posner J. Intramedullary spinal cord metastases. Clinical and radiographic findings in nine cases. Neurology. 1972;22(12):1222–31.
14. Tognetti F, Lanzino G, Calbucci F. Metastases of the spinal cord from remote neoplasms. Study of five cases. Surg Neurol. 1988;30(3):220–7.
15. Diehn F, Rykken J, Wald J, Wood C, Eckel L, Hunt C, et al. Intramedullary spinal cord metastases: prognostic value of MRI and clinical features from a 13-year institutional case series. AJNR Am J Neuroradiol. 2015;36(3):587–93.
16. Goyal A, Yolcu Y, Kerezoudis P, Alvi M, Krauss W, Bydon M. Intramedullary spinal cord metastases: an institutional review of survival and outcomes. J Neuro-Oncol. 2019;142(2):347–54.
17. Lv J, Liu B, Quan X, Li C, Dong L, Liu M. Intramedullary spinal cord metastasis in malignancies: an institutional analysis and review. Onco Targets Ther. 2019;12:4741.
18. Rykken J, Diehn F, Hunt C, Schwartz K, Eckel L, Wood C, et al. Intramedullary spinal cord metastases: MRI and relevant clinical features from a 13-year institutional case series. AJNR Am J Neuroradiol. 2013;34(10):2043–9.
19. Sung W, Sung M, Chan J, Manion B, Song J, Dubey A, et al. Intramedullary spinal cord metastases: a 20-year institutional experience with a comprehensive literature review. World Neurosurg. 2013;79(3–4):576–84.
20. Dam-Hieu P, Seizeur R, Mineo J-F, Metges I-P, Meriot P, Simon H. Retrospective study of 19 patients with intramedullary spinal cord metastasis. Clin Neurol Neurosurg. 2009;111(1):10–7.
21. Shin D, Huh R, Chung S, Rock J, Ryu S. Stereotactic spine radiosurgery for intradural and intramedullary metastasis. Neurosurg Focus. 2009;27(6):E10–E.
22. Hashii H, Mizumoto M, Kanemoto A, Harada H, Asakura H, Hashimoto T, et al. Radiotherapy for patients with symptomatic intramedullary spinal cord metastasis. J Radiat Res (Tokyo). 2011;52(5):641–5.
23. Hoover J, Krauss W, Lanzino G. Intradural spinal metastases: a surgical series of 15 patients. Acta Neurochir. 2012;154(5):871–7; discussion 7
24. Flanagan E, O'Neill B, Habermann T, Porter A, Keegan B. Secondary intramedullary spinal cord non-Hodgkin's lymphoma. J Neuro-Oncol. 2012;107(3):575–80.
25. Jellinger K, Kothbauer P, Sunder-Plassmann E, Weiss R. Intramedullary spinal cord metastases. J Neurol. 1979;220(1):31–41.
26. Olson M, Chernik N, Posner J. Infiltration of the leptomeninges by systemic cancer. A clinical and pathologic study. Arch Neurol. 1974;30(2):122–37.
27. Price R, Johnson W. The central nervous system in childhood leukemia. I. The arachnoid. Cancer. 1973;31(3):520–33.
28. Batson OV. The role of the vertebral veins in metastatic processes. Ann Intern Med. 1942;16(1):38–45.
29. Grem J, Burgess J, Trump D. Clinical features and natural history of intramedullary spinal cord metastasis. Cancer. 1985;56(9):2305–14.
30. Winkelman M, Adelstein D, Karlins N. Intramedullary spinal cord metastasis. Diagnostic and therapeutic considerations. Arch Neurol. 1987;44(5):526–31.
31. Iwata H. Future treatment strategies for metastatic breast cancer: curable or incurable? Breast Cancer (Tokyo, Japan). 2012;19(3):200–5.

32. Dunne J, Harper C, Pamphlett R. Intramedullary spinal cord metastases: a clinical and pathological study of nine cases. Q J Med. 1986;61(235):1003–20.

33. Samartzis D, Gillis C, Shih P, O'Toole J, Fessler R. Intramedullary spinal cord tumors: Part I-epidemiology, pathophysiology, and diagnosis. Global Spine J. 2015;5(5):425–35.

34. Bauer H, Wedin R. Survival after surgery for spinal and extremity metastases. Prognostication in 241 patients. Acta Orthop Scand. 1995;66(2):143–6.

35. Chao S, Koyfman S, Woody N, Angelov L, Soeder S, Reddy C, et al. Recursive partitioning analysis index is predictive for overall survival in patients undergoing spine stereotactic body radiation therapy for spinal metastases. Int J Radiat Oncol Biol Phys. 2012;82(5):1738–43.

36. Kalayci M, Cağavi F, Gül S, Yenidünya S, Açikgöz B. Intramedullary spinal cord metastases: diagnosis and treatment-an illustrated review. Acta Neurochir. 2004;146(12):1347–54; discussion 54

37. Koeller K, Rosenblum R, Morrison A. Neoplasms of the spinal cord and filum terminale: radiologic-pathologic correlation. Radiographics. 2000;20(6):1721–49.

38. Wein S, Gaillard F. Intradural spinal tumours and their mimics: a review of radiographic features. Postgrad Med J. 2013;89(1054):457–69.

39. Rudnicki S, Dalmau J. Paraneoplastic syndromes of the spinal cord, nerve, and muscle. Muscle Nerve. 2000;23(12):1800–18.

40. Dropcho E. Neurologic paraneoplastic syndromes. J Neurol Sci. 1998;153(2):264–78.

41. Flanagan E, McKeon A, Lennon V, Kearns J, Weinshenker B, Krecke K, et al. Paraneoplastic isolated myelopathy: clinical course and neuroimaging clues. Neurology. 2011;76(24):2089–95.

42. Schultheiss T, Stephens L, Maor M. Analysis of the histopathology of radiation myelopathy. Int J Radiat Oncol Biol Phys. 1988;14(1):27–32.

43. Murphy K, Feld R, Evans W, Shepherd F, Perrin R, Sima A, et al. Intramedullary spinal cord metastases from small cell carcinoma of the lung. J Clin Oncol. 1983;1(2):99–106.

44. Kosmas C, Koumpou M, Nikolaou M, Katselis J, Soukouli G, Markoutsaki N, et al. Intramedullary spinal cord metastases in breast cancer: report of four cases and review of the literature. J Neuro-Oncol. 2005;71(1):67–72.

45. Stranjalis G, Torrens M. Successful removal of intramedullary spinal cord metastasis: case report. Br J Neurosurg. 1993;7(2):193–5.

46. Findlay J, Bernstein M, Vanderlinden R, Resch L. Microsurgical resection of solitary intramedullary spinal cord metastases. Neurosurgery. 1987;21(6):911–5.

47. Potti A, Abdel-Raheem M, Levitt R, Schell DA, Mehdi SA. Intramedullary spinal cord metastases (ISCM) and non-small cell lung carcinoma (NSCLC): clinical patterns, diagnosis and therapeutic considerations. Lung Cancer. 2001;31(2–3):319–23.

48. Fakih M, Schiff D, Erlich R, Logan T. Intramedullary spinal cord metastasis (ISCM) in renal cell carcinoma: a series of six cases. Ann Oncol. 2001;12(8):1173–7.

49. Noureldine MHA, Shimony N, Ahdab R, Jallo GI. Brainstem and spinal cord mapping. In: Quinones-Hinojosa A, Chaichana KL, Mahato D, editors. Brain mapping: indications and techniques. 1st ed. New York: Thieme Medical Publishers, Inc; 2020. p. 143–53.

50. Hazenfield JM, Gaskill-Shipley MF. Neoplastic and paraneoplastic involvement of the spinal cord. Semin Ultrasound CT MR. 2016;37(5):482–97.

51. Fenton DS. Post radiation effects. In: Czervionke LF, Fenton DS, editors. Imaging painful spine tumors. Philadelphia: Saunder; 2011. p. 450–5.

Part III

Adjuvant Treatment

Radiotherapy for Extramedullary Tumors

8

Joseph P. Weiner

Abbreviations

AAPM	American Association of Physics in Medicine
CSF	Cerebrospinal fluid
CSI	Craniospinal irradiation
CT	Computed tomography
CTV	Clinical target volume
Dmax	Maximum point dose
EQ D_2	Equivalent dose in 2 Gy fractions
GTV	Gross tumor volume
IGRT	Image-guided radiation therapy
IMRT	Intensity-modulated radiation therapy
ITV	Internal target volume
KPS	Karnofsky Performance Scale
LMD	Leptomeningeal disease
MLC	Multi-leaf collimator
MPNST	Malignant peripheral nerve sheath tumor
MRI	Magnetic resonance imaging
NST	Nerve sheath tumors
OAR	Organ at risk
PET	Positron emission tomography
PTV	Planning target volume
SABR	Stereotactic ablative body radiotherapy
SBRT	Stereotactic body radiation therapy
SRS	Stereotactic radiosurgery
WHO	World Health Organization

J. P. Weiner (✉)
Rutgers Cancer Institute of New Jersey, Department of Radiation Oncology, New Brunswick, NJ, USA
e-mail: weinerjp@cinj.rutgers.edu

Introduction

The diagnosis of a benign or malignant spine tumor is a life-changing event for any patient. Thoughts of prognosis, outcomes, side effects, and subsequent quality of life are at the forefront of the patient's concerns. In line with current trends in medicine, as a field we are moving closer to more targeted and less invasive treatment options. Radiation therapy is a powerful, focal treatment that can be delivered with extreme accuracy due to an ever-increasing sophistication in planning, target delineation, dose delivery, and quality assurance. Advancements in the treatment platforms we use, and in the way we deliver dose, have contributed to a steady improvement in cancer-related outcomes.

Though radiation itself is unseen and unfelt by the patient during delivery, the ensuing side effects can very much be. Just like any other medical procedure, successful outcomes and the mitigation of adverse events are based on the radiation oncologist's grasp of many aspects in a demanding discipline. In order to properly "speak the language," one must be versed in the appropriate vocabulary, which includes knowledge of medical physics and radiation biology. In addi-

© Springer Nature Switzerland AG 2021
S. Hanft, P. C. McCormick (eds.), *Tumors of the Spinal Canal*,
https://doi.org/10.1007/978-3-030-55096-7_8

tion, thorough understanding and review of various medical imaging modalities are essential for treatment decision-making, target and organ-at-risk delineation, dose selection, and fractionation. Thus, practitioners must be well versed in neuroanatomy and pathophysiology to deliver high-quality treatment.

Gone are the days of providing care in a vacuum. Given the complex decision-making we routinely encounter in the clinic, treatment in the modern era is a collaborative effort among radiation oncologists, neurosurgeons, and medical oncologists. With the adoption of radiation therapy, the neurosurgeon's armamentarium has expanded to include treatments for inoperable tumors, microscopic residual disease, or even as definitive treatment in lieu of open surgery. This cooperative spirit is best exemplified in the joint field of radiosurgery, where a special bond between the neurosurgeon and radiation oncologist is maintained given the close intersection in judgment and treatment planning.

A Brief History of Radiotherapy

Through the use of radioactive isotopes or ionizing beams, radiotherapy has been used as a tool to treat cancer for over a century [1]. While working on cathode ray tubes, a chance observation by the German physicist Wilhelm Conrad Röntgen led to the discovery of an invisible yet penetrating form of light which he named "X-rays" in 1895 [2]. Though first used for rudimentary diagnostic imaging, within 1 year X-rays were repurposed for therapeutic applications in the treatment of breast cancer [3].

Subsequent work was directed at the phenomenon of radioactivity, which is the emission of ionizing radiation due to the spontaneous disintegration of atomic nuclei. Led by work from Henri Becquerel, and then Marie Curie, radium was discovered as a source of natural radiation [4]. From this discovery, the field of brachytherapy was born. As the early part of the twentieth century progressed, advances in radiation biology led to reduced normal tissue toxicity with multiple small fractions rather than one large fraction.

Still, treatment quality assurance was primitive at this time, as the use of "erythema dose" was a method of estimating the strength of one's radiation device. This was crudely calculated by having the treating physician expose their own skin and determine how long it took for it to appear sunburnt. At this time radiation was not yet known to be carcinogenic, a point that was eventually learned as early practitioners became sick from the very tool they used to fight disease.

The ability to quantify the amount of delivered radiation was made widely available with the invention of the ionizing chamber in 1932 [5]. This, plus the development of supervoltage X-ray tubes, allowed for the treatment of deeper-seated tumors with more confidence. Then in 1956, the field of radiation therapy changed forever with the novel use of a tool previously limited to physicists, the linear accelerator. The following decades found new applications in the treatment of a whole variety of human cancers with the linear accelerator.

By the late 1970s, the implementation of proton beam therapy was successful due to breakthroughs in imaging and computing. This technology has more desirable dosimetric properties compared to photon or electron beam therapy and is an active area of research to this day. In the 1990s, more powerful computing allowed for a switch to 3D-based treatment planning which resulted in more conformal treatment plans. With the advent of the multi-leaf collimator, a variable radiation beam-shaping device located in the treatment head, it was only a matter of time before an even more advanced radiation modality was developed, intensity-modulated radiation therapy (IMRT) [6]. This treatment now allowed for an even more highly conformal treatment plan with the ability to treat irregular or even concave targets.

At the tail end of the 1990s, the ability to deliver high-dose, limited fraction treatment with extreme precision, known as stereotactic body radiation therapy (SBRT), was introduced in several centers in Europe, Japan, and the USA. Results from these early reports showed promising results with increased control and acceptable toxicity [7]. Since the turn of the century, radiation therapy continues to develop, now with the routine use of dedicated imaging at the time of treatment for added treatment confidence, known as image-guided radiation therapy.

Fundamentals of Radiation Oncology

Radiation is the transmission of energy in wave or particle form through a medium. The field of radiation oncology utilizes ionizing radiation, which has the ability to break chemical bonds at the DNA level, for the treatment of benign or malignant tumors. Both tumor and normal cells within the radiation beam are subject to the effects of this treatment. However, we are able to exploit the superior repair of normal tissues compared to tumor cells, which results in preferential tumor damage from radiation. At a certain dose of radiation, which is inherent to each tumor histology and experimentally derived, a certain percentage of control can be expected. Independent of this, normal tissues do have their own maximum and volumetric doses which they can withstand, with an expected probability of acute or chronic injury at that dose. This leads to the principle of normal tissue tolerance which will be explored later in the chapter.

With increasing cumulative doses of radiation, the percentage of tumor control rises. However, the risk of normal tissue damage also rises. The most basic goal of the radiation oncologist is to maximize tumor control while minimizing normal tissue complication, a concept referred to as the therapeutic ratio. In the last century, as radiation techniques have become more sophisticated and conformal, we have seen a concordant gain in the therapeutic ratio.

Radiation can be delivered via external beam radiation (teletherapy), focal internal radiation via sealed radioactive isotopes (brachytherapy), or via the introduction of a systemic form of radiation into the body (unsealed source radionuclide therapy). In the treatment of intradural, extramedullary tumors of the spine, the vast majority of radiation therapy is via external beam radiation therapy, which will therefore be the focus of

this chapter. Brachytherapy [8, 9] and unsealed isotopes [10] have been mainly limited to the treatment of extradural spine tumors, which is outside of the scope of this chapter.

Radiation is an extremely common treatment modality, with approximately 50% of oncology patients receiving some type of radiation during their life [11]. Treatment can range in duration from a single treatment session up to 8 weeks of daily radiation. The intent of treatment with radiation can be for curative or palliative purposes. Depending on the indication, radiation can be used for monotherapy with definitive intent or in conjunction with surgery and/or systemic therapy via a neoadjuvant, concurrent, or adjuvant sequencing. For tumors of the extramedullary space, all of these options may apply, though broadly the most common treatments would include focal definitive or adjuvant postoperative treatment for benign tumors and post operative for malignant. Decisions with respect to which intent, or even whether to offer radiation at all, can depend on factors such as extent of resection and concern for gross or microscopic residual disease.

The workflow in radiation oncology is unique compared to that of any other field in medicine. After consultation, patients will undergo a "simulation" session when immobilization devices and patient imaging are acquired. Once the simulation is complete, this information is loaded into a treatment planning system, and the radiation oncologist, who is sometimes aided by the treating neurosurgeon, physically draws targets and avoidance regions for the radiation. Then begins the iterative process of plan calculation and dose evaluation. Once an acceptable plan is created, this plan undergoes quality control and quality assurance procedures [12]. This generally involves verifying that the treatment machine is within a certain tolerance for variation in dose and spatial delivery accuracy. In addition, depending on the modality used, special checks using a patient "phantom" can be performed to make sure that the delivered plan is accurately represented by the calculated plan. Only after all of these steps can a patient be treated with radiation therapy.

Patient Simulation and Immobilization

Once the decision has been made to offer radiation therapy to a patient, many steps must be taken before the delivery of any radiation. After consultation and informed consent, a patient will be offered a "radiation planning simulation" on a CT simulator. Lasting generally 30–60 min depending on case complexity, this short outpatient encounter allows for the radiation oncologist to obtain detailed CT imaging of the treatment site. This in turn enables the delineation of the target as well as the nearby organs at risk. All relevant structures will be contoured and this information passed on to a professional dosimetrist or physicist who can calculate a customized radiation plan.

But the purpose of the simulation is not just to obtain the imaging of the patient, which could have been obtained from dedicated diagnostic quality imaging instead. Additionally, simulation results in the placement of either temporary or permanent ink (i.e., tattoo) marks on the skin of the patient, which allows for a reproducible setup for each intended fraction. This is completed through the use of a laser localization system which projects an image on the patient which is then marked. Subsequently this helps to minimize change in position from day to day, which is defined as "interfraction" motion.

Another purpose of simulation is the careful immobilization of the patient for the duration of any one radiation treatment. Without proper immobilization, setup margins would need to be larger, and thus a larger volume of healthy tissue would be within the irradiated field. The consequence of this would be increased treatment toxicity and a decrease in the therapeutic ratio. Thus, simulation helps to minimize this "intrafraction" motion. Such movement can be due to involuntary patient movement, which is a concern for spine radiation. Movement can also be physiologic, such as breathing or peristalsis. Though techniques exist to minimize physiologic movement, they are seldom employed for spine radiation given the fixed surrounding bony vertebrae.

Immobilization devices range from simple, interchangeable aides such as plastic neck rests and knee wedges to custom-created pieces depending on the location in the spine or the treatment intent. For example, treatment of the cervical spine and uppermost thoracic spine is generally aided by a custom-molded Aquaplast mask to minimize neck movement (Fig. 8.1a). Likewise, any planned process that would involve millimeter precision, such as radiosurgery, would generally be performed with a full spine custom mold that the patient rests within (Fig. 8.1b).

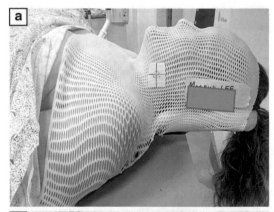

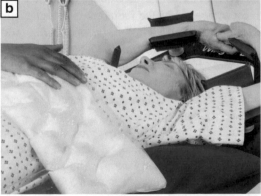

Fig. 8.1 Panel "**a**" shows Aquaplast mask with neck and shoulder immobilization used in the treatment of a target spanning the upper thoracic and the lower cervical spine. Panel "**b**" shows custom full body immobilizing device for radiosurgery plan in the lower thoracic spine

Target Delineation

Prior to the advent of three-dimensional treatment planning aided by CT images, delineation of the target would be based on surface anatomy or plain X-rays. This had clear limitations on the conformality of treatment plans, and thus cumulative dose was limited. In the modern era, once simulation has been completed, the CT images are loaded into a radiation treatment planning system. Though most radiation simulators use solely CT-based imaging, combination simulators with same-time MRI or PET images are now available. Since this technology has not gained widespread implementation yet, traditional CT-based simulation can be aided by the fusion of outside MRI or PET imaging to help with target delineation, though there can be challenges with accurate fusion if the patient was in a different position at the time of simulation.

The goal of target delineation, often referred to as contouring, is to outline both the target that requires radiation therapy and the nearby critical structures to which radiation should be minimized. A logical concern with individual practitioners subjectively outlining structures is variation among different users in the field. Therefore, contouring guidelines have been created from experts and national organizations, as well as the creation of a universally used system to reproducibly outline and communicate both target volumes and avoidance structures [13, 14]. Depending on the tumor histology and the radiation modality chosen, one or all of these concepts may be used. The gross tumor volume (GTV) is the position and extent of any gross disease as noticeable on physical exam or imaging. Accurate contouring of the GTV is aided by using multiple imaging planes (axial, coronal, and sagittal) from simulation with oral or IV contrast, or the fusion of diagnostic imaging. The clinical target volume (CTV) is a margin around the GTV which accounts for real or possible microscopic spread of tumor that cannot be seen on imaging. The internal target volume (ITV) is the addition of the CTV plus any change in position of that CTV due to internal motion such as respiration. The planning target volume (PTV) is a margin around the ITV to account for uncertainty in planning or treatment delivery. An organ at risk (OAR) is any normal organ or tissue in close proximity to the target or in the path of the radiation beam.

Conventionally Fractionated Radiation Versus Stereotactic Radiosurgery (SRS/SBRT)

In the beginning of the twentieth century, radiation was only superficially penetrating, resulting in highest doses to the skin [15]. Therefore, the treatment of a deep-seated tumor was limited by a patient's development of skin toxicity. In the 1920s it was observed that by delivering the radiation in multiple smaller doses, separated by hours to days between each treatment, patients were able to better tolerate treatment compared to single-session delivery [16]. Thereby, in breaking the dose into a smaller "fraction" of the intended total dose, the concept of "fractionation" was born. This eventually led way to the modern concept of "conventionally fractionated" radiotherapy, which is the backbone of contemporary treatment.

Conventionally fractionated radiotherapy is the delivery of a small dose of radiation given daily on the order of 25–30 fractions spaced over 5–6 weeks. The utility of such treatment is that by using smaller dose per fraction with 24 h between treatments, normal tissue repair is possible, even if a large target volume is treated. Tissue repair allows for a higher total dose of radiation safely deliverable to normal tissues while still permitting a dose that is tumoricidal. Given technical limitations of the time, this was the only way to safely treat some tumors and to achieve a successful outcome without excess toxicity.

Cranial radiosurgery, or the treatment with a single or few high-dose fractions, was the first site amenable to such treatment due to the lack of target movement and early frame-based fixation techniques to the skull. Recent developments in patient immobilization and targeting now allows for the delivery of a higher dose per fraction safely to the body, setting the stage for the introduction of stereotactic body radiation therapy (SBRT). The American Association of Physics in Medicine (AAPM) Task Group 101 has set up the formal definition for SBRT [17]. This stipulates that SBRT is a method of external beam radiation that must employ extremely accurate delivery of high-dose radiation in one to five fractions to an extra-cranial target. Treatment can be via a traditional linear accelerator-based platform, as long as they are equipped with proper image-guidance technology, or via a platform specifically adapted for SBRT. SBRT is often interchangeably used with the term SRS (stereotactic radiosurgery, which is more commonly utilized in reference to cranial targets and one single session) as well as SABR (stereotactic ablative radiotherapy). Please refer to Table 8.1 for a summary view of the radiotherapy approaches discussed in this section.

Radiosurgery differs from conventionally fractionated radiation in more than just the number of treatments. Patient immobilization is critically important and coupled to integrated image guidance for a level of accuracy in radiosurgery that supersedes conventional fractionated paradigms. Moreover, the effect of a large radiation dose in a short time leads to a more tumoricidal effect; while the overwhelming source of cell death with conventional radiation is apoptosis, alternative modes of cell kill are thought to exist with radiosurgery, such as endothelial collapse and radiation-induced tumor antigen-specific immune response [18]. It is proposed that these sources of cell kill might allow for greater tumor response and increased control based on the fundamental concept of a high radiation dose per treatment fraction. Not to be ignored, there is the significant convenience factor for patients undergoing SBRT as there are only a few treatment sessions compared to conventional treatment plans that often extend for weeks.

Fractionated radiosurgery, also referred to as hypofractionated radiation, is the use of 2–5 high doses of radiation. This modality strikes a middle ground between single fraction treatment and conventional radiation and theoretically should allow for the use of radiosurgery on tumors that would have otherwise been excluded due to concern for toxicity. Specifically, the treatment of large targets or targets near critical organs at risk (e.g., spinal cord) may be considered via fractionated radiosurgery as studies have shown an improved balance of tumor control and toxicity compared with single fraction radiosurgery [19].

Radiation Delivery Platforms

Isocentric Linear Accelerator

By far, the workhorse for spine radiation is the linear particle accelerator, colloquially referred to as the "LINAC." The majority of platforms are

Table 8.1 Comparison of the three fundamental radiotherapy approaches to tumors of the spinal canal

	Conventional	Hypofractionated SBRT	Single fraction SBRT (SRS)
Number of fractions	28–33	2-5	1
Dose per fraction	1.8–2.0 Gy	5–12 Gy	14–16 Gy benign, 15–24 Gy malignant
Duration of therapy	5–6 weeks	2–5 days	1 day
Platform	LINAC, Proton, CyberKnife (rare)	LINAC, Proton, CyberKnife, Gamma Knife (Icon only)	LINAC, Proton (rare), CyberKnife, Gamma Knife (all models)
Degree of patient immobilization and image guidance	Moderate (3–5 mm)	Strict (</=2 mm)	Strictest (</=1 mm)
Desired dose heterogeneity	Low	High	High
Tumoricidal impact (dose to fraction ratio)	Medium	High	Highest
Mechanism of cell death	Apoptosis	Vascular damage, tumor-specific immune response	Similar to hypofractionated

designed to use an "isocentric technique," meaning that they are constructed in a way to have all axes of machine rotation based on a fixed point in space. This point, known as the isocenter, is the location in space where the central axis of the radiation beam passes through and is generally planned to be the "focal point" for the delivered radiation. Examples of some systems include the TrueBeam (Varian Medical Systems Inc.), Novalis Tx (BrainLab), and Axesse (Elekta Inc.). Treatments can include both conventionally fractionated treatment and radiosurgery.

Non-Isocentric Linear Accelerator: CyberKnife

The CyberKnife stereotactic radiosurgery system uses a compact 6 MeV linear accelerator, a computer-controlled robotic arm with six degrees of freedom, and an image-guidance technology that does not depend on a rigid stereotactic frame and thereby enables treatment of extracranial sites. Because of this, there are some advantages to this platform. These include an enhanced ability to avoid critical structures, ability to treat lesions throughout the body, delivery of highly conformal dose distributions either via single fraction or fractionated approach, and finally the potential to target multiple tumors at different locations during a single treatment. Further, because the system does not require the use of a stereotactic head frame temporarily attached to the patient's head, patient comfort is maximized.

The CyberKnife obtains stereotactic localization in a different manner than isocentric linear accelerators. It uses an image-guidance technology that depends on the skeletal structure of the body as a reference frame. In addition, it continually monitors and tracks patient position during treatment. It is most often used for treatment with radiosurgical intent, though conventional treatment is possible.

Isotope-Based Unit: Gamma Knife

Though commonly thought to be limited to treating disorders of the brain, with proper frame placement the Gamma Knife platform can be used to treat the upper cervical spine, generally from C1 to C4 depending on patient anatomy. The origin of radiosurgery can be traced to 1949 when Dr. Lars Leksell proposed the use of high-dose radiation in the treatment of small targets in the brain unable to undergo surgery [20]. The simple but elegant solution to converge beams of radiation from multiple entry points to spread out low dose to healthy tissues while obtaining a lethal dose at the center of the target has persisted for over 80 years now. After years of refinement, in 1968 Dr. Leksell presented the world the first Gamma Knife, installed at the Karolinska Institute [21]. The concept is surprisingly similar to the most recent iteration of this platform, the Gamma Knife Icon (Fig. 8.2). With this platform, immobilization can be via standard frame placement or, for the first time, a mask-based frameless alternative. Due to its less invasive nature, the mask-based system allows for the ability to offer frameless single fraction and multi-fractionated radiosurgery, similar to LINAC-based radiosurgical systems like CyberKnife.

Proton Beam Therapy

Though much more complicated and costly to run compared to a photon linear accelerator, proton beam cyclotrons are gaining wider use due to the many theoretical benefits of this modality. The main advantage to proton beam radiation includes the unique absorption profile compared to standard photon-based radiation. This pattern, known as the Bragg peak, allows for the maximum deposition of energy at a specified depth and the resultant complete sparing of dose deep to this area. In a standard photon plan, though some energy is deposited along the tissue and the beam is attenuated as it travels deeper in a patient, there is at least some deposition of dose deep to the intended target, which results in healthy tissue irradiation. Proton beam radiation can largely spare surrounding organs at risk, which may result in an improved therapeutic ratio and in theory less side effects. This makes proton beam radiation particularly attractive in the treatment

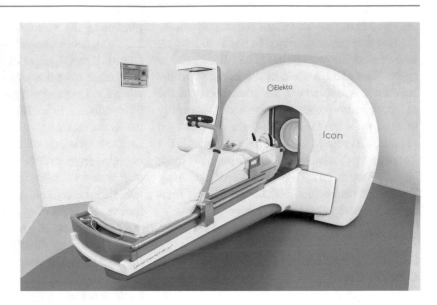

Fig. 8.2 The Elekta Gamma Knife Icon with patient on treatment couch with frameless mask immobilization. Though generally thought of as limited solely to the brain, the Gamma Knife Icon can treat tumors of the upper cervical spine. Infrared camera visible in front of the patient and cone beam CT arm lateral to the patient. Image courtesy of Elekta. All rights reserved

of pediatric tumors, patients requiring re-irradiation, and for tumors that are intimately involved with critical structures such as the spinal cord. Another possible benefit is the higher linear energy transfer (LET) and biological effectiveness with proton beam therapy, which may result in more effective cell kill in radioresistant cancers like melanoma or sarcoma [22].

Normal Tissue Tolerance

Delivered radiation dose and volume irradiated are correlated with a certain probability for the development of a normal tissue toxicity. The most commonly used summary of this is the Quantitative Analysis of Normal Tissue Effects in the Clinic (QUANTEC) [23]. It is broken down by specific organ and correlates a certain dose to the likelihood of a toxicity endpoint occurring for conventionally fractionated radiation (1.8–2.0 Gy, daily). Given heterogeneity in normal tissue tolerance based on an individual's inherent radiosensitivity, it is only useful in predicting percentages. Regardless, the goal of the radiation oncologist is to keep normal tissue exposure as low as reasonably achievable, given that no excess dose of radiation is totally safe. QUANTEC helps guide the radiation oncologist to safely deliver treatment, though the benchmarks set by

it may not be clinically appropriate for every case.

Radiation dose is not simply additive. For example, biologically the effect in tissue from a daily 2 Gy dose given 3 days in a row which equals a cumulative of 6 Gy is very different from the biological effect of a single 6 Gy dose given all at once. Therefore, a series of constraints has been created for radiosurgical doses and fractionation as well. The AAPM came out with Task Group 101 in 2010 which systematically categorized dose constraints for individual tissue based on maximum point dose and volume thresholds into single, three, or five fraction regimens [17]. Since this time, additional constraints have been released with the general United Kingdom Consensus on Normal Tissue Dose Constraints for Stereotactic Radiotherapy report [24].

Most recently, the AAPM has commissioned a series of updated papers on radiosurgical doses, specific for each individual organ based on prior reported data and models. In 2019 the most recent manuscript on spinal cord dose tolerance was released by Sahgal et al. [25] Current dose recommendations for the radiation-naïve patient treated with SBRT include the following spinal cord maximum point doses (Dmax): 12.4–14.0 Gy in one fraction, 17.0 Gy in two fractions, 20.3 Gy in three fractions, 23.0 Gy in four fractions, and 25.3 Gy in five fractions. If these constraints are met, they are associated with an estimated 1–5% risk of radiation myelopathy. For directly overlapping radiation fields ("re-irradiation") treated with SBRT, a lower risk of radiation myelopathy includes cumulative thecal sac equivalent dose in 2 Gy fractions (EQD_2) to meet the following constraints: Dmax $\leq$70 Gy, SBRT thecal sac EQD_2 Dmax $\leq$25 Gy, thecal sac SBRT EQD_2 Dmax to cumulative EQD_2 Dmax ratio $\leq$0.5, and a minimum time interval to re-irradiation of $\geq$5 months. These constraints assume an alpha/beta ratio of 2 in order to model late responding tissue.

Treatment of Extramedullary Tumors

The purpose of this chapter is to review the radiation treatment options for intradural extramedullary tumors of the spine. These are mainly benign tumors such as meningiomas, schwannomas, and neurofibromas, though there are rare instances of malignant entities in this domain [26]. There are three general circumstances in which radiation is utilized for these tumors: (1) upfront treatment for asymptomatic patients; (2) adjuvant treatment following subtotal and gross total resections; and (3) radiographic progression following surgical resection. Multiple radiation platforms can be utilized in all of these clinical settings. The general trend has overwhelmingly been toward radiosurgical approaches, as these confer greater tumor control with fewer side effects to the spinal cord and surrounding tissues. These treatments can also be delivered over a few fractions as compared to conventional plans which often take many weeks. The convenience factor for patients cannot be overstated. We present a total of five cases here that incorporate new-age platforms, such as proton beam therapy, in the three general conditions noted above. In addition, we have included a case of drop metastases or leptomeningeal metastases (LMD, leptomeningeal disease) treated with palliative radiation. Our goal was to include multiple radiotherapy delivery platforms in the treatment of diverse pathology. In this fashion, we hope to provide a representative view of radiotherapeutic options for both benign and malignant extramedullary tumors.

Case #1: Cervical Meningioma, Upfront SRS via Gamma Knife

Presentation and Treatment Plan

A 56-year-old female presented with progressively worsening headaches involving the right occipital region. MRI of the brain with and without contrast followed by a cervical MRI revealed a 2 cm craniocaudal mass in the ventral right aspect of the spinal canal at C1 (Fig. 8.3). Given the degree of dural thickening especially rostral to the lesion, a presumed diagnosis of meningioma was made. The mass was abutting and very slightly deforming the spinal cord. Based on the patient's age, the ventral and therefore more challenging location of the mass, lack of severe cord compression, and favorable volume of the mass, we elected to treat this with upfront SRS via the Gamma Knife radiosurgical platform. The patient underwent standard treatment of 14 Gy to the 50% isodose line without any neurologic issues. Point dose (0.035 cc) to the cervical spinal cord was limited to less than 14 Gy.

Discussion

Radiosurgical platforms have allowed neurosurgeons to consider primary treatment of spinal meningiomas with SRS. The underlying precondition is the lack of spinal cord compression and significant symptoms. Therefore, incidental meningiomas or those with very mild symptom profiles represent the most suitable targets. Patients who are older, who have elevated surgical risk, or who have meningiomas in difficult to access surgical locations are also considered for SRS in lieu of open surgical resection. But these criteria are typically part and parcel with the smaller, less symptomatic meningioma varieties. The majority of spinal meningiomas, especially in the grade 1 category, demonstrate an indolent growth pattern and typically come to clinical attention in the spinal canal after they have reached a fairly large size and have begun to cause symptoms of spinal cord compression.

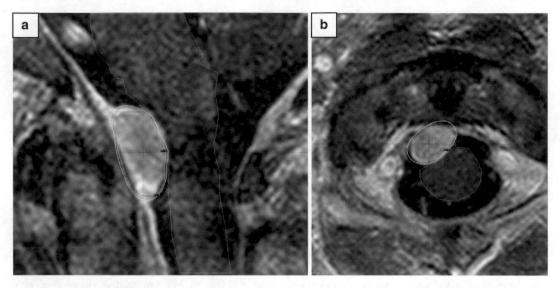

Fig. 8.3 Case #1: Cervical meningioma, upfront SRS via Gamma Knife. (**a**) Sagittal T1 postcontrast MRI showing ventral C1 meningioma, with gross tumor volume con- toured in red and radiation treatment isodose line in yel- low. (**b**) Axial T1 postcontrast MRI view of the same lesion

SRS comes into play before these dimensions and symptoms have been realized.

Based largely on the location of the tumor in our patient, surgical treatment was deferred in favor of upfront radiotherapy. Both conventionally fractionated radiation and radiosurgery can be used in the primary treatment setting for meningiomas. Conventional radiation is generally dosed from 50.4 to 54 Gy in 1.8 Gy daily doses depending on location. Spinal meningiomas are usually limited to <52 Gy given concerns about radiation dosing to the spinal cord.

Due to the proximity of the spinal cord and dose limits with conventionally fractionated radiation, radiosurgery has long been an attractive option for treatment of spinal meningiomas. With the ability for sharp dose falloff, single fraction radiosurgery has revolutionized the use of radiation in the treatment of small- to moderately sized tumors of the spinal canal. Common dosing ranges from 14 to 16 Gy in one fraction using the Gamma Knife, with de-escalated single dose down to 9–12 Gy in more recent literature using other platforms. A recent study by Lee et al. had 100% local control in 11 patients treated with SRS for spinal meningioma over a median 4-year follow-up period [27]. The Stanford experience

reported on 39 spinal meningiomas over a similar median 4-year period, as well as other benign spinal tumors, and showed a 3-, 5- and 10-year cumulative local failure rate of 1%, 2%, and 8%, respectively [28]. Tumors larger than 3 cm in maximum dimension or > 10 cc in total volume may be better suited to a fractionated approach to spare toxicity. Common dosing includes 25 Gy delivered over five fractions. A study by Marchetti reviewed single and multi-fraction treatment of benign spinal tumors, including 11 meningiomas [29]. With a median follow-up of 43 months, none of these cases showed progression.

Case #2: Recurrent Thoracic Meningioma, Conventionally Fractionated Proton Beam Therapy

Presentation and Treatment Plan

A 48-year-old female underwent initial open surgical resection of a circumferential grade 1 meningioma extending from C5 to T6. Adequate spinal cord decompression with improvement of symptoms was achieved. On surveillance MRI imaging, there was regrowth of the mass. The patient also had developed some mild worsening of numbness in her hands and arms. Due to the multisegment and en plaque nature of the meningioma, its circumferential location, and the current lack of severe cord compression, the decision was made to proceed with conventionally fractionated radiotherapy instead of repeat surgery or radiosurgery. Proton beam was recommended as we felt it would provide significant conformal advantage with respect to anterior organs at risk and in reduced heterogeneity to the spinal cord compared to photon-based IMRT. The patient was treated with 50.4 Gy from C5 to T6 over five and a half weeks (Fig. 8.4). She tolerated her treatment with no

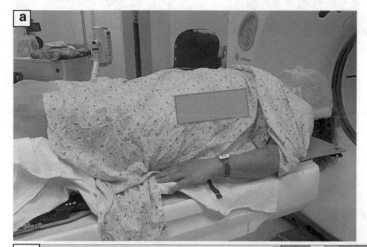

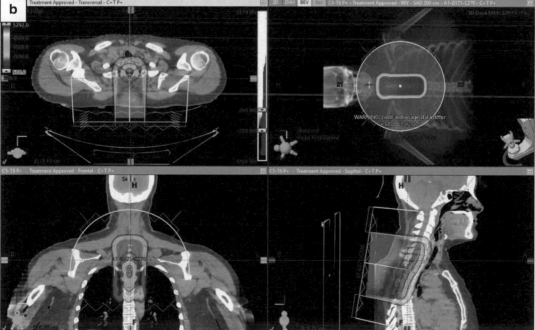

Fig. 8.4 Case #2: Recurrent thoracic meningioma, SBRT via proton beam. (**a**) Patient immobilized for pretreatment simulation. (**b**) Treatment planning system layout showing axial, coronal, and sagittal view showing target in the red contour. Dose is represented via color wash and is delivered to the C5-T6 with sparing of the anterior structures. (**c**) Sagittal T1 postcontrast. Pretreatment regrowth of meningioma. (**d**) Sagittal T1 postcontrast 1 year from radiation showing slight interval reduction in tumor mass. Notice posttreatment changes to the vertebral body marrow signal compared to pretreatment. (**e**) Sagittal T1 postcontrast 2 years from radiation showing stability

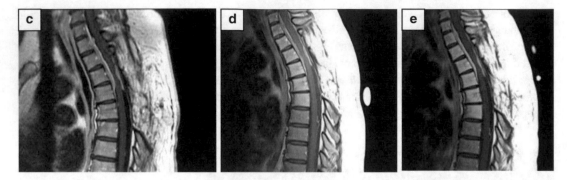

Fig. 8.4 (continued)

major side effects and was found to have a favorable response to treatment on follow-up imaging.

Discussion

Proton beam therapy is available at our institution, and we have been able to prescribe it in select spinal tumor cases beyond the more obvious indications for chordoma. Despite the elevated cost of proton compared to traditional photon-based platforms, and the resulting difficulty in getting insurance agencies to approve its use, we have pursued it for select cases such as the above, where a fairly large tumor volume exists in close proximity to the spinal cord. The rapid dose falloff at the periphery of the treatment field is theoretically advantageous in this circumstance though the literature remains scant. As more proton centers open nationally, we expect outcomes data to support its use for tumors in the extramedullary space. The general expectation is that there will be more long-term control of the tumor due to the increased tumoricidal impact of proton as opposed to photon therapy and also less of a deleterious impact to the spinal cord given its highly conformal delivery.

As is the case with their intracranial counterparts, there is no role for adjuvant radiation in the case of a gross totally resected grade 1 meningioma of the spinal canal. For patients who undergo a subtotal resection, many will not have progression or will progress slowly and thus can avoid the toxicity of adjuvant radiation therapy. Therefore, we recommend 6–12-month MRI surveillance after subtotal resection of a grade 1 meningioma, and then radiation can be considered upon radiographic progression. Repeat surgery is absolutely a viable option for recurrences as well, and some neurosurgeons would opt for that approach since radiation can make future surgery more complicated in the event of local failure. Similar to upfront treatment, when adjuvant radiation is offered to a subtotally resected meningioma, conventional doses are still limited to 50.4–54 Gy (in 1.8 Gy daily).

Grade II (atypical) meningiomas represent an interesting problem. They are exceedingly rare in the spinal canal, and accordingly recommendations are largely lacking regarding the use of adjuvant treatment. In addition, nearly all neurosurgeons leave behind the dural origin of the meningioma, as dural resection and patch grafting can potentiate a CSF leak, whereas the dura can be resected with impunity in most cranial meningioma cases. Therefore, most resected spinal meningiomas are inherently a Simpson grade 2 resection. We advocate for long-term surveillance only, even after subtotally resected grade 2 meningiomas (Simpson grades 2 and 3) as their growth profile appears to be fairly indolent in the more recent literature. As in cases of subtotally resected grade 1 meningiomas, adjuvant radiation should be withheld and then considered for cases of recurrence (typically 5% of cases though there are older reports of higher rates) or radiographic progression of known residual disease [30]. The recommended approach is the same as above, between 50.4 and 54 Gy in conventional fractions. Data supporting an improvement in overall survival remains lacking for adjuvant radiation, and so we will likely continue to withhold radiotherapy until there is more compelling evidence [31]. Other factors such as ki67 index along with Simpson grade and preoperative neurologic status (McCormick scale) may impact overall survival and therefore might influence the utilization of adjuvant radiation in subtotally resected grade 2 meningiomas, but again, given the paucity of data, we tend toward close surveillance in most cases [32].

Case #3: Primary CNS Melanoma, Adjuvant SBRT via TrueBeam (LINAC)

Presentation and Treatment Plan

A 53-year-old female presented with progressive worsening of left neck and arm pain over one month. There was also a component of imbalance and left arm weakness. MRI of the cervical spine with and without contrast revealed a largely intradural mass at C2–C3 causing cord deflection with compression. The mass also appeared to exit through the left C2–C3 foramen consistent with a schwannoma appearance. She underwent a C2–C3 laminectomy for resection of the intradural component. The foraminal disease was intentionally left behind. The mass appeared exceptionally dark, consistent with either a melanotic schwannoma or other pathology. Final pathology revealed a malignant melanoma, representing a primary CNS melanoma of the extramedullary space, an exceptionally rare disease entity. The tumor was negative for BRAF, NRAS, and KIT mutations, making it less likely to respond to immunotherapy. Given the aggressive nature of the tumor, the presence of residual foraminal disease, the patient's young age and high performance status, and the negative mutation status, she underwent SBRT delivered as 35 Gy in five fractions (Fig. 8.5).

Discussion

This case represents a rare, unexpected finding on pathology, but the treatment approach can be extrapolated to all intradural extramedullary metastatic tumors. Primary central nervous system melanoma comprises less than 0.1% of all melanoma diagnoses. Understanding the treatment principles in radiation, with respect to the necessary dose to sterilize melanoma cells while respecting the spinal cord tolerance, helped us to formulate a plan for this unusual situation. Knowing that upfront gross total resection could result in a suboptimal clinical outcome, the patient was operated on with the expectation that postoperative SBRT would be delivered to residual disease with the intent of preserving her neurological function. The patient was able to complete radiation treatment with minimal side effects and with preservation of function. Though rare, intradural extramedullary malignant disease, which is overwhelmingly metastatic in origin, should be treated with adjuvant radiation even in cases of gross total resection. The dosing scheme for a more typical metastasis, say from breast or lung origin, would be similar to what was given in this case, perhaps with a dose de-escalation to 30 Gy if a gross total resection was achieved.

Case #4: Cervical Neurofibroma, Adjuvant SBRT via TrueBeam (LINAC)

Presentation and Treatment Plan

A 47-year-old female presented with severe neck pain, left arm pain, and imbalance, all of which became progressively severe over one month. MRI of the cervical spine with and without contrast revealed a large intradural mass compressing the spinal cord with significant extension through the left C6–C7 foramen into the anterior neck region. She underwent a C6–C7 laminectomy for resection of the intradural tumor with some removal of the foraminal component via

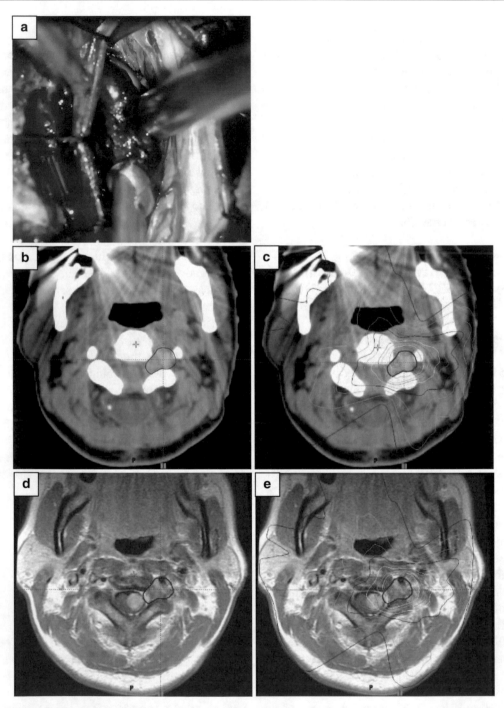

Fig. 8.5 Case #3: Primary CNS melanoma, adjuvant SBRT via TrueBeam (LINAC). Intraoperative image showing a darkly pigmented mass upon entering the dura (**a**). Axial CT reconstruction showing left C2–C3 foraminal tumor with gross tumor volume contoured (**b**) and with treatment isodose lines (**c**). Postoperative axial T1 postcontrast MRI showing greater definition of the foram- inal tumor with a clear view of the intradural component with gross tumor volume in thick red contour (**d**). Isodose levels in thin colored contours (**e**), all in cGy: light pink = 3675, yellow = 3500, cyan = 3100, dark green = 2700, yellow = 2300, orange = 1900, pur- ple = 1500, pink = 1100, green = 700, blue = 300

the exiting nerve root sleeve. Final pathology revealed a neurofibroma with an elevated ki67 index of 10%. Due to the significant amount of residual tumor, the patient's young age, and the final diagnosis with elevated ki67, we recommended adjuvant SBRT via LINAC platform (Fig. 8.6). This was done in three fractions with 21 Gy total. 3D reconstruction illustrates the impressive extent of the residual tumor into the brachial plexus, a highly complicated surgical domain that we feel was best treated using this adjuvant SBRT approach.

Discussion

Nerve sheath tumors (NST) comprise 25% of tumors arising in the extramedullary compartment. The majority of NSTs are schwannomas, consisting of 65% of all NSTs, while neurofibromas represent nearly all of the remainder. Less than 5% of such tumors are an aggressive, malignant variant known as malignant peripheral nerve sheath tumors (MPNST).

The treatment of NSTs is primarily surgical resection, though small and asymptomatic tumors may be observed to assess for stability. Upfront SBRT (via LINAC as in this case or CyberKnife) has become more prevalent for incidental schwannomas especially for those contained within the foramen or extraforaminal in location. Typically these schwannomas are followed for growth or symptom development before SBRT is pursued. The popularity of SBRT for these foraminal and extraforaminal schwannomas has increased with the proven success rate in the literature, in particular the studies from the Stanford and Pittsburgh groups. For those schwannomas couched within the foramen, bony resection of the facet is often necessary for exposure, and instrumented fusion is therefore required. Large extraforaminal schwannomas can necessitate multidisciplinary surgical teams for high morbidity approaches depending on the paraspinal location of the schwannoma. SBRT represents an effective and convenient alternative, often dosed in the three-fraction 21 Gy format utilized in this case, but there are variations on this radiosurgical

theme as we discuss below [33, 34]. Surgery can be pursued as a salvage for radiation failures, and occasionally re-irradiation is an option as well.

Larger or symptomatic NSTs will generally be offered resection, with gross total resection often curative. As these tumors generally have a slow growth velocity, the ability to spare function and preserve nervous tissue is key, even if this results in subtotal resection. With the advent of the treatment platforms described throughout this chapter, neurosurgeons have become more accepting of subtotal resections given the established efficacy of radiotherapy in controlling residual disease. For residual schwannomas and neurofibromas, conventional radiation and SBRT are considered, especially in cases of an elevated ki67 index. Though conventional radiation is highly effective, it is quite cumbersome in delivery as it usually lasts almost 6 weeks requiring daily administration. Doses are similar to those in the treatment of meningioma with 50.4–54 Gy utilized depending on doses to nearby organs.

The movement in radiotherapy has clearly been toward targeted radiosurgery (SBRT/SRS) for these tumors. Goals include escalating dose in the tumor and avoiding dose to the spinal cord and nerve roots. SBRT of such benign entities was first attempted in 1999, with the first report on fractionated SBRT shortly thereafter in 2001. In these initial reports, higher doses such as 16–24 Gy, similar to malignant tumor radiosurgical doses, were used. This resulted in excellent control outcomes with Gerszten et al. reporting their experience with 25 neurofibromas and 35 schwannomas showing 100% local control at median follow-up of 37 months and a long-term pain improvement in 73% of cases [35].

Due to concerns over toxicity, more contemporary manuscripts report a de-escalation of dose for benign spine tumors [36]. Doses generally in the range of 14–16 Gy in single fraction (down to 9 Gy in some very recent cases), 20 Gy in two fractions, 21 Gy in three fractions, or 25 Gy in five fractions are now more commonly used compared to the older dosing schemes. Even with this dose de-escalation, local control has been excellent. Shin et al. report on 65 benign neurogenic tumors treated with spinal SBRT with a median

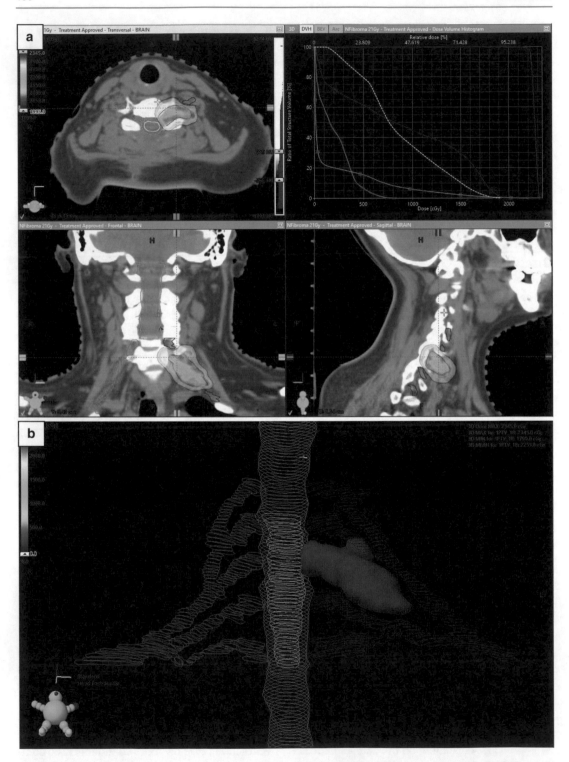

Fig. 8.6 Case #4: Cervical neurofibroma, adjuvant SBRT via TrueBeam (LINAC). (**a**) Axial, coronal, and sagittal view of CT-based fractionated SBRT plan with dose volume histogram. Contours include the tumor (red), while organs at risk include the spinal canal (pink), the partial spinal cord (cyan), the left brachial plexus (dark blue), and the right brachial plexus (dark green). (**b**) 3D projection of gross residual tumor (red), the spinal canal (pink), the partial spinal cord (cyan), the left brachial plexus (dark blue), and the right brachial plexus (dark green)

Table 8.2 Overview of most commonly utilized radiosurgical doses to benign and malignant intradural extramedullary tumors

Tumor Type	SRS (single fraction)	Hypofractionated SBRT	Conventional
Benign: Meningioma Schwannoma Neurofibroma	**14–16 Gy**	10 Gy × 2 fractions (20 Gy) **7–8 Gy × 3 fractions (21–24 Gy)** 5 Gy × 5 fractions (25 Gy)	1.8–2.0 Gy × 28–30 fractions (50.4–54 Gy)
Malignant: Metastasis Primary tumor	15–24 Gy	12 Gy × 2 fractions (24 Gy) 8–9 Gy × 3 fractions (24–27 Gy) **6-7 Gy × 5 fractions (30-35 Gy)**	1.8–2.0 Gy × 30–33 fractions (54–59.4 Gy)

These doses are intended to be general guidelines based on our experience and the most current literature. The bolded schemes represent our preferred approach in most cases

follow-up of 44 months and a local control of 95.4% [37]. Similarly, another report on SBRT with single fraction radiosurgery for both schwannomas and meningioma reports 100% local control at a median of 18 months, with MRI stability in 51% of lesions and decrease in 49% of lesions [38]. Table 8.2 contains an overview of the most commonly utilized dosages for treatment of the tumor types discussed in the above cases.

Case #5: Leptomeningeal Disease, Palliative Hypofractionated Treatment via TrueBeam (LINAC)

Presentation and Treatment Plan

A 60-year-old female with metastatic breast cancer and brain metastases treated with Gamma Knife radiosurgery 2 years prior to the development of leptomeningeal disease (LMD). She presented with increasing lower back pain without other neurological comprise and was very high functioning with Karnofsky Performance Scale (KPS) index of 90. The patient was treated with palliative radiation to partial spine, 20 Gy in five fractions, with a linear accelerator-based treatment. Treatment was directed at sites of gross disease (Fig. 8.7). The patient was started on intrathecal chemotherapy sequentially at the conclusion of her spine radiation.

Discussion

Leptomeningeal disease, or neoplastic meningitis, is the widespread seeding of the leptomeninges by cancerous cells. This is a relatively rare event, and incidence is thought be limited to 5% of all cancer patients [39]. Interestingly, as treatment improves and patients are experiencing increased survival, the incidence of LMD has been on the rise. The source of these malignant tumors in the extramedullary space (though there can be associated intramedullary invasion, blurring the line between the two compartments) can include metastatic tumors (e.g., breast cancer, lung cancer), medulloblastoma, ependymoma (typically high grade), glioblastoma, and pineal region tumors (e.g., pineoblastoma, germinoma), among other rare entities. It is a condition that is not typically in the domain of the neurosurgeon, as there is no role for neurosurgical intervention in the treatment of this diffuse disease. However, neurosurgeons are often consulted when such lesions are found, and in very rare circumstances where an LP is negative and there is a need for tissue, an open biopsy may be in order. Once a tumor cell has obtained access to the leptomeninges, the cerebrospinal fluid (CSF) disseminates these cells throughout the neuraxis with spinal symptoms including lower extremity weakness, imbalance, sensory disturbances, low back pain, and radicular pain. The diagnosis of LMD is grave, with median survival <3 months from diagnosis [40].

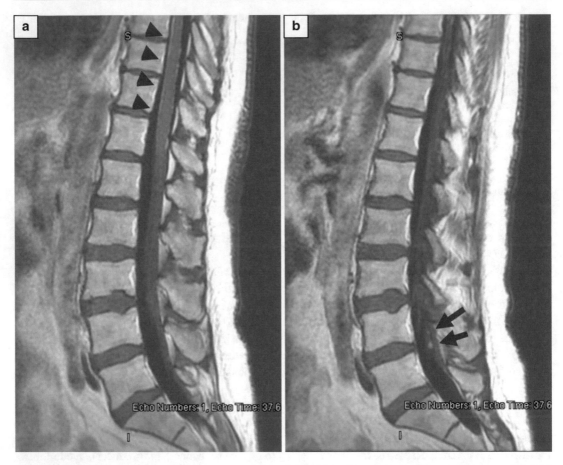

Fig. 8.7 Case #5: Leptomeningeal disease, palliative hypofractionated treatment via TrueBeam (LINAC). Sagittal T1 postcontrast images through two different planes are shown (**a, b**). Red arrowheads show linear enhancement lining the ventral spinal cord, while red arrows show nodular metastases in the cauda equina nerve roots

Given overall prognosis, the goals of treatment of LMD are to resolve or stabilize any current neurologic dysfunction, to prevent further neurologic deficits from unfolding, and to prolong survival. Unfortunately, current literature is lacking with respect to the randomized comparison of different treatments. Therefore, decision-making with each treatment modality is based more on practitioner judgment than evidence-based medicine. To aid in this, patients are commonly divided into "good-risk" or "poor-risk" groups, with the latter being defined as KPS < 60, multiple serious neurological deficits, extensive systemic disease, or poor treatment options. Such patients are generally offered only supportive care. If radiation is considered, it is directed only at symptomatic locations in the body, and one should avoid prolonged courses of palliative radiation.

For "good-risk" patients, treatment may be directed toward treatment of the entire neuraxis. This is usually via systemic or intrathecal drug administration. Craniospinal irradiation (CSI), which is treatment of the entire brain and spine with radiation, is extremely toxic and is typically not recommended for patients with LMD. Thus, for those who may be offered radiation, the main goal of this treatment is in the focal alleviation of symptoms such as low back pain, leg pain, or motor weakness. Radiation can improve these functions due to the reduction of visible tumor or the correction of CSF flow. Therefore, radiation treatment in patients with LMD should be limited to focal areas of the neuraxis that have either gross disease or a corresponding neurological sign.

Conclusions

Radiotherapy, both conventionally fractionated and radiosurgery, has rapidly become an integral consideration in the neurosurgical management of intradural extramedullary tumors. Whether being utilized in the upfront setting as primary treatment for a tumor that presents elevated surgical risk, or given in adjuvant fashion to provide long-term disease control, or as salvage in recurrent disease, radiotherapy must be incorporated into the neurosurgeon's treatment paradigm for these rare spinal tumors. The progress in this field has allowed neurosurgeons to reconsider goals of surgery; the imprimatur for a gross total resection has now transitioned into a more conservative approach where residual and recurrent disease can be treated with the appropriate form of radiotherapy. Rapid evolution in radiation platforms has led to improvements in accuracy, target delineation, and dose delivery while minimizing damage to adjacent critical structures. Though data is lacking for progression-free and overall survival in many of these rare tumor types, we strongly believe that there will be more compelling evidence to support radiotherapy as its use becomes more widespread. The utilization of radiotherapy is a multidisciplinary decision, though often initiated by the neurosurgeon who is the gatekeeper for these rare tumors. It remains the responsibility of all involved physicians to provide a balanced view as to the relative risks and benefits of observation, open surgery, conventional radiation, and stereotactic radiosurgery or a combination of these methods.

References

1. Tward JD, Anker CJ, Gaffney DK, Bowen GM. "Radiation Therapy and Skin Cancer." Modern practices in radiation therapy, edited by Gopishankar Natanasabapathi, InTechOpen, 2012, pp. 207–46.
2. Rontgen WC. Uber eine neue Art von Strahlen. Vorl äufige Mitteilung. In: Sitzungsberichte der physikalisch-medicinischen Gesellschaft zu Wüurzburg, Sitzung 1985. 30. p. 132–41.
3. Grubbe EH. Priority in the therapeutic use of X-rays. Radiology. 1933;21:156–62.
4. Becquerel AH, Curie P. Action physiologique des rayons de radium. C R Acad Sci. 1901;132:1289–91.
5. Thoraeus RA. A study of ionization method for measuring the intensity and absorption of roentgen rays and of the efficiency of different filters used in therapy. Acta Radiol. 1932;15:1–86.
6. Hong TS, Ritter MA, Tomé WA, et al. Intensity-modulated radiation therapy: emerging cancer treatment technology. Br J Cancer. 2005;92:1819–24.
7. Nagata Y. "Introduction and history of stereotactic body radiation therapy (SBRT)." Stereotactic Body Radiation Therapy, edited by Yasushi Nagata, Springer Japan, 2015, pp. 3–8.
8. Folkert MR, Bilsky MH, Cohen GN, et al. Intraoperative and percutaneous iridium-192 high-dose-rate brachytherapy for previously irradiated lesions of the spine. Brachytherapy. 2013;12:449–56.
9. Zuckerman SL, Lim J, Yamada Y, et al. Brachytherapy in spinal tumors: a systematic review. World Neurosurg. 2018;118:235 44.
10. Parker C, Nilsson S, Heinrich D, et al. Alpha emitter radium-223 and survival in metastatic prostate cancer. N Engl J Med. 2013;18:213–23.
11. Delaney G, Jacob S, Featherstone C, et al. The role of radiotherapy in cancer treatment: estimating optimal utilization from a review of evidence-based clinical guidelines. Cancer. 2005;104:1129–37.
12. Ishikura S. Quality assurance of radiotherapy in cancer treatment: toward improvement of patient safety and quality of care. Jpn J Clin Oncol. 2008;38:723–9.
13. ICRU Report 50. Prescribing, Recording, and Reporting Photon Beam Therapy, International Commission on Radiation Units and Measurements, Bethesda, MD; 1993.
14. ICRU Report 62. Prescribing, recording, and reporting photon beam therapy (supplement to ICRU report 50), international commission on radiation units and measurements, Bethesda, MD; 1999.
15. Lederman M. The early history of radiotherapy: 1895–1939. Int J Radiat Oncol Biol Phys. 1981;7:639–48.
16. Coutard H. Principles of X-ray therapy of malignant disease. Lancet. 1934;2:1–12.
17. Benedict SH, Yenice KM, Followill D, et al. Stereotactic body radiation therapy: the report of AAPM Task Group 101. Med Phys. 2010;37:4078.
18. Brown JM, Carlson DJ, Brenner DJ. The tumor radiobiology of SRS and SBRT: are more than the 5 Rs involved? Int J Radiat Oncol Biol Phys. 2014;88:254–62.
19. Kirkpatrick JP, Soltys SG, Lo SS, et al. The radiosurgery fractionation quandary: single fraction or hypofractionation? Neuro-Oncology. 2017;19:38–49.
20. Leksell L. The stereotaxic method and radiosurgery of the brain. Acta Chir Scand. 1951;102(4):316–9.
21. Leksell L. Stereotactic radiosurgery. J Neurol Neurosurg Psychiatry. 1983;46(9):797–803.
22. Schulz-Ertner D, Tsujii H. Particle radiation therapy using proton and heavier ion beams. J Clin Oncol. 2007;25:953–64.

23. Marks LB, Yorke ED, Jackson A, et al. Use of normal tissue complication probability models in the clinic. Int J Radiat Oncol Biol Phys. 2010;76:S10–9.
24. Hanna GG, Murray L, Patel R, et al. UK consensus on normal tissue dose constraints for stereotactic radiotherapy. R Coll Radiol. 2018;30(1):5–14.
25. Sahgal A, Chang J, Ma L, et al. Spinal cord dose tolerance to stereotactic body radiation therapy. Int J Radiat Oncol Biol Phys. 2019;S0360-3016(19):33862–3.
26. Simmons ED, Zheng Y. Vertebral tumors: surgical versus nonsurgical treatment. Clin Orthop Relat Res. 2006;443:233–47.
27. Lee ME, Hwang YJ, Sohn MJ, et al. Assessment of the treatment response of spinal Meningiomas after radiosurgery focusing on serial MRI findings. Jpn J Radiol. 2015;33(9):547–58.
28. Chin AL, Fujimoto D, Kumar KA, et al. Long-term update of stereotactic radiosurgery for benign spinal tumors. Neurosurgery. 2019;85(5):708–16.
29. Marchetti M, De Martin E, Milanesi I, et al. Intradural extramedullary benign spinal lesions radiosurgery. Medium- to long-term results from a single institution experience. Acta Neurochir. 2013;155(7):1215–22.
30. Sun SQ, Cai C, Ravindra VM, et al. Simpson grade I-III resection of spinal atypical (world health organization grade II) meningiomas is associated with symptom resolution and low recurrence. Neurosurgery. 2015;76(6):739–46.
31. Yolcu YU, Goyal A, Alvi MA, Moinuddin FM, Bydon M. Trends in the utilization of radiotherapy for spinal meningiomas: insights from the 2004-2015 national cancer database. Neurosurg Focus. 2019;46(6):1–10.
32. Noh SH, Kim KH, Shin DA, et al. Treatment outcomes of 17 patients with atypical spinal meningioma, including 4 with metastases: a retrospective observational study. Spine J. 2019;19(2):276–84.
33. Dodd RL, Ryu MR, Kamnerdsupaphon P, et al. CyberKnife radiosurgery for benign intradural extramedullary spinal tumors. Neurosurgery. 2006;58:674–85.
34. Ryu SI, Chang SD, Kim DH, et al. Image-guided hypo-fractionated stereotactic radiosurgery to spinal lesions. Neurosurgery. 2001;49:838–46.
35. Gerszten PC, Burton SA, Ozhasoglu C, et al. Radiosurgery for benign Intradural spinal tumors. Neurosurgery. 2008;62(4):887–95.
36. Kalash R, Glaser SM, Flickinger JC, et al. Stereotactic body radiation therapy for benign spine tumors: is dose de-escalation appropriate? J Neurosurg Spine. 2018;29(2):220–5.
37. Shin DW, Sohn MJ, Kim HS, et al. Clinical analysis of spinal stereotactic radiosurgery in the treatment of neurogenic tumors. J Neurosurg Spine. 2015;23(4):429–37.
38. Kufeld M, Wowra B, Muacevic A, et al. Radiosurgery of spinal meningiomas and schwannomas. Technol Cancer Res Treat. 2012;11(1):27–34.
39. Pavlidis N. The diagnostic and therapeutic management of leptomeningeal carcinomatosis. Ann Oncol. 2004;15(Suppl 4):iv285–91.
40. Clarke JL, Perez HR, Jacks LM, et al. Leptomeningeal metastases in the MRI era. Neurology. 2010;74:1449–54.

Radiotherapy for Intramedullary Tumors

Hima B. Musunuru, John C. Flickinger, and Peter C. Gerszten

Introduction

Primary spinal tumors are rare, comprising only 4–8% of all CNS tumors [1]. The majority of primary spinal tumors are nonmalignant, with only 22% categorized as malignant. The most common site of primary spinal tumors is the spinal cord (60.5%), followed by spinal meninges and lastly cauda equina. The location of the tumor is commonly used to classify spinal tumors into extradural lesions, which comprise 60% of all spinal tumors, and the rare intradural subset that comprise the remaining 30%. Intradural tumors are further subdivided into extramedullary tumors and intramedullary tumors (IMSCTs), with the latter comprising only 10% of all spinal tumors [2].

Ependymomas constitute the most common IMSCTs in adults, followed by astrocytic tumors and hemangioblastomas [2]. In the pediatric population, astrocytoma is the most common IMSCT

H. B. Musunuru
University of Pittsburgh School of Medicine,
Departments of Radiation Oncology,
Pittsburgh, PA, USA

J. C. Flickinger · P. C. Gerszten (✉)
University of Pittsburgh School of Medicine,
Departments of Radiation Oncology,
Pittsburgh, PA, USA

University of Pittsburgh School of Medicine,
Departments of Neurological Surgery,
Pittsburgh, PA, USA
e-mail: gersztenpc@upmc.edu

[3]. Other less common histologies include ganglioglioma, subependymoma, neurocytoma, lipoma, lymphomas, and PNETs [4].

Management of IMSCTs

First-line treatment for most IMSCT is surgery [5, 6], while radiotherapy is usually reserved for patients with malignant tumors. However, resection of IMSCT necessitates a clear plane of dissection. While this is feasible for ependymomas, astrocytomas tend to be more infiltrative and challenging. Any attempt at GTR for intramedullary astrocytomas may damage spinal pathways, leading to residual neurological deficits. In this situation, radiotherapy (RT) is utilized either in the definitive setting or as adjuvant therapy following resection.

Spinal Ependymomas

Approximately 30–45% of intramedullary spinal cord tumors in adults are ependymomas, making this the most common histology [2]. According to the World Health Organization (WHO) classification, ependymomas are divided into three different types: Grade I, which includes myxopapillary ependymoma (MPE) and subependymomas; Grade II, which includes the cellular, clear cell, tanycytic, and papillary subtypes; and finally Grade III, anaplastic ependymomas (AE). Ependymomas cause neurological symptoms by compression of adjacent critical structures. Surgery remains the cornerstone in the management of spinal ependymomas [7, 8].

Lin et al. evaluated outcomes for 1353 spinal ependymoma patients using information from SEER database. On multivariate analysis (MVA), histology and extent of surgery were associated with OS. At 5 years, mortality was 2.4% for MPE patients, 19.7% for low-grade non-MPE, and it was highest (30.8%) for patients with AE. Compared to patients who had GTR, patients who underwent subtotal resection (HR 2.2, $p = 0.01$) or biopsy alone (HR 2.05, $p = 0.03$) had worse overall survival (OS) [9]. In a literature review by Oh et al., PFS was longer for patients with tumors in the upper spinal cord (cervicomedullary, cervical, and cervicothoracic) when compared to thoracic, thoracolumbar, and conus/cauda equina location, despite the lower cord tumors being Grade I [10].

Myxopapillary Ependymomas

Myxopapillary ependymomas (MPE) have good prognosis and occur almost exclusively in the filum terminale [11]. In a SEER analysis performed by Bates et al., surgery, adjuvant RT, age <30 years, and Caucasian race were associated with better prognosis on MVA. A 10-year OS exceeding 90% was confirmed in this study for MPE. In a retrospective review of 51 spinal MPEs by MDACC [12], the 10-year OS, progression-free survival (PFS), and local control (LC) were 93%, 63%, and 67%, respectively. Recurrences were noted in 37% of the patients, and most of these (79%) were local recurrences. Among patients with GTR, adjuvant RT increased the time to local recurrence (4.75 years vs. 10.5 years $p = 0.03$). Similarly, 10-year local control following STR was better if patients received adjuvant RT (0% vs. 65%, $p = 0.008$). On MVA, adjusting for the type of resection, age >35 years, and receipt of adjuvant RT were associated with better LC and PFS. This was also seen in an earlier study done at Cleveland Clinic. Their report on

37 patients with spinal ependymomas has shown that recurrence-free survival time was longer for patients that received adjuvant RT (9.6 years vs. 1.1 years, $p = 0.0093$). Presacral MPE tend to have worse outcome when compared to MPE at filum terminale/cauda equina region [13].

In an earlier case series from Mayo Clinic, all MPE patients ($n = 12$) received adjuvant RT following GTR/STR. When their data was examined for RT dose relationship, 5-year LC rates were 100% for RT doses exceeding 50Gy and lower (67%) for RT doses less than 50Gy [14].

Grade II and Grade III Ependymomas

The role of adjuvant radiotherapy in general for ependymomas has remained controversial due to the small number of studies with limited patient numbers. In patients where GTR is not feasible due to infiltration of critical neurological structures, adjuvant radiotherapy is commonly used to improve disease outcomes. NCCN guidelines endorse adjuvant radiotherapy for Grade II ependymomas following subtotal resection and for all anaplastic ependymomas irrespective of extent of resection. Yeboa et al. reviewed current patterns of care for 1345 Grade II–III spinal ependymoma patients. Surgery was performed in majority of the patients (78.2%), more so in Grade II patients when compared to Grade III. On the contrary, RT was administered to 60.9% of Grade III patients, whereas only 15.3% of Grade II patients received RT [15]. In another recent NCDB analysis by Brown et al., the impact of adjuvant radiotherapy on OS was assessed for 1058 Grade II–III spinal ependymoma patients. Most of the cohort (85.9%) underwent either subtotal resection (STR) or biopsy alone. Grade III comprised only 3.7% of the cohort. Patients with either Grade III ependymomas or STR/biopsy alone were more likely to receive adjuvant radiotherapy. On MVA, factors associated with worse OS were increasing age and higher grade. Adjuvant RT was not associated with better OS in the entire cohort or for patients with Grade II tumors. This analysis could not be repeated separately for Grade III tumors due to limited patient numbers. Limitations of this study include lack of data pertaining to recurrence and PFS [8]. In a recent SEER analysis done by Ryu et al., age≥65 years, histology, metastatic disease at presentation, multiple lesions, RT, and GTR were found to be independent predictors of OS. In this study, patients who received adjuvant RT had worse OS when compared to surgery alone (HR 2.02, $p < 0.001$). This could have been due to selection bias as most of the patients who received adjuvant RT had Grade III tumors and metastatic lesions, and fewer patients had GTR [16]. Limitations once again include lack of data about recurrence patterns, neurological morbidity related to recurrence, and PFS.

Oh et al. performed individual patient data analysis on 348 patients with Grade II–III spinal ependymomas. Patients with GTR had the best 5-year PFS and OS. The 5-year PFS for GTR, STR + adjuvant radiotherapy, and STR groups was 97.9%, 65.3%, and 45.1%, respectively. Adjuvant RT improved 5-year PFS by 20.2% following STR. In contrast, adjuvant RT did not improve OS. The 5-year OS for GTR, STR + adjuvant radiotherapy, and STR groups was 98.8%, 79.3%, and 73.7%, respectively [8]. Small retrospective studies reported differing outcomes due to small patient numbers in combination with significant heterogeneity related to histology, extent of resection, and adjuvant RT.

The optimal dose for adjuvant RT is a matter of debate. One of the earlier studies reported that among patients with adjuvant radiotherapy dose ≤50Gy, there were 35% failures, whereas there was only one failure (20%) in patients treated with adjuvant RT dose >50Gy. The majority (86%) of failures occurred within the initial RT field [17]. In a more recent study, patients were divided into two different adjuvant RT cohorts: <50Gy vs. ≥50Gy. There was no difference in the number of recurrences, PFS, or OS between the two RT groups [8].

Spinal Astrocytomas

Spinal cord gliomas account for approximately 80% of intramedullary spinal tumors. Ependymomas comprise the majority of these gliomas (70%), whereas astrocytomas comprise the

remaining 30% [18]. The majority (75%) of spinal astrocytomas are WHO low grade (Grades I–II), and only 25% are high grade (WHO Grades III and IV) when compared to cranial astrocytomas [19].

Though surgical resection is the standard of care for spinal astrocytomas, achieving GTR in high-grade tumors is often not feasible [20].

In a multicenter retrospective review, receipt of adjuvant RT was associated with better PFS for low- and intermediate-grade astrocytomas (HR 0.24, $p = 0.02$). There was no evidence of benefit with adjuvant RT for patients with higher-grade tumors (HR 1.42, $p = 0.67$). Extent of surgery was also associated with better PFS, with GTR patients having a lower risk of progression (HR 0.16, $p = 0.01$). On MVA, the only factor that was associated with OS was grade of the tumor ($p < 0.01$). Overall survival at 5, 10, and 15 years for spinal astrocytoma was 59%, 53%, and 32%, respectively [21]. Minehan et al. reported on 136 patients with spinal astrocytomas treated at Mayo Clinic between 1962 and 2005 [22]. Postoperative RT doses varied from 11.1Gy to 66.6Gy, prescribed at cord depth. The most common radiotherapy field arrangement was a single posterior field, encompassing the tumor with two vertebrae above and below the tumor. Fifty-one percent of the cohort had pilocytic astrocytomas. Biopsy alone was done in 59% of the tumors. RT was used in 75% of the study population with the majority receiving doses higher than 35Gy. On UVA, age ≤20 years and thoracic cord involvement were associated with better OS for pilocytic astrocytomas. In this cohort, receipt of RT was associated with better median OS for patients with pilocytic astrocytomas, but this finding did not reach statistical significance. In patients with infiltrative astrocytomas, duration of symptoms >180 days, Grade II, receipt of RT, and RT dose>35Gy were associated with longer median OS. When MVA was performed for all astrocytomas, pilocytic histology, symptom duration>180 days, postoperative RT, and minimal surgery were all associated with better OS. In a more recent but smaller ($n = 16$) retrospective review of astrocytoma patients following definitive or adjuvant RT, patients had either primary spinal astrocytomas or drop metastases from cranial astrocytomas [23]. On univariate analysis, surgical resection, primary spinal astrocytomas, and RT dose ≥45Gy were associated with improved OS.

Hemangioblastomas

Hemangioblastomas are benign vascular neoplasms originating from embryonic remnant tissues of mesodermal origin [24]. They present either as sporadic lesions in 70–80% of the patients or can be manifestations of von Hippel-Lindau disease (VHL) due to a loss of function mutation in the VHL tumor suppressor gene. VHL-related lesions can occur anywhere along the neuraxis, including the cerebellum, brain stem, and spinal cord [25]. Spinal cord lesions are usually symptomatic and present with pain followed by sensory impairment or motor loss [24]. Historically surgical resection had been the treatment of choice for these tumors [26]. In addition to surgery, conventionally fractionated radiotherapy was also used in the management of hemangioblastomas, either in the definitive, adjuvant, or salvage setting [27]. In one such paper from Mayo Clinic treating patients with CNS hemangioblastomas, in-field disease control was improved when patients received adjuvant EBRT dose ≥50Gy [27]. In a retrospective study evaluating patients with diffuse VHL-related hemangioblastomas, infratentorial craniospinal radiotherapy to a dose of 43.2Gy in 24 fractions was used successfully to slow the growth rate of tumors, with minimal treatment-related toxicity [28].

Due to the highly vascularized nature of hemangioblastomas, surgical resection can carry a significant complication risk for spinal lesions [29]. Therefore, in patients with multiple hemangioblastomas in the setting of VHL disease, nonsurgical options might be preferable in the definitive management of these patients needing multiple intracranial and extracranial treatments. Dose escalation using conventional EBRT is limited by spinal cord tolerance, as radiation field arrangements cannot preferen-

tially spare spinal cord adjacent to the tumor. On the contrary, SRS can deliver highly localized radiation with a steep dose gradient that leads to a significant reduction in the volume of adjacent critical structures like spinal cord irradiated to high radiation doses (Fig. 9.1). Recent studies investigating SRS for spinal hemangioblastomas have reported favorable outcomes. In a recent review by Hernández-Durán et al., 10 studies that included 52 patients with 70 primary or metastatic intramedullary lesions treated with SRS were evaluated [30]. Most tumors (67%) were primary spinal tumors. Hemangioblastoma was the most common histology followed by ependymoma. Most patients had de novo SRS, whereas 13% had prior therapy in the form of either surgery or external beam radiotherapy. The majority of the lesions (87%) were treated on the CyberKnife® platform.

In the studies treating primary tumors, SRS schedules consisted of 20.65Gy–25.75Gy in 2–3 fractions [31–34]. Most of the lesions (94%) showed tumor stabilization on imaging correlating with clinical improvement. Overall grade 1–2 treatment-related complication rate was 4%. No grade 3 toxicities were reported.

A recent prospective study from Stanford reported outcomes after de novo definitive CyberKnife®-based SRS for 46 spinal hemangioblastomas in 28 patients, of which 50% had VHL disease. Mean SRS prescription dose to the periphery was 21.6Gy. The actuarial control rate at 5 years was 92.3%, with no treatment-related toxicity [35].

In an interesting paper evaluating the SRS dose effect on benign spine lesions, seven patients (18.4%) had hemangioblastomas, while the remaining patients had extramedullary tumors. Majority of the patients (70%) in this study received prior therapy in the form of surgery or radiotherapy. SRS consisted of 9–21Gy in 1–3 fractions delivered using CyberKnife® or Linac-based platforms. At a median follow-up of 54 months, the local control rate was 76% in this heavily pretreated population. No grade 3 or higher acute or late toxicity was noted. The authors also found no differential effect of dose

$(BED_{10} \leq 30Gy$ vs. $BED_{10} > 30Gy)$ on local control, pain flare, or toxicity [36].

Intramedullary Spinal Cord Metastases (ISCM)

ISCMs constitute 1–3% of all intramedullary tumors and 0.6% of all spinal cord tumors. The most common histology is lung cancer, followed by breast cancer [37]. There is controversy in the literature about the most common anatomical location of ISCMs: cervical cord, thoracic, or conus medullaris. The majority of the patients with ISCMs have concomitant brain metastases, and this portends a poor prognosis [38].

Microsurgical resection, especially complete removal of ISCMs, is associated with a substantial risk of neurological deficits given the critical location of tumors in combination with poorly defined resection plane. This, in combination with poor overall survival [38] for patients with ISCMs, makes definitive radiotherapy a favorable treatment option. There are no studies directly comparing surgery with definitive radiotherapy for ISCMs. In one of the early case reports, Vindlacheruvu et al. described using EBRT at a dose of 20Gy in five fractions to treat a metastatic small-cell lung cancer patient who presented with ISCM [39]. This patient noted improvement in lower limb function following treatment completion and maintained ambulatory status till death. In a single institution series from the Mayo Clinic, 35 patients with ISCMs were treated with EBRT and five patients with surgery. Of the patients who were ambulatory at ISCM diagnosis, 91% remained ambulatory at their last follow-up [40].

Conill et al. reported their experience treating six lung cancer ISCM patients with EBRT, with doses ranging from 27Gy in 5 fractions to 40Gy in 20 fractions. Improvement in neurological symptoms was noted in 83% of the treated patients at a median time interval of 17.2 days following radiotherapy [41].

In a Korean series by Lee et al., 11 out of 12 ISCM patients secondary to lung or breast cancer were treated with EBRT doses ranging from 20Gy to 30Gy. Neurological deterioration was noted rapidly in all patients following treatment, which is most likely due to aggressive disease biology, reflected by a shorter median overall survival of 3.9 months [42].

More recently, SRS has gained popularity due to its convenience when compared to conventional EBRT and less morbidity when compared to surgery. In the largest series to date reported by Veeravagu et al., 11 ISCMs were treated with SRS doses ranging from 14 to 27Gy in 1–3 fractions. At the last follow-up, there were no local recurrences, and none of the patients had worsening neurological status [43]. Follow-up MRI was available for only four patients, and this showed either stable disease or regression. In the next largest series by Shin et al., 7 out of the 11 spinal lesions were ISCMs. SRS doses ranged from 10 to 16Gy, with a mean dose of 13.8Gy. Following SRS, 78% remained ambulatory, and radiographic response/stable changes were noted in 88% of the lesions [44]. SRS-related toxicity was not noted in either of these studies, with follow-up limited by poor median overall survival of 4.1–8 months.

Advances in Radiotherapy

In the past decade, RT has seen tremendous progress in all aspects of treatment, including patient immobilization, imaging, treatment planning, and delivery. A few of these include image-guided radiotherapy (IGRT), intensity-modulated radiotherapy (IMRT), volumetric modulated arc therapy (VMAT), and stereotactic radiosurgery (SRS) or fractionated stereotactic radiotherapy (FSRT). These advances improved the accuracy of radiotherapy dose delivery, thereby increasing the probability of tumor control while limiting dose to the adjacent normal tissues. Particle therapy, including protons, has gained popularity due to its ability to selectively deposit radiotherapy dose in the target with a very steep dose gradient outside the target, thereby sparing critical organs at risk.

Fractionated EBRT for Spinal Cord Gliomas

Kahn et al. reported on long-term outcomes of 32 spinal glioma patients treated with modern conformal RT techniques [45]. Most of the patients had either astrocytoma (53%) or ependymoma (44%), with only one patient diagnosed with oligodendroglioma. Twenty-one percent of ependymoma patients and 56% of astrocytoma patients had biopsy alone without resection. Of the patients treated with radiotherapy, 22 patients (68.75%) were treated with IMRT and the remaining 10 patients with protons. Patients underwent CT-based simulation. Diagnostic MRI and planning CT were used to define target volumes. Residual postoperative tumor volume, resection cavity, and T2 FLAIR abnormality were encompassed with a 1.5 cm margin to define PTV. Median RT dose was 51Gy using mostly 1.8Gy per fraction, with a range of 50–55Gy for 26 patients and 45–50Gy for the remaining 6 patients. The 5-year OS for the entire cohort was 65%. On MVA, younger patients (age < 54 years), ependymoma histology, and photon vs. proton RT patients had better OS. The 5-year OS for ependymoma patients was superior at 86% when compared to 52% for astrocytoma and oligodendroglioma. Most common RTOG/EORTC acute toxicity was fatigue (41%) followed by nausea/vomiting (28%) and skin irritation (25%). No RT myelopathy was reported.

In a subsequent report from Korea [46], 45 spinal cord astrocytoma patients treated with adjuvant or definitive radiotherapy were reviewed. Fifty-six percent of the cohort had high-grade astrocytomas. The majority had surgical intervention, with biopsy alone patients comprising only 7% of the cohort. Radiotherapy was utilized in the adjuvant setting for 85% of the cohort, as definitive treatment for 11%, and as a salvage option for the remaining 4%. Very few patients (9%) received craniospinal RT. Median dose of RT was 50.4Gy, with 73% receiving RT dose greater than 45Gy. 3DCRT was utilized in majority of the patients (64%), while IMRT was used in the remaining 36%. T1-weighted MRI was used to define GTV for high-grade gliomas, and T2-weighted sequence was used for low-grade gliomas. A 5 cm craniocaudal margin encompassing at least two vertebral bodies was used around GTV to define CTV1; this was coned down to a 2 cm expansion for CTV2. A 5 mm margin around CTVs was used to define PTV1 and PTV2. 45Gy was usually prescribed to PTV1 with an optional sequential boost of 5.4Gy–9.0Gy to PTV2. The 2-year and 5-year PFS were 52% and 38%, respectively, whereas the 2-year and 5-year OS were 71% and 49%, respectively. On MVA, only grade was associated with worse PFS and OS.

Two other smaller series have used RT margins ranging from 2 cm to 5 cm for spinal cord gliomas [23, 47]. Cross comparison across studies is very challenging given significant heterogeneity with respect to histology, extent of surgery, and RT techniques/fields/dose.

Unlike intracranial gliomas, local failure patterns in relation to RT field and RT dose have not been reported for spinal gliomas, and as such, no standard guidelines exist to guide RT target definition and prescription doses.

SRS

Since its inception in the 1970s, stereotactic radiosurgery (SRS) has become an important tool in the management of intracranial neoplasms [48]. The application of SRS for spinal tumors was first described by Hamilton et al. in 1995 [49] and has since gained significant popularity mainly for the treatment of metastatic lesions [50]. Concerns about radiation myelopathy (RM) have limited the application of SRS to extradural metastatic lesions, and as such, there is a paucity of data on its utilization for intramedullary lesions. Ryu et al. published the first report investigating the role of SRS for benign spine lesions [51]. Following this, multiple studies have reported favorable outcomes following SRS for benign spine tumors [52–54].

In regard to SRS for exclusively intramedullary lesions, a recent review article by Hernández-Durán et al. evaluated 10 SRS studies that included 52 patients with 70 primary or metastatic intramedullary lesions [30]. Most tumors (67%) were primary spinal tumors. Hemangioblastoma was the most common histology followed by ependymoma. In patients with intramedullary metastatic tumors (33%), breast was the most common histology. Most patients had de novo SRS, whereas 13% had prior therapy in the form of either surgery or external beam radiotherapy. Most lesions (87%) were treated on the CyberKnife® platform.

In the studies treating primary tumors, 20.65Gy–25.75Gy in 2–3 fractions was used [31–34]. Most of the lesions (94%) showed tumor stabilization on imaging correlating with clinical improvement. The overall grade1–2 treatment-related complication rate was 4%. No grade 3 toxicities were reported.

SRS schedules using 15.0Gy–39.75Gy in 2–11 fractions were employed in the studies treating metastatic lesions [43, 44, 55–58]. In this subgroup, all studies reported radiological and clinical stabilization or improvement. Toxicity data was not available.

Technical Considerations of SRS

With the rapid adoption of SBRT for spine lesions across many centers, there has been ever-increasing focus on the safety of these complex radiotherapy techniques with respect to image guidance, immobilization, target delineation, SBRT planning, and delivery.

The first critical step in spine SBRT is patient immobilization while acquiring SBRT planning CT scan. A recent MRI-based analysis of spinal cord motion has shown that the physiologic motion of the spinal cord is less than 0.5 mm when compared to gross patient motion without immobilization that has resulted in maximal displacements of 2.21 mm, 2.87 mm, and 3.90 mm in the anteroposterior, lateral, and superior-inferior direction, respectively [59]. Multiple immobilization devices are in use, including BodyFIX (Elekta, Stockholm, Sweden), which has increased setup accuracy to within 1.2 mm translational and 0.9° rotational error [60].

SPIne response assessment in Neuro-Oncology (SPINO) guidelines [61] that were developed for extramedullary spine SBRT can also be applied to certain aspects of intramedullary SBRT/SRS. As per these guidelines, CT simulation scan thickness should be ideally 1 mm and not exceed 2 mm. Volumetric MRI should be acquired on thin slices in order to facilitate accurate registration with the planning CT. Due to steep dose gradient associated with SBRT, accurate delineation of target volume and critical structures like the spinal cord is very important. Comprehensive volumetric diagnostic imaging including T1-weighted and T2-weighted MRI acquired around the time of SBRT planning is of utmost importance to facilitate this process [62]. In the postoperative setting, spinal hardware can create significant artifacts and distortions on MRI imaging. In this situation, CT myelogram should be performed prior to CT simulation. At the time of target delineation, the spinal cord is usually defined on diagnostic MRI fused with planning CT. This approach can result in fusion errors of the order of 2 mm [63] and should be evaluated carefully as part of SBRT QA process.

With the advent of newer-generation Linacs that have sensitive feedback systems allowing control of gantry speed, collimator angles, flattening-free filter mode to reduce treatment time, 6 degrees of freedom couch to correct positioning errors [64], in combination with effective onboard imaging like cone beam CT(CBCT), volumetric modulated arc therapy (VMAT) is being used more commonly to deliver spine SBRT/SRS. Compared to conventional 3D conformal radiotherapy, IMRT/VMAT plans have steep dose gradient with detrimental consequences if there were to be a geometric miss. As such, stringent QA is essential during treatment planning and delivery [65].

Image guidance is a critical component of SBRT delivery. Linear accelerator platforms have a kilovoltage source and detector mounted onto the gantry, to acquire cone beam CT (CBCT). CBCT provides three-dimensional volume and anatomy that aids accurate target registration and comparison. In recent single institution series, evaluation of intra-treatment CBCT and post-treatment CBCT for intradural spine SRS has shown translational and rotational variations as small as 1 mm and 1°, respectively [66] (Fig. 9.1).

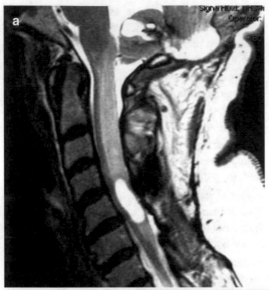

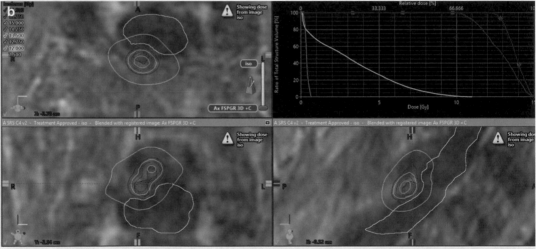

Fig. 9.1 A 41-year-old woman with a history of von Hippel-Lindau syndrome. She initially underwent surgery to remove a solitary hemangioblastoma at the C5 level. One year after surgery, she was found to have a second ventral tumor associated with a syrinx on T2-weighted MR imaging (**a**). It was felt that the tumor was not amenable to open surgical resection, and she was referred for

SRS. It was elected to treat the tumor with SRS using a fusion of a fine-cut MRI with the CT simulation. The GTV was 0.1 ml with a prescription dose of 12 Gy delivered in a single fraction (**b**). The D_{max} to the GTV was 15 Gy, and the D_{min} was 12 Gy. The D_{max} to a single voxel of the spinal cord was 11 Gy

CyberKnife®

CyberKnife® delivers multiple radiation beams to the target via a 6MV Linac mounted on a robotic arm. It has an integrated KV imaging system that can track targets through bony anatomy for targets such as spine or through fiducials for soft tissue targets like liver. Shifts resulting from real time tracking are used to adjust the robotic Linac arm accordingly for accurate dose delivery. Given that the traditional CyberKnife® units had to rely on circular collimators to deliver highly conformal SBRT/SRS treatments, higher monitor units were required to deliver the same SRS prescription dose when compared to linear accelerators [67]. Modern CyberKnife® units have high-definition MLCs that can deliver SRS to large fields and reduce treatment delivery time and also total monitor units [68].

MR-Linac

The advantage of MR-guided radiotherapy is the superior soft tissue contrast inherent to MR imaging when compared to traditional CT image guidance. This in turn improves the quality of target delineation, patient setup, image localization, and real-time gating, all of which have the potential to translate into clinically meaningful benefit by improving treatment efficacy while reducing toxicity [69]. Another interesting avenue that is being explored by MR-Linac teams is the ability to adapt daily treatment to tumor or anatomical changes (adaptive radiotherapy) [70].

The first commercial MRI-guided cobalt radiation therapy system "MRIdian®" or "ViewRay" treated patients at Washington University, St Louis, MO. The next version (MRIdian Linac™) combined a 0.345 T field strength split-bore magnet MRI with a 6 MV flattening filter-free linear accelerator (Linac). The TRUFI imaging sequence on the ViewRay MRIdian Linac™ platform enables real-time visualization of the spinal cord and surrounding cerebrospinal fluid, thereby making MRIdian an attractive modality for spine SRS [71]. Several other MR-Linacs from other manufacturers have since started treating patients throughout the world [72].

RT Complications

Radiation-induced spinal cord injury, also known as radiation myelopathy (RM), though rare, can result in significant morbidity including pain, paresthesia, sensory disturbances, weakness/paralysis, and bladder/bowel dysfunction [73]. RM, which is a diagnosis of exclusion, is considered when highly suspicious clinical findings are supported by characteristic MRI findings. MRI findings include hypointense changes on T1-weighted (T1W) images and high signal intensity on T2W images, with areas of focal contrast enhancement in the region of irradiation [74].

With conventional radiotherapy fractionation using 2 Gy per day, 50 Gy, 60 Gy, and ~69 Gy radiotherapy doses to complete cross section of cord are associated with a 0.2%, 6%, and 50% risk of myelopathy [75]. The latent time to develop RM with conventional radiation is 18 months after de novo radiotherapy and 11 months after reirradiation [74, 76].

With SBRT, the latent time to develop RM was 12 months after de novo SBRT [77, 78] and 6 months following reirradiation [79, 80]. In a recent paper by Sahgal et al., mathematical and biological modeling was performed to derive SBRT recommendations for spinal cord dose constraints [81]. In the de novo SBRT setting using 1–5 fractions, Dmax values of 12.4–14.0 Gy in one fraction, 17.0 Gy in two fractions, 20.3 Gy in three fractions, 23.0 Gy in four fractions, and 25.3 Gy in five fractions appear to be associated with an estimated risk of RM ranging from 1% to 5%. The 14 Gy single-fraction constraint was based on a myelogram-determined spinal cord, while the remaining constraints generally refer to the thecal sac, which is usually used as a surrogate for cord PRV. In the SBRT reirradiation scenario, the following dose constraints were proposed: cumulative thecal sac $EQD2_2$ Dmax not greater than 70 Gy, reirradiation SBRT thecal sac $EQD2_2$ Dmax not greater than 25 Gy, reirradiation SBRT thecal sac EQD2$_2$ Dmax to cumulative EQD2$_2$ Dmax ratio not greater than 0.5, and, finally, the minimum time interval from first course of RT to reirradiation should be at least 5 months [81]. This paper also specified standards for reporting SBRT treatment parameters, treatment outcomes, and toxicity.

Last of all, bevacizumab has emerged as an effective therapy in reducing radiation injury to spinal cord and brain [82]. Psimaras reported on the use of bevacizumab in four patients with late-onset myelopathy after radiotherapy that was unresponsive to corticosteroids. They saw imaging improvement in all four and stabilization in neurological deficits in three of four. The availability of bevacizumab to treat radiation myelopathy can diminish or limit the risks of radiotherapy in the management of intramedullary tumors when reasonable treatment doses are used.

Conclusion

Because intramedullary tumors are relatively rare and studies of radiotherapy for these tumors can be affected by selection bias, the medical literature regarding radiotherapy for management of intramedullary tumors has limitations and some areas of controversy. Overall there is reasonable evidence supporting radiotherapy in the management of ependymomas of the spinal cord and cauda equina, astrocytomas of the spinal cord, and intramedullary spinal cord metastases. There is also reasonable evidence supporting radiosurgery for managing hemangioblastomas of the spinal cord and cauda equina when complete resection cannot be achieved with low morbidity.

References

1. Schellinger KA, Propp JM, Villano JL, McCarthy BJ. Descriptive epidemiology of primary spinal cord tumors. J Neuro-Oncol. 2008;87(2):173–9.
2. Duong LM, McCarthy BJ, McLendon RE, Dolecek TA, Kruchko C, Douglas LL, et al. Descriptive epidemiology of malignant and nonmalignant primary spinal cord, spinal meninges, and cauda equina tumors, United States, 2004–2007. Cancer. 2012;118(17):4220–7.
3. Townsend N, Handler M, Fleitz J, Foreman N. Intramedullary spinal cord astrocytomas in children. Pediatr Blood Cancer. 2004;43(6):629–32.
4. Ostrom QT, Gittleman H, Truitt G, Boscia A, Kruchko C, Barnholtz-Sloan JS. CBTRUS statistical report: primary brain and other central nervous system tumors diagnosed in the United States in 2011–2015. Neuro-Oncology. 2018;20(suppl_4):iv1–iv86.
5. Bostrom A, von Lehe M, Hartmann W, Pietsch T, Feuss M, Bostrom JP, et al. Surgery for spinal cord ependymomas: outcome and prognostic factors. Neurosurgery. 2011;68(2):302–8. discussion 9
6. Mandigo CE, Ogden AT, Angevine PD, McCormick PC. Operative management of spinal hemangioblastoma. Neurosurgery. 2009;65(6):1166–77.
7. Volpp PB, Han K, Kagan AR, Tome M. Outcomes in treatment for intradural spinal cord ependymomas. Int J Radiat Oncol Biol Phys. 2007;69(4):1199–204.
8. Oh MC, Ivan ME, Sun MZ, Kaur G, Safaee M, Kim JM, et al. Adjuvant radiotherapy delays recurrence following subtotal resection of spinal cord ependymomas. Neuro-Oncology. 2013;15(2):208–15.
9. Lin Y, Smith ZA, Wong AP, Melkonian S, Harris DA, Lam S. Predictors of survival in patients with spinal ependymoma. Neurol Res. 2015;37(7):650–5.
10. Oh MC, Kim JM, Kaur G, Safaee M, Sun MZ, Singh A, et al. Prognosis by tumor location in adults with spinal ependymomas. J Neurosurg Spine. 2013;18(3):226–35.
11. Akyurek S, Chang EL, Yu TK, Little D, Allen PK, McCutcheon I, et al. Spinal myxopapillary ependymoma outcomes in patients treated with surgery and radiotherapy at M.D. Anderson Cancer Center. J Neuro-Oncol. 2006;80(2):177–83.
12. Tsai CJ, Wang Y, Allen PK, Mahajan A, McCutcheon IE, Rao G, et al. Outcomes after surgery and radiotherapy for spinal myxopapillary ependymoma: update of the MD Anderson Cancer Center experience. Neurosurgery. 2014;75(3):205–14; discussion 13–4.
13. Chao ST, Kobayashi T, Benzel E, Reddy CA, Stevens GH, Prayson RA, et al. The role of adjuvant radiation therapy in the treatment of spinal myxopapillary ependymomas. J Neurosurg Spine. 2011;14(1):59–64.
14. Schild SE, Wong W, Nisi K. In regard to the radiotherapy of myxopapillary ependymoma. Int J Radiat Oncol Biol Phys. 2002;53(3):787.
15. Yeboa DN, Liao KP, Guadagnolo BA, Rao G, Bishop A, Chung C, et al. National patterns of care in the management of World Health Organization Grade II and III Spinal Ependymomas. World Neurosurg. 2019;124:e580–94.
16. Ryu SM, Lee SH, Kim ES, Eoh W. Predicting survival of patients with spinal Ependymoma using machine learning algorithms with the SEER database. World Neurosurg. 2018;124:e331–39.
17. Shaw EG, Evans RG, Scheithauer BW, Ilstrup DM, Earle JD. Radiotherapeutic management of adult

intraspinal ependymomas. Int J Radiat Oncol Biol Phys. 1986;12(3):323–7.

18. Milano MT, Johnson MD, Sul J, Mohile NA, Korones DN, Okunieff P, et al. Primary spinal cord glioma: a surveillance, epidemiology, and end results database study. J Neuro-Oncol. 2010;98(1): 83–92.

19. Chamberlain MC, Tredway TL. Adult primary intradural spinal cord tumors: a review. Curr Neurol Neurosci Rep. 2011;11(3):320–8.

20. Raco A, Piccirilli M, Landi A, Lenzi J, Delfini R, Cantore G. High-grade intramedullary astrocytomas: 30 years' experience at the Neurosurgery Department of the University of Rome "Sapienza". J Neurosurg Spine. 2010;12(2):144–53.

21. Abdel-Wahab M, Etuk B, Palermo J, Shirato H, Kresl J, Yapicier O, et al. Spinal cord gliomas: a multi-institutional retrospective analysis. Int J Radiat Oncol Biol Phys. 2006;64(4):1060–71.

22. Minehan KJ, Brown PD, Scheithauer BW, Krauss WE, Wright MP. Prognosis and treatment of spinal cord astrocytoma. Int J Radiat Oncol Biol Phys. 2009;73(3):727–33.

23. Corradini S, Hadi I, Hankel V, Ertl L, Ganswindt U, Belka C, et al. Radiotherapy of spinal cord gliomas : a retrospective mono-institutional analysis. Strahlenther Onkol. 2016;192(3):139–45.

24. Dornbos D 3rd, Kim HJ, Butman JA, Lonser RR. Review of the neurological implications of von Hippel-Lindau disease. JAMA Neurol. 2018;75(5):620–7.

25. Maher ER, Yates JR, Ferguson-Smith MA. Statistical analysis of the two stage mutation model in von Hippel-Lindau disease, and in sporadic cerebellar haemangioblastoma and renal cell carcinoma. J Med Genet. 1990;27(5):311–4.

26. Yasargil MG, Antic J, Laciga R, de Preux J, Fideler RW, Boone SC. The microsurgical removal of intramedullary spinal hemangioblastomas. Report of twelve cases and a review of the literature. Surg Neurol. 1976;(3):141–8.

27. Smalley SR, Schomberg PJ, Earle JD, Laws ER Jr, Scheithauer BW, O'Fallon JR. Radiotherapeutic considerations in the treatment of hemangioblastomas of the central nervous system. Int J Radiat Oncol Biol Phys. 1990;18(5):1165–71.

28. Simone CB 2nd, Lonser RR, Ondos J, Oldfield EH, Camphausen K, Simone NL. Infratentorial craniospinal irradiation for von Hippel-Lindau: a retrospective study supporting a new treatment for patients with CNS hemangioblastomas. Neuro-Oncology. 2011;13(9):1030–6.

29. Li X, Wang J, Niu J, Hong J, Feng Y. Diagnosis and microsurgical treatment of spinal hemangioblastoma. Neurol Sci. 2016;37(6):899–906.

30. Hernandez-Duran S, Hanft S, Komotar RJ, Manzano GR. The role of stereotactic radiosurgery in the treatment of intramedullary spinal cord neoplasms: a systematic literature review. Neurosurg Rev. 2016;39(2):175–83; discussion 83

31. Chang SD, Meisel JA, Hancock SL, Martin DP, McManus M, Adler JR Jr. Treatment of hemangioblastomas in von Hippel-Lindau disease with linear accelerator-based radiosurgery. Neurosurgery. 1998;43(1):28–34; discussion -5

32. Daly ME, Choi CY, Gibbs IC, Adler JR Jr, Chang SD, Lieberson RE, et al. Tolerance of the spinal cord to stereotactic radiosurgery: insights from hemangioblastomas. Int J Radiat Oncol Biol Phys. 2011;80(1):213–20.

33. Ryu SI, Kim DH, Chang SD. Stereotactic radiosurgery for hemangiomas and ependymomas of the spinal cord. Neurosurg Focus. 2003;15(5):E10.

34. Chang UK, Rhee CH, Youn SM, Lee DH, Park SQ. Radiosurgery using the Cyberknife for benign spinal tumors: Korea Cancer Center Hospital experience. J Neuro-Oncol. 2011;101(1):91–9.

35. Pan J, Ho AL, D'Astous M, Sussman ES, Thompson PA, Tayag AT, et al. Image-guided stereotactic radiosurgery for treatment of spinal hemangioblastoma. Neurosurg Focus. 2017;42(1):E12.

36. Kalash R, Glaser SM, Flickinger JC, Burton S, Heron DE, Gerszten PC, et al. Stereotactic body radiation therapy for benign spine tumors: is dose de-escalation appropriate? J Neurosurg Spine. 2018;29(2):220–5.

37. Payer S, Mende KC, Westphal M, Eicker SO. Intramedullary spinal cord metastases: an increasingly common diagnosis. Neurosurg Focus. 2015;39(2):E15.

38. Sung WS, Sung MJ, Chan JH, Manion B, Song J, Dubey A, et al. Intramedullary spinal cord metastases: a 20-year institutional experience with a comprehensive literature review. World Neurosurg. 2013;79(3–4):576–84.

39. Vindlacheruvu RR, McEvoy AW, Kitchen ND. Intramedullary thoracic cord metastasis managed effectively without surgery. Clin Oncol (R Coll Radiol). 1997;9(5):343–5.

40. Schiff D, O'Neill BP. Intramedullary spinal cord metastases: clinical features and treatment outcome. Neurology. 1996;47(4):906–12.

41. Conill C, Marruecos J, Verger E, Berenguer J, Lomena F, Domingo-Domenech J, et al. Clinical outcome in patients with intramedullary spinal cord metastases from lung cancer. Clin Transl Oncol. 2007;9(3):172–6.

42. Lee SS, Kim MK, Sym SJ, Kim SW, Kim WK, Kim SB, et al. Intramedullary spinal cord metastases: a single-institution experience. J Neuro-Oncol. 2007;84(1):85–9.

43. Veeravagu A, Lieberson RE, Mener A, Chen YR, Soltys SG, Gibbs IC, et al. CyberKnife stereotactic radiosurgery for the treatment of intramedullary spinal cord metastases. J Clin Neurosci. 2012;19(9):1273–7.

44. Shin DA, Huh R, Chung SS, Rock J, Ryu S. Stereotactic spine radiosurgery for intradural and intramedullary metastasis. Neurosurg Focus. 2009;27(6):E10.

45. Kahn J, Loeffler JS, Niemierko A, Chiocca EA, Batchelor T, Chakravarti A. Long-term outcomes of patients with spinal cord gliomas treated by modern

conformal radiation techniques. Int J Radiat Oncol Biol Phys. 2011;81(1):232–8.

46. Choi SH, Yoon HI, Yi S, Park JW, Cho J, Shin DA, et al. Treatment outcomes of radiotherapy for primary spinal cord glioma. Strahlenther Onkol. 2019;195(2):164–74.

47. McLaughlin MP, Buatti JM, Marcus RB Jr, Maria BL, Mickle PJ, Kedar A. Outcome after radiotherapy of primary spinal cord glial tumors. Radiat Oncol Investig. 1998;6(6):276–80.

48. Santacroce A, Kamp MA, Budach W, Hanggi D. Radiobiology of radiosurgery for the central nervous system. Biomed Res Int. 2013;2013:362761.

49. Hamilton AJ, Lulu BA, Fosmire H, Stea B, Cassady JR. Preliminary clinical experience with linear accelerator-based spinal stereotactic radiosurgery. Neurosurgery. 1995;36(2):311–9.

50. Gerszten PC, Burton SA, Ozhasoglu C, Welch WC. Radiosurgery for spinal metastases: clinical experience in 500 cases from a single institution. Spine (Phila Pa 1976). 2007;32(2):193–9.

51. Ryu SI, Chang SD, Kim DH, Murphy MJ, Le QT, Martin DP, et al. Image-guided hypo-fractionated stereotactic radiosurgery to spinal lesions. Neurosurgery. 2001;49(4):838–46.

52. Gerszten PC, Quader M, Novotny J Jr, Flickinger JC. Radiosurgery for benign tumors of the spine: clinical experience and current trends. Technol Cancer Res Treat. 2012;11(2):133–9.

53. Dodd RL, Ryu MR, Kamnerdsupaphon P, Gibbs IC, Chang SD Jr, Adler JR Jr. CyberKnife radiosurgery for benign intradural extramedullary spinal tumors. Neurosurgery. 2006;58(4):674–85. discussion -85

54. Marchetti M, De Martin E, Milanesi I, Fariselli L. Intradural extramedullary benign spinal lesions radiosurgery. Medium- to long-term results from a single institution experience. Acta Neurochir. 2013;155(7):1215–22.

55. Chamberlain MC, Eaton KD, Fink JR, Tredway T. Intradural intramedullary spinal cord metastasis due to mesothelioma. J Neuro-Oncol. 2010;97(1):133–6.

56. Koga T, Morita A, Maruyama K, Tanaka M, Ino Y, Shibahara J, et al. Long-term control of disseminated pleomorphic xanthoastrocytoma with anaplastic features by means of stereotactic irradiation. Neuro-Oncology. 2009;11(4):446–51.

57. Lieberson RE, Veeravagu A, Eckermann JM, Doty JR, Jiang B, Andrews R, et al. Intramedullary spinal cord metastasis from prostate carcinoma: a case report. J Med Case Rep. 2012;6:139.

58. Parikh S, Heron DE. Fractionated radiosurgical management of intramedullary spinal cord metastasis: a case report and review of the literature. Clin Neurol Neurosurg. 2009;111(10):858–61.

59. Tseng CL, Sussman MS, Atenafu EG, Letourneau D, Ma L, Soliman H, et al. Magnetic resonance imaging assessment of spinal cord and cauda equina motion in supine patients with spinal metastases planned for spine stereotactic body radiation therapy. Int J Radiat Oncol Biol Phys. 2015;91(5):995–1002.

60. Hyde D, Lochray F, Korol R, Davidson M, Wong CS, Ma L, et al. Spine stereotactic body radiotherapy utilizing cone-beam CT image-guidance with a robotic couch: intrafraction motion analysis accounting for all six degrees of freedom. Int J Radiat Oncol Biol Phys. 2012;82(3):e555–62.

61. Thibault I, Chang EL, Sheehan J, Ahluwalia MS, Guckenberger M, Sohn MJ, et al. Response assessment after stereotactic body radiotherapy for spinal metastasis: a report from the SPIne response assessment in Neuro-Oncology (SPINO) group. Lancet Oncol. 2015;16(16):e595–603.

62. Kirkpatrick JP, Kelsey CR, Palta M, Cabrera AR, Salama JK, Patel P, et al. Stereotactic body radiotherapy: a critical review for nonradiation oncologists. Cancer. 2014;120(7):942–54.

63. Sharpe M, Brock KK. Quality assurance of serial 3D image registration, fusion, and segmentation. Int J Radiat Oncol Biol Phys. 2008;71(1 Suppl):S33–7.

64. Ma L, Sahgal A, Hossain S, Chuang C, Descovich M, Huang K, et al. Nonrandom intrafraction target motions and general strategy for correction of spine stereotactic body radiotherapy. Int J Radiat Oncol Biol Phys. 2009;75(4):1261–5.

65. Gerszten PC, Sahgal A, Sheehan JP, Kersh R, Chen S, Flickinger JC, et al. A multi-national report on methods for institutional credentialing for spine radiosurgery. Radiat Oncol. 2013;8:158.

66. Monserrate A, Zussman B, Ozpinar A, Niranjan A, Flickinger JC, Gerszten PC. Stereotactic radiosurgery for intradural spine tumors using cone-beam CT image guidance. Neurosurg Focus. 2017;42(1):E11.

67. Ding C, Chang CH, Haslam J, Timmerman R, Solberg T. A dosimetric comparison of stereotactic body radiation therapy techniques for lung cancer: robotic versus conventional linac-based systems. J Appl Clin Med Phys. 2010;11(3):3223.

68. Furweger C, Prins P, Coskan H, Heijmen BJ. Characteristics and performance of the first commercial multileaf collimator for a robotic radiosurgery system. Med Phys. 2016;43(5):2063.

69. Henke L, Kashani R, Robinson C, Curcuru A, DeWees T, Bradley J, et al. Phase I trial of stereotactic MR-guided online adaptive radiation therapy (SMART) for the treatment of oligometastatic or unresectable primary malignancies of the abdomen. Radiother Oncol. 2018;126(3):519–26.

70. Henke LE, Olsen JR, Contreras JA, Curcuru A, DeWees TA, Green OL, et al. Stereotactic MR-guided online adaptive radiation therapy (SMART) for ultracentral thorax malignancies: results of a phase 1 trial. Adv Radiat Oncol. 2019;4(1):201–9.

71. Yadav P, Musunuru HB, Witt JS, Bassetti M, Bayouth J, Baschnagel AM. Dosimetric study for spine stereotactic body radiation therapy: magnetic resonance guided linear accelerator versus volumetric modulated arc therapy. Radiol Oncol. 2019;53(3):362–8.

72. Pollard JM, Wen Z, Sadagopan R, Wang J, Ibbott GS. The future of image-guided radiotherapy will be MR guided. Br J Radiol. 2017;90(1073):20160667.

73. Schultheiss TE, Kun LE, Ang KK, Stephens LC. Radiation response of the central nervous system. Int J Radiat Oncol Biol Phys. 1995;31(5):1093–112.

74. Wong CS, Fehlings MG, Sahgal A. Pathobiology of radiation myelopathy and strategies to mitigate injury. Spinal Cord. 2015;53(8):574–80.

75. Kirkpatrick JP, van der Kogel AJ, Schultheiss TE. Radiation dose-volume effects in the spinal cord. Int J Radiat Oncol Biol Phys. 2010;76(3 Suppl):S42–9.

76. Schultheiss TE, Higgins EM, El-Mahdi AM. The latent period in clinical radiation myelopathy. Int J Radiat Oncol Biol Phys. 1984;10(7):1109–15.

77. Gerszten PC, Chen S, Quader M, Xu Y, Novotny J Jr, Flickinger JC. Radiosurgery for benign tumors of the spine using the synergy S with cone-beam computed tomography image guidance. J Neurosurg. 2012;117 Suppl:197–202.

78. Sahgal A, Weinberg V, Ma L, Chang E, Chao S, Muacevic A, et al. Probabilities of radiation myelopathy specific to stereotactic body radiation therapy to guide safe practice. Int J Radiat Oncol Biol Phys. 2013;85(2):341–7.

79. Thibault I, Campbell M, Tseng CL, Atenafu EG, Letourneau D, Yu E, et al. Salvage Stereotactic Body Radiotherapy (SBRT) following in-field failure of initial SBRT for spinal metastases. Int J Radiat Oncol Biol Phys. 2015;93(2):353–60.

80. Sahgal A, Ma L, Weinberg V, Gibbs IC, Chao S, Chang UK, et al. Reirradiation human spinal cord tolerance for stereotactic body radiotherapy. Int J Radiat Oncol Biol Phys. 2012;82(1):107–16.

81. Sahgal A, Chang JH, Ma L, Marks LB, Milano MT, Medin P, et al. Spinal cord dose tolerance to stereotactic body radiation therapy. Int J Radiat Oncol Biol Phys. 2019;In Press, Corrected proof.

82. Psimaras D, Tafani C, Ducray F, Leclercq D, et al. Bevacizumab in late-onset radiation-induced myelopathy. Neurology. 2016;86(5):454–7.

Part IV

New Age Surgical Approaches

Minimally Invasive Surgery for Intradural Tumors

10

R. Nick Hernandez, Sertac Kirnaz,
Franziska Schmidt, and Roger Härtl

Introduction

The traditional approach for resection of intradural spinal tumors is an open laminectomy. This approach provides a wide, bilateral exposure to the spinal column. However, in order to achieve this exposure, the surgeon must strip the bilateral musculature from the posterior bony anatomy and disrupt the posterior ligamentous complex. Other potential detrimental effects are disruption of the facet joint complex and potential for disconnection of the pars interarticularis. Such an exposure can result in significant postoperative pain and iatrogenic instability. Minimally invasive spine surgery (MISS) has gained increasing popularity and use over the past two decades. Since the introduction of the tubular retractor and microendoscopic discectomy (MED) by Foley and Smith in 1997 [1], and with the subsequent application of the microscope in 2002 by Palmer [2, 3], MISS approaches utilizing tubular retractors have been applied to all levels of the spinal canal for the performance of microdiscectomy, laminectomy, foraminotomy, and fusions [4].

The philosophy of MISS is to minimize trauma to and disruption of the native anatomy. In this manner, MISS aims to leave the smallest operative footprint possible, while still achieving the same operative goals as traditional open approaches. The hypothesized advantages of such MISS techniques over open procedures include decreased postoperative pain and less postoperative narcotic use, faster recovery and return to daily activity, shorter hospitalization, less intraoperative blood loss, smaller incisions, fewer overall complications, and less iatrogenic instability. In fact, each of these hypothesized advantages has been demonstrated in the scientific literature [4]. The use of tubular retractors to access the spinal column has already expanded its use to include resection of intradural spinal tumors, as will be discussed in this chapter. Even prior to the advent of the tubular retractor, in the 1980s and early 1990s, Eggert and colleagues [5, 6] and Yasargil et al. [7] reported a less invasive hemilaminectomy approach for resection of both intradural extramedullary (IDEM) and intramedullary (IM) spinal tumors and noted patients who underwent the less invasive hemilaminectomy experienced fewer complications and shorter hospital stays than patients who underwent a traditional open laminectomy [6]. A key concept of MISS is achieving bilateral decompression via a unilateral laminotomy, thus providing an exposure to the spinal canal similar to that described by Eggert and Yasargil. In this chapter, we will

R. N. Hernandez (✉)
Neurosurgery, Rutgers New Jersey Medical School, Newark, NJ, USA

S. Kirnaz · F. Schmidt · R. Härtl
Neurological Surgery, Weill Cornell Brain and Spine Center, New York-Presbyterian Hospital, Weill Cornell Medicine, New York, NY, USA

© Springer Nature Switzerland AG 2021
S. Hanft, P. C. McCormick (eds.), *Tumors of the Spinal Canal*,
https://doi.org/10.1007/978-3-030-55096-7_10

discuss our technique for resection of intradural spinal tumors using a tubular retractor and discuss the MISS outcomes as reported in the literature.

Indications

The indications for surgical resection of intradural tumors are addressed in a separate chapter. We will focus this discussion on how to select a patient for MISS once the decision to operate has been made. Patient selection is of the utmost importance for the success of MISS techniques. As such, a thorough patient history and physical examination and careful study of the imaging are necessary to identify patients who will benefit from an MISS approach versus a traditional open approach. Workup should include advanced imaging, which at minimum should include magnetic resonance imaging (MRI) with and without contrast to evaluate the tumor. For tumors that extend laterally into or out of the foramen, if one is planning for complete resection, necessitating facetectomy and posterolateral fusion, we also recommend obtaining standing AP and lateral XR and computed tomography (CT) scan.

We consider two main factors when making the determination on a tubular retractor approach versus an open approach: tumor size and tumor location. In our practice, we utilize non-expandable (or fixed diameter) tubular retractors of at least 24 mm diameter for intradural tumor resection. There also exist a variety of expandable retractors that, when expanded, offer a larger operative corridor; however, this comes at the expense of greater trauma to the surrounding tissues. One must consider the exposure one can obtain through tubular retractors prior to choosing an MISS technique for tumor resection. When considering the size of a tumor amenable to an MISS approach, tumors that can be accessed via a single level laminotomy and that fit within the diameter of the tubular retractor are ideal. "Wanding" of a non-expandable tubular retractor or expansion of an expandable tubular retractor allow the surgeon a larger area that can be accessed, but if a tumor measures greater than

3 cm in diameter, this is likely quite difficult to access via a single tubular retractor port. We, therefore, would not select a tumor larger than 3 cm in diameter for resection through a tubular retractor. Similarly, multiple other groups performing intradural tumor resection through tubular retractors (expandable and non-expandable) report they would not apply MISS approaches to tumors spanning more than 2 vertebral segments [8–11].

The location of a tumor is also crucial for selecting an MISS approach to ensure safe resection and minimal risk of nerve or spinal cord injury. Location refers to both the location of the tumor within the thecal sac (e.g., dorsal, dorsolateral, lateral, ventrolateral, ventral) and the level of the spinal column (e.g., cervical, thoracic, lumbosacral). Tumors of the lumbosacral spine below the conus medullaris can be accessed regardless of the location within the thecal sac as there is no concern regarding spinal cord manipulation. IDEM tumors within the cervical and thoracic spine require a greater degree of preoperative examination. Small IDEM tumors located dorsal or dorsolateral may be considered for an MISS approach; however, it is our preference to perform open resection when operating at the level of the spinal cord to minimize any risk of injury to normal spinal cord tissue. Tumors that lie ventral are not recommended to be resected via an MISS approach due to concerns regarding manipulation of the spinal cord in order to access and resect the tumor. These tumors are more safely approached using an open technique to allow the surgeon a wide lateral-to-medial working trajectory to avoid spinal cord injury and permanent neurologic deficit. There do exist in the literature reports of MISS resection of cervical and thoracic IDEM tumors, at all locations within the thecal sac; however, in our practice, we would not select such tumors for an MISS approach.

With regard to IM tumors, it is not our practice to perform resection through a tubular retractor due to the limited space for maneuvering instruments within the spinal cord safely and the higher risk of inadvertent injury to normal spinal cord tissue. Additionally, some key instruments that assist with IM tumor resection, such as ultrasonic aspiration for tumor resection and ultrasound for lesion localization, do not fit within the operative corridor afforded by the non-expandable tubular retractors we utilize. Again, however, there are surgeons who are performing intramedullary tumor resection via MISS approaches and we will mention these in our discussion of the literature.

Instrumentation

There are several instruments that are critical for resection of intradural spine tumors through a tubular retractor listed below. In general, extended, bayoneted instruments are required when working down the surgical corridor afforded by the tubular retractor to allow adequate visualization of the target anatomy.

- Non-expandable tubular retractor set, 24 mm or greater tubular diameter (Fig. 10.1).
- Bayoneted instruments (Fig. 10.2).
- Curved, extended shaft, high-speed drill (we utilize a matchstick drill bit with a blunt tip) (Fig. 10.3).
- Bayoneted bipolar electrocautery.
- Operative microscope.
- MIS dural closure set (will be discussed later in the chapter; Fig. 10.10a).

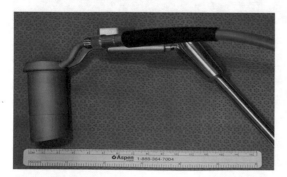

Fig. 10.1 Photograph of a non-expandable (fixed diameter) tubular retractor attached to the rigid table arm. A light source can be attached to the tubular retractor for illumination, or, as we utilize, the operative microscope is used for magnification and illumination

Intraoperative neuromonitoring (IOM) is utilized for all intradural tumors regardless if approached via MISS versus open. For IDEM tumors at the level of the spinal cord, motor evoked potentials (MEPs), somatosensory evoked potentials (SSEPs), and triggered electromyography (tEMG) are utilized. For lumbar tumors below the level of the conus medullaris, only tEMG is used. For IM tumors, MEPs, SSEPs, and epidural MEP (D-wave) are utilized.

Surgical Technique

All intradural spinal tumors are accessed via a unilateral laminotomy through a tubular retractor. Our technique for unilateral laminotomy for bilateral decompression has been previously described and will be summarized in this chapter [12, 13]. There are many types of tubular retractors on the market, including specular retractors, expandable blade retractors, expandable tubular retractors, and non-expandable (or fixed diameter) tubular retractors. As mentioned above, our technique utilizes a non-expandable tubular retractor of at least 24 mm in diameter. In general, the microsurgical principles and techniques for the definitive tumor resection are consistent between MISS and open procedures. It is the approach and dural exposure and dural closure that must be adapted for MISS.

Localization/Incision

Localization of the target level is a critical portion of any MISS procedure and must not be overlooked. The orientation afforded by the surrounding anatomy visualized in open procedures is not present through the narrow working corridor of a tubular retractor, and thus one must place more reliance on intraoperative imaging for localization and orientation. The two methods for intraoperative localization are fluoroscopy and/or computer assisted navigation (CAN). Using fluoroscopy, a metal instrument is placed perpendicular to the patient's spine and lateral fluoroscopy is used to identify the target level. Alternatively, if

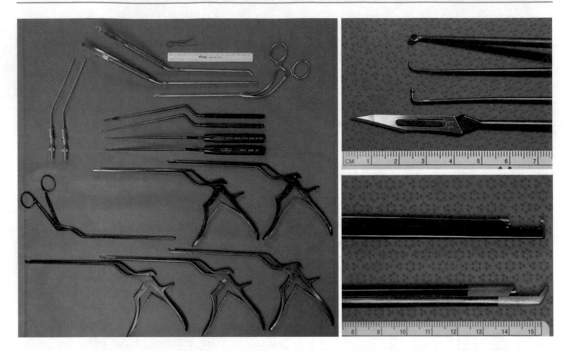

Fig. 10.2 Photograph of instruments used for procedures through the tubular retractor. Note the instruments are bayonetted to allow visualization down the tubular retractor when working

Fig. 10.3 Photograph of the curved, extended drill with a matchstick drill tip

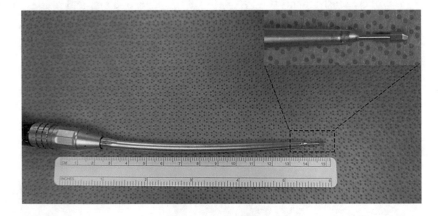

CAN is available, an intraoperative CT (or 3D fluoroscopy depending on the system) is obtained and merged with a preoperative MRI. The navigated probe is then used for incision localization. The incision should be centered directly over the midpoint of the tumor. A linear incision is marked 2 cm to the left or right of midline, depending upon the eccentricity of the tumor (e.g., if the tumor is eccentric to left, then a left-sided incision is used). A 15-blade scalpel is used to make a linear incision and monopolar electrocautery is used to dissect through the soft tissue until fascia

is encountered. The fascia is incised sharply using the 15-blade to facilitate closure at the conclusion of the case.

Serial Dilation and Tubular Retractor Placement

The first dilator is passed through the incised fascia and paraspinal musculature directly onto the lamina. We never use K-wires for laminar docking at any spinal level. Using the dilator, one

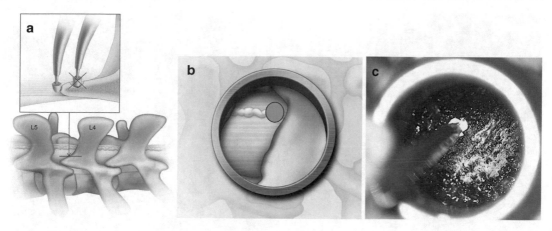

Fig. 10.4 Illustrations (**a**, **b**) and intraoperative photograph (**c**) depicting the starting point for bony drilling in the lumbar spine. Note the drill tip rests atop the ligamen-tum flavum just caudal to the target lamina and drilling proceeds cranially using the side-cutting surface of the drill bit

should palpate the base of the spinous process and inferior edge of the lamina. Medial-lateral and cranial-caudal sweeping of the first dilator is performed to scrape soft tissue away from the bone. Dilators of sequentially enlarging diameter are then passed to the desired final diameter. A twisting motion should be performed when passing each dilator to facilitate muscle fiber splitting. The tubular retractor depth is determined by depth marks on the side of the final dilator and the desired diameter retractor is passed, again using a twisting motion. The tubular retractor is then secured in place with the rigid table arm. The tube diameter should be determined by measurement of the tumor diameter on sagittal MRI, ideally measuring at least a few millimeters larger than the tumor diameter. We typically use a 24 mm or greater diameter tube. Fluoroscopy or CAN is used to confirm the retractor has been docked at the correct level prior to bony drilling. At this point, the microscope is brought into the field. The extended tip monopolar electrocautery is used to remove any remaining soft tissue to expose the bony surfaces of the target spinous process base and lamina.

Laminotomy

Once the anatomy has been clearly defined, drilling begins atop the ligamentum flavum (LF) just caudal to the junction of the spinous process and inferior edge of the lamina to be removed. This starting point is a key technical point for efficiency of the bony decompression. The match-stick drill bit used for drilling has a blunt tip that can safely rest atop the LF, while the side-cutting edges remove the bone (Fig. 10.4). The drilling proceeds cranially to identify the cranial attachment of the LF, indicated by the presence of epidural fat. The LF is left intact during drilling to act as a protective layer from dural injury (Fig. 10.5a). Once epidural fat is identified, a Kerrison rongeur is used to remove the remainder of the thinned lamina until dura is identified. Drilling also extends laterally to expose the ipsilateral leaflet of the LF. Care should be taken not to violate the pars interarticularis and to avoid excessive drilling of the medial ipsilateral facet to avoid iatrogenic instability. A ball-tip probe is used to strip the ipsilateral leaflet of LF from its cranial attachment (Fig. 10.5b). The ipsilateral and contralateral leaflets of LF are divided in the midline by epidural fat and can be defined with the ball-tip probe. A Kerrison rongeur is used to resect the ipsilateral LF, exposing the underlying dura. The LF should be resected from its cranial attachment to its caudal attachment. Bony drilling can extend cranially or caudally as needed for adequate exposure of the intradural tumor. The tubular retractor is then "wanded" medially (e.g., away from the surgeon) and the operating table is

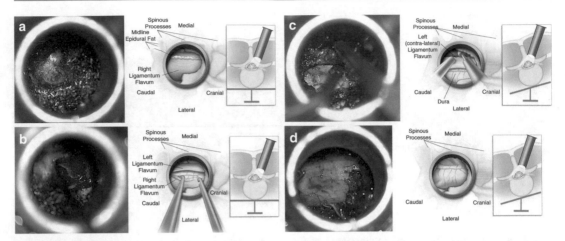

Fig. 10.5 Intraoperative photographs and illustrations depicting the steps for bilateral decompression via unilateral laminotomy through a tubular retractor in the lumbar spine. (**a**) The bony drilling has been completed, exposing the underlying ligamentum flavum (LF). (**b**) A ball-tip probe is used to strip the LF from its bony attachments and define the midline raphe between leaflets of the LF. (**c**) Contralateral drilling of the lamina atop the contralateral LF. D) Final exposure of the dura

tilted away from the surgeon to perform the contralateral laminotomy. A ball-tip probe is used to create a plane between the contralateral LF and the dura. A number 9 metal suction tip is used to retract the dura away from the LF, while drilling begins at the base of the spinous process and continues in a medial to lateral direction. In the lumbar spine, this retraction can be liberal. The ventral aspect of the contralateral lamina is then drilled away. Once again, the LF is left intact to serve as a protective layer from dural injury (Fig. 10.5c). One may drill the contralateral lamina directly atop the LF, or, alternatively, one may drill a trough into the contralateral lamina leaving a thin rim of bone atop the LF, which can be removed later with an upgoing curette. Drilling extends contralaterally until the LF in the lateral recess is encountered. Drilling in the cranial-caudal direction extends until the cranial and caudal attachments of LF are identified and can continue as needed to obtain wide enough exposure to encompass the intradural tumor. A ball-tip probe is used to create a plane between the LF and dura and Kerrison rongeurs are used to resect the contralateral LF. The decompression is extended in the cranial-caudal direction until adequate exposure of the thecal sac is achieved (Fig. 10.5d). The tubular retractor is then "wan-

ded" laterally (e.g., toward the surgeon) and the operating table is returned to the neutral position.

Intradural Extramedullary Tumor Resection

Once adequate exposure of the dura is obtained, tumor resection proceeds in a similar fashion to that of an open procedure with two notable exceptions. The first is that ultrasonic aspiration will be limited or impossible through a non-expandable tubular retractor, unless the current devices are modified for MISS approaches (e.g., bayonetted or curved with a slim, extended shaft to allow surgeon visualization). The second is that ultrasound for tumor localization prior to dural opening is not possible with a non-expandable tubular retractor because the ultrasound cannot physically fit down the tubular retractor. This is where CAN alone, or with the use of augmented reality, which will be discussed later in this chapter, can be useful. Once the dura is opened, the same microsurgical principles used for traditional open resection of intradural tumors apply. An illustrative case of an L3-L4 intradural schwannoma is presented (Fig. 10.6). The dura is

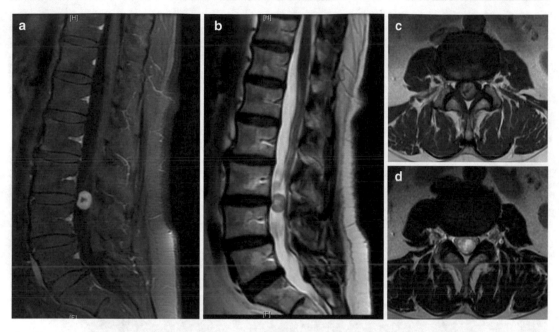

Fig. 10.6 Preoperative MR images demonstrating an intradural extramedullary tumor localized to the L3-L4 level. (**a**) Sagittal T1-weighted with contrast. (**b**) Sagittal T2-weighted. (**c**) Axial T1-weighted with contrast. (**d**) Axial T2-weighted

opened sharply in the midline with an 11-blade on a long handle (Fig. 10.8a) after CAN was used to confirm the location of the tumor at the level of the dura (Fig. 10.7). A blunt tip nerve hook is inserted under the dura and used to extend the dural opening cranially and caudally. Dural tack-ups are placed (Fig. 10.8b). The arachnoid is opened and the tumor is identified (Fig. 10.8c). The cranial and caudal nerve rootlet attachments are identified (Figs. 10.8d, f and 10.9a) and stimulated with tEMG (Fig. 10.9a) to rule out any motor rootlet involvement. If the rootlet is silent (i.e., sensory), bipolar electrocautery is used to cauterize the rootlet at its entry into the tumor (Figs. 10.8e and 10.9b) and it is incised sharply with microscissors. The tumor can then be delivered from the surgical bed (Fig. 10.9f) and the resection cavity is inspected (Fig. 10.9c). In the rare instance when the rootlet has motor function according to tEMG, we attempt to dissect it away from the tumor. If the rootlet cannot be dissected from the tumor, a small amount of residual tumor is left attached to the motor rootlet. Meningiomas are dissected away from any neural tissue attachments and, as able, from the dura. The involved dura is coagulated, not resected. If there is any

trouble manipulating the tumor within the thecal sac or delivering from the surgical bed, one may internally debulk the tumor, staying within the tumor capsule to protect the surrounding neural elements.

Intramedullary Tumor Resection

Safe and effective tumor resection should always be the paramount goal of surgery. Therefore, the threshold to perform resection of an IM spinal cord tumor through an MISS approach should be much higher. Concern includes the limited ability to maneuver within the spinal canal safely and the higher risk of inadvertent injury to normal spinal cord tissue. Additionally, ultrasound cannot be used to determine the exact location of dural opening or midline myelotomy because the ultrasound cannot fit down the tubular retractor. Another hurdle to adopting MISS techniques for IM tumor resection is that current ultrasonic aspiration devices on the market are not amenable to MISS as the current designs do not allow surgeon visualization down the tubular retractor while using the devices. One may consider resec-

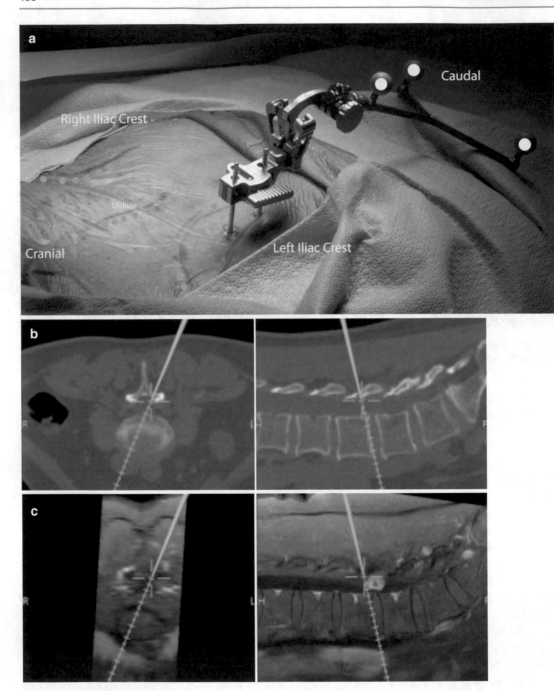

Fig. 10.7 (a) Photograph of the computer-assisted navigation (CAN) reference array secured to the patient's iliac crest. (b, c) Screenshots from the computer navigation system demonstrating real-time navigation of an intraoperative CT (b) merged to the preoperative MRI (c) for tumor localization at the level of the dura

tion of small lesions or biopsies using MISS techniques; however, for the abovementioned reasons, we generally prefer open laminectomy for IM tumors.

Dural Closure

A hesitation of many surgeons to adopting MISS approaches to intradural tumors is the dural clo-

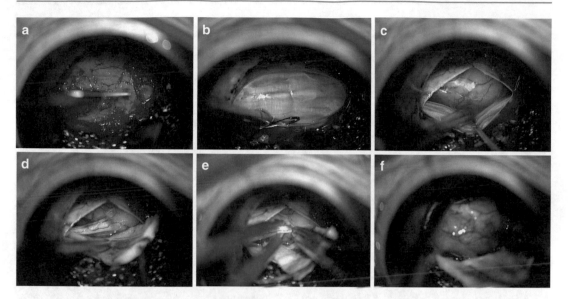

Fig. 10.8 Intraoperative photographs. (a) An 11-blade is used to make the durotomy. (b) Dural tack-ups are placed. (c) The arachnoid is dissected to expose the tumor. (d) The cranial rootlet entering the tumor is identified and (e) coagulated. (f) The tumor is mobilized into the dorsal aspect of the spinal canal

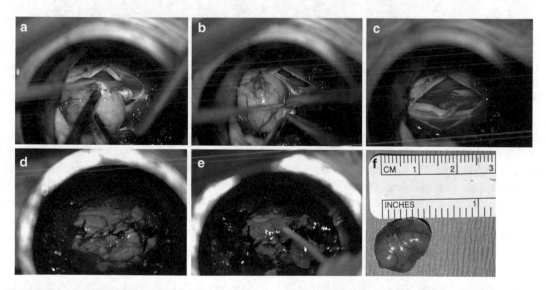

Fig. 10.9 Intraoperative photographs. (a) The caudal rootlet is identified and stimulated and (b) coagulated. (c) Gross total resection of the tumor. (d) The dura has been closed using a running 4–0 neurolon suture. (e) Fibrin sealant is applied over the suture line. F) Gross specimen

sure. While the task may seem daunting to those who are just adopting MISS techniques, with the correct instruments, dural closure is easily achieved. Prior to dural closure, strict hemostasis within the intradural space must be achieved and any blood within the intradural space should be irrigated out. The instruments necessary for dural closure through a non-expandable tubular retractor must be extended and bayoneted. Tan et al., described the use of a modified needle driver, bayoneted knot pusher, modified suture scissors, and fibrin glue to achieve primary dural closure

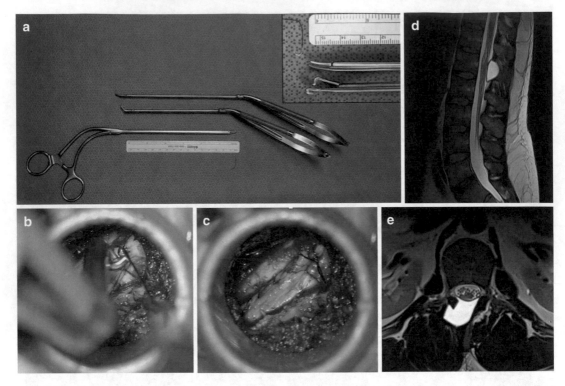

Fig. 10.10 (**a**) The Scanlan dural closure instruments including a needle holder, knot pusher, and microscissors. The 4-0 Nurolon fishhook needle is visualized in the upper right panel. (**b**) The knot pusher is used to tie the suture. (**c**) Final dural closure. (**d, e**) T2-weighted MRI demonstrating a small pseudomeningocele. Note the fluid collection is "sealed" within the surgical cavity by the paraspinal muscle fibers that fall back into place after the muscle-splitting tubular retractor is removed

after intended durotomy with no instances of symptomatic pseudomeningocele in a case series of 23 patients [14]. We have adopted a similar technique for dural closure using the SCANLAN® minimally invasive dural closure kit (Scanlan International, Inc., St. Paul, MN, USA; Fig. 10.10a) and reported our technique for unintended lumbar durotomy using a 4–0 Nurolon® TF-5 (Ethicon, Inc., Somerville, NJ, USA) "fishhook" running, locked suture (Fig. 10.9d) [12]. However, we noticed that due to the larger needle diameter relative to thread diameter, there can be continued CSF egress even after primary closure. More recently, we have been utilizing with success the CV-5 GORE-TEX® suture (Gore Medical, Flagstaff, AZ, USA), which has a thread diameter that more closely approximates the needle diameter. The modified needle driver is used to suture the dura in a running, locked fashion (Fig. 10.10c) and the knot pusher is used to

tightly lock down the suture knots (Fig. 10.10b). A Valsalva maneuver is then performed and any points of significant CSF egress are addressed with additional suture or muscle patch. Fibrin sealant is then applied over the suture line (Fig. 10.9e). Postoperatively, we keep patients on flat bedrest overnight (<24 hours) with early mobilization the morning following surgery. Patients are monitored for signs of CSF leakage, such as positional headache, nausea, vomiting, or blurry vision. In our experience, the rate of symptomatic pseudomeningocele is extremely low. We believe this can be attributed to the minimally invasive, muscle fiber splitting approach that maintains the paraspinal musculature attachments intact. Upon removal of the tubular retractor, the split muscle fibers fall back into place, thus "sealing" the surgical bed. If there does happen to be a small CSF leak, we have found that the muscular layer functions to contain the small pseudomeningocele (Fig. 10.10d, e). In contrast, with an open approach, the musculature is stripped from its attachments to the bony anatomy, creating dead space into which CSF can egress to the fascial layer.

Closure

The tubular retractor is removed slowly under direct visualization and any bleeding from the soft tissue is addressed with bipolar electrocautery. We ensure adequate hemostasis as we do not use subfascial drains in the wound. The fascia is closed in a water-tight fashion followed by dermal stitches and a subcutaneous stitch for the skin.

Complication Avoidance/Technical Considerations

There are several technical points to consider when planning for a tubular tumor resection that will aid in realizing the surgical goal and avoid complications.

Conversion to an Open Approach

MISS approaches for IDEM tumors are safe and effective. However, if there is an unforeseen complication during surgery or if the surgery becomes more challenging than expected, one should not hesitate to convert an MISS approach to an open approach. The safety and outcome of the patient must be the priority. This may be especially applicable as a surgeon is overcoming the learning curve of MISS techniques.

Iatrogenic Instability

At the upper lumbar segments (e.g., L1-L2, L2-L3, L3-L4), the lamina are less wide, the facet joints are in a more sagittal orientation, and the pars interarticularis is thinner compared to the lower segments (e.g., L4-L5, L5-S1). Therefore, to avoid iatrogenic instability of the upper lumbar segments, the incision should be placed more medially (about 1 cm from the midline versus 2–3 cm) and the tubular retractor should be ori-

ented more vertically to avoid excessive ipsilateral facet removal or pars violation. One must be cognizant of the part interarticularis in the lumbar spine to avoid disconnection and resultant iatrogenic instability.

Intraoperative Localization

Localization of the correct level is a critical portion of any spine procedure, but it is especially important in MISS to facilitate the goals of surgery and avoid complications [15]. This can be accomplished in the simplest way with fluoroscopy. This task is relatively straightforward in the lumbar spine where one counts up from the sacrum. If a surgeon is considering an MISS approach for a cervical or thoracic tumor, localization in the upper cervical spine is straightforward with fluoroscopy counting down from C2, but can be challenging in the lower cervical and thoracic spine, depending upon body habitus, anatomic variations, and bone quality. As part of the preoperative workup, one should obtain imaging to facilitate intraoperative localization. Identification of any bony abnormalities that could complicate localization should be identified. This includes radiographic examination of the lumbosacral spine (e.g., lumbarized S1, sacralized L5) and ribs (e.g., number of ribs). Alternatively, if CAN is available, the task of target localization becomes much easier. Nevertheless, when utilizing CAN, one must be cognizant of the anatomy and correlate the gross anatomy to what is being relayed by the CAN system. If there is any concern regarding accuracy of the CAN system, one must take steps to verify the correct level.

Augmented Reality

As CAN technology advances, we have begun implementing augmented reality (AR) into our operative workflow. Figure 10.11 provides an illustrative case of a sacral schwannoma resected using AR technology. A preoperative MRI with contrast is merged with the intraoperative CT (Fig. 10.12). The CAN system, using a patient reference array and a reference array attached to the operative microscope, can then project a computer-generated representation of the tumor

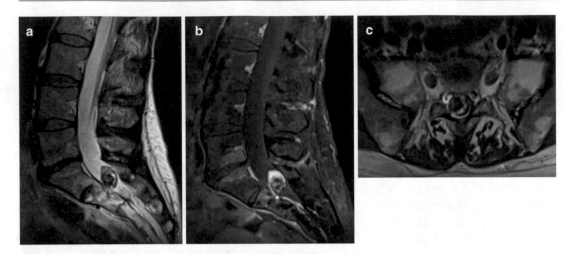

Fig. 10.11 Preoperative MR images demonstrating an IDEM tumor at S1-S2. (**a**) Sagittal T2-weighted. (**b**) Sagittal T1-weighted with contrast. (**c**) Axial T2-weighted

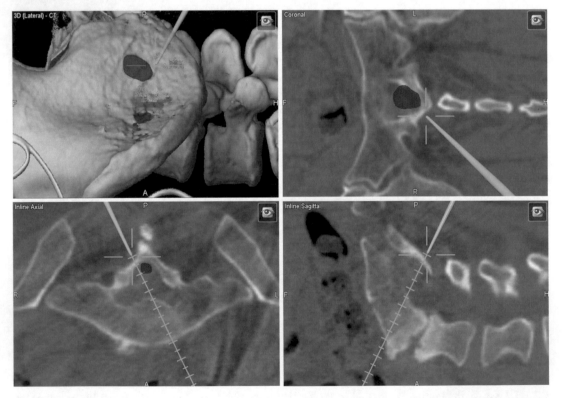

Fig. 10.12 Screenshot of the computer-assisted navigation display demonstrating the location of the tumor by merging the preoperative MRI to an intraoperative CT and overlaying the tumor onto the CT

onto the operative view through the optics of the microscope (Fig. 10.13). In this manner, the surgeon can identify the location of the tumor throughout the case and perform exactly the bony removal and dural opening required for resection. This aids to further facilitate a key aspect of MISS: leave the smallest operative footprint possible. This technology may substitute for intraoperative ultrasound and, therefore, may be particularly attractive for surgeons who would

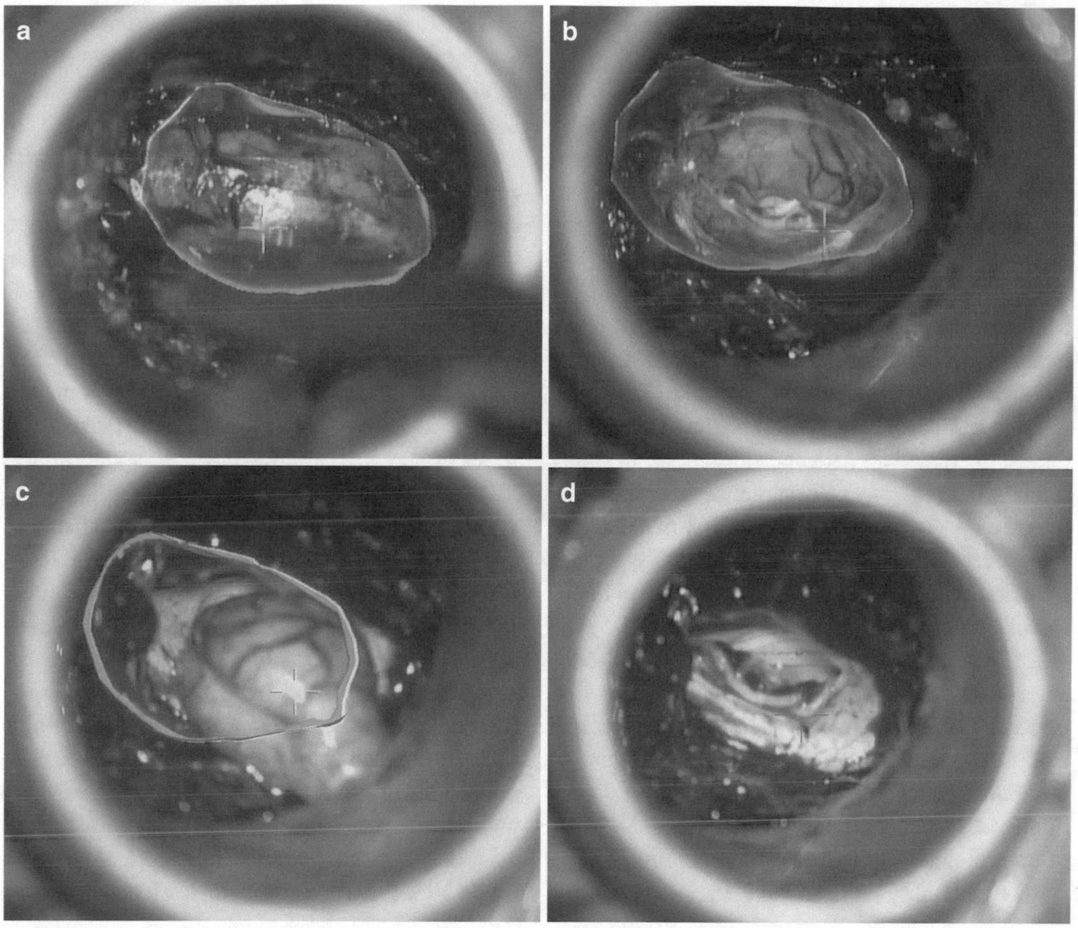

Fig. 10.13 Intraoperative photographs demonstrating the augmented reality display through the optics of the microscope. (**a**) The dura is exposed and an overlay of the tumor is displayed, identifying the location of the tumor within the intradural space. (**b**) The dura has been opened and the tumor can be grossly visualized with the AR overlay. (**c**) The tumor has been dissected and is being delivered from the cavity. (**d**) Gross total resection

like to adopt MISS techniques but are hesitant to do so due to the inability to reliably use ultrasound through a tubular retractor for tumor localization prior to dural opening.

Outcomes According to the Literature

The application of MISS techniques for intradural tumor resection began with open, unilateral hemilaminectomy approaches in the 1980s and early 1990s [5–7]. These studies demonstrated that tumor resection through a unilateral approach was safe and effective. More recently, Turel and colleagues reported on 164 patients who underwent unilateral hemilaminectomy for IDEM tumor resection with good results. GTR was achieved in 92% of cases with a complication rate of 4.9% (3 patients with symptomatic CSF leak, 5 patients with worse spasticity/power postoperatively) [16]. Pompili et al. examined 77 patients who underwent the same approach for spinal meningiomas and schwannomas. GTR was achieved in 98.7% of cases with a complication rate of 3.9% (2 pseudomeningoceles requiring reoperation, 1 patient with worsened motor deficit postoperatively) [17].

This approach, however, still requires subperiosteal stripping of the unilateral musculature from the bony attachments. The use of a tubular retractor allows for splitting of the muscle fibers, while leaving the muscular attachments intact and achieves the same hemilaminectomy exposure afforded by the above-mentioned open hemilaminectomy technique. There are numerous reports in the literature on MISS approaches using tubular retractors primarily for IDEM spinal tumors [9, 10, 14, 15, 18–29]. These reports demonstrate that MISS techniques are both as safe and as effective relative to traditional open approaches, with complication rates ranging from 0% to 18.2% and GTR rates ranging from 66.6% to 100%. Of these studies, the largest examined 83 patients with intradural spinal tumors, including 49 schwannomas, 18 meningiomas, 10 ependymomas, and 6 tumors of other histology, treated with either an expandable tubular retractor or specular retractor. A single level hemilaminectomy was adequate for exposure in 75% of cases, whereas the remaining 25% required two-level hemilaminectomy. GTR was achieved in 87% of patients. The surgery-related complication rate was 11%, including 2 CSF leaks, 1 asymptomatic pseudomeningocele, 2 superficial surgical site infections, 1 venous sinus thrombosis, and 4 cases of neurologic deterioration postoperatively. The surgical mortality rate was 0% [10].

The literature on MISS techniques for IM tumors is more sparse, and many of the studies that do include IM tumors are case series examining predominantly IDEM tumors with a few IM tumors interspersed [9, 10, 20, 22, 29]. Ogden and Fessler described the resection of a thoracic ependymoma via expandable tubular retractor with a good outcome (Fig. 10.14) [30]. Soriano-Sánchez and colleagues described their case series and technique for intradural tumor resection utilizing non-expandable tubular retractors, which included a cervical hemangioblastoma and a thoracic astrocytoma [29]. The largest reported series of an MISS approach for IM spinal tumors examined 18 patients with hemangioblastomas. The authors utilized either a non-expandable or expandable tubular retractor to achieve a 100% GTR rate on follow-up MRI obtained within 1 year after surgery. One patient (5.5%) developed worsening neurologic symptoms that did not improve during follow-up [28].

While there are several case series describing MISS techniques for intradural spinal tumors, there are very few studies that directly compare MISS to traditional open approaches. The studies that do exist only report on IDEM tumors. Lee and colleagues examined 6 patients treated via tubular

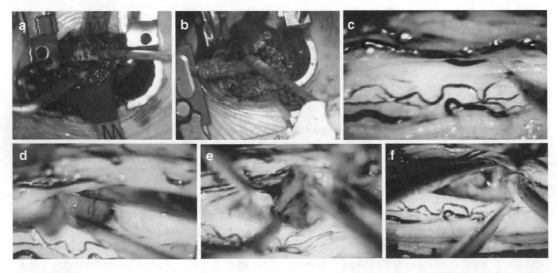

Fig. 10.14 Minimally invasive resection of a thoracic ependymoma utilizing an expandable tubular retractor. Intraoperative images. (**a**) subperiosteal dissection; (**b**) contralateral osseous exposure; (**c**) midline myelotomy; (**d**) tumor dissection, caudal pole; (**e**) tumor removal; (**f**) inspection of resection bed. (With permission from Ogden AT and Fessler RG. Minimally invasive resection of intramedullary ependymoma: case report. Neurosurgery 2009;65:E1203-E1204)

retractor, 25 patients via open unilateral hemilaminectomy, and 18 patients via traditional open laminectomy, with the tubular retractor and unilateral
hemilaminectomy cohorts grouped together into
the "MISS" label. While this combined MISS label
does not represent a true, muscle preserving MISS
approach, they reported shorter operative time, less
blood loss, and shorter hospital length of stay

(LOS) in the MISS group compared to the open
group. A limitation of this study is that the MISS
mean tumor size was significantly smaller than that
of the open cohort [23]. Mummaneni has reported
his experience using a transspinous mini-open
approach for intradural spinal pathology
(Fig. 10.15) [24, 31, 32]. In their most recent publication examining this topic, the authors compared

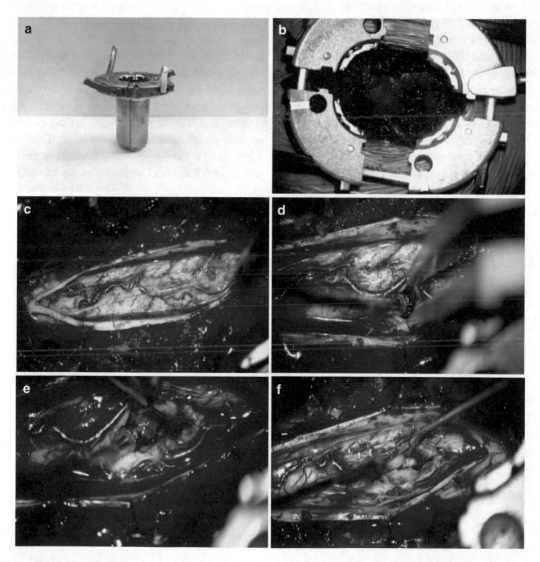

Fig. 10.15 Minimally invasive transspinous approach
for resection of a spinal cavernous malformation. (**a, b**)
The tubular retractor system utilized is 6 cm in depth and
2.5 cm wide. With expansion, the retractor system may
reach lesions up to 9 cm deep and provides a surgical corridor which is 5 cm in width. This provides sufficient dorsal midline visualization to perform a multilevel
laminectomy for intradural pathologies up to 3-spinal segments (image, lamina of T11 & T12; (**b**)). (**c**) Following
dural opening, a dorsal developmental venous anomaly

was noted. Just lateral to the vein a small hemosiderin
blush was observed. (**d**) A small subcentimeter myelotomy was made over the hemosiderin staining and the
hematoma cavity was entered. Blood products were
removed with gentle suction. (**e**) After evacuation of the
hematoma, the cavernous malformation was visualized
and carefully removed with sharp dissection and a pitu-
itary rongeur. (**f**) Apparent gross total resection of the cavernous malformation and of the intramedullary hematoma.
(With permission from Winkler et al. [35])

25 patients with IDEM tumors treated via the mini-open approach to 26 patients treated via an open laminectomy. They found no difference in operative time, extent of resection, hospital LOS, ASIA score improvement, or complication or recurrence rates. The mini-open group had less blood compared to the open cohort. CSF leak or pseudomeningocele was encountered in 1 (4%) mini-open patient and in 3 (11.5%) open patients [31]. Wong et al. examined 27 patients treated via expandable tubular retractors and 18 patients treated via open approach for IDEM tumors. The authors similarly discovered no difference in operative time, complication or reoperation rates, or extent of resection between the groups with less blood loss and shorter hospital LOS in the MISS group. Interestingly, while the dural closure may seem more challenging in MISS approaches due to the narrow working corridor, there was a significantly greater rate of postoperative CSF leak in the open group (16.6%) compared to the MISS group (3.7%) [25]. Lastly, in a cost savings analysis, Fontes et al. compared MISS to open resection of IDEM tumors in a group of 35 patients (17 MISS, 18 open). There were no differences between the groups in operative time, blood loss, complications, or rate of CSF leak. The MISS patients had mean shorter ICU and floor stays relative to patients treated via open approaches [26]. While the N of these studies is relatively small, limiting the conclusions that can be taken away from the publications individually, these studies, taken together, at least support that MISS approaches for intradural spinal tumors are as safe and effective as traditional open approaches. Larger studies that directly compare MISS to open approaches are needed to better quantify the advantages and disadvantages of MISS in this patient population. Table 10.1 summarizes the abovemen-

Table 10.1 Studies comparing MISS approaches to open approaches for intradural spinal tumor resection

Study	MISS/ Open (N)	MISS technique	Tumor size	Operative time (min)	Blood loss (ml)	Complication rate	CSF leak rate	Extent of resection (% GTR)	LOS
Lee et al. (2015)	31/18	Non-expandable tubular retractor ($n = 6$), unilateral hemilaminectomy ($n = 25$)	MISS 16.0 mm[a] Open 23.3 mm[a]	MISS 127.4[a] Open 174.0[a]	MISS 207.0[a] Open 426.6[a]	MISS 0% Open 5.5%	MISS 0% Open 5.5%	MISS 100% Open 88.9%	MISS 3.8 days[a] Open 6.8 days[a]
Raygor et al. (2015)	25/26	Transspinous expandable retractor	MISS 1.9 cm[b] Open 3.0 cm[b]	MISS 188.9 Open 218.6	MISS 142[a] Open 320[a]	MISS 8.0% Open 19.2%	MISS 4% Open 11.5%	MISS 92% Open 88.5%	MISS 6.9 days Open 7.2 days
Wong et al. (2015)	27/18	Expandable tubular retractor	–	MISS 256.3 Open 241.1	MISS 133.7[a] Open 558.8[a]	MISS 11.1% Open 22.2%	MISS 3.7%[a] Open 16.6%[a]	MISS 92.6% Open 94.4%	MISS 3.9 days[a] Open 6.1 days[a]
Fontes et al. (2016)	17/18	Expandable or non-expandable tubular retractor	MISS 1.76 ml Open 2.51 ml	MISS 162.1 Open 170.8	MISS 90.3 Open 135	MISS 0% Open 16.6%	MISS 0% Open 11.1%	–	*ICU* MISS 7.1 hrs Open 23.3 hrs *Floor* MISS 62.1 hrs Open 102.4 hrs

cm centimeters, *GTR* gross total resection, *hrs* hours, *LOS* length of stay, *MISS* minimally invasive spine surgery, *min* minutes, *ml* milliliters, *mm* millimeters
[a]Reached statistical significance $p < 0.05$
[b]Reached statistical trend $p < 0.10$

tioned studies comparing MISS to open approaches for IDEM tumor resection.

Additional Benefits of Tubular Retractors

Iatrogenic Instability

A key concept of MISS is to limit the amount of tissue disruption, achieving the surgical goal with the smallest possible operative footprint. Tubular retractor approaches allow preservation of the muscular and ligamentous attachments to the spi-

nous processes and limit the bony removal by performing a unilateral laminotomy for bilateral exposure of the thecal sac. Figure 10.16 illustrates the differences in exposure between the tubular retractor unilateral laminotomy versus a traditional open approach in the lumbar spine. A hypothesized benefit of this MISS approach is decreased iatrogenic instability compared to open techniques. Multiple biomechanical studies support this hypothesis insofar as unilateral laminotomy/laminectomy, as performed through a tubular retractor, has been shown to result in less biomechanical instability compared to traditional open laminectomy [33–36].

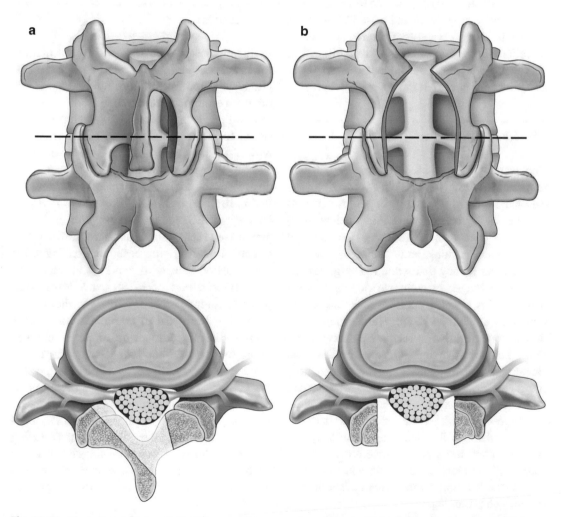

Fig. 10.16 Illustration depicting the exposure and decompression achieved with a tubular retractors approach (**a**) versus an open approach (**b**) in the lumbar spine

Cost Savings

Cost savings of MISS has been well reported in the literature. Multiple studies and systematic reviews have demonstrated the increased cost-effectiveness of MISS relative to open procedures. These savings are often attributed to the decreased length of stay, decreased blood loss, and decreased rates of postoperative complications, particularly surgical site infections, observed in the MISS population [37–39]. While these studies performed cost analyses of transforaminal lumbar interbody fusion procedures [37, 38], Fontes et al. examined the cost of MISS versus open surgery for IDEM tumors. The authors reported MISS resulted in a 29.5% reduction in acute perioperative costs and a 24.5% reduction in hospital charges when compared to open tumor resection. These cost savings were attributed to shorter hospital ICU and floor stays and fewer complications in the MISS group [26].

The Learning Curve

The learning curve is a well-documented phenomenon in MISS [40, 41]. While operative time, estimated blood loss, and postoperative time to ambulation have been shown to be increased, while surgeons are overcoming the learning curve, complications and outcomes are not affected; suggesting that while the surgeries initially take longer to complete due to surgeon learning, this learning period is safe and patient outcomes are not affected. These studies also demonstrate negative correlations between experience and operative time and complication rates. Because MISS techniques are becoming more prevalent as an increasing number of surgeons add such skills to their armamentarium, trainees are exposed to MISS earlier in their surgical careers and more often than the generations prior. As a result, spine surgeons entering the workforce will be more comfortable and may even surpass the learning curve during their residency or fellowship training.

A survey conducted to evaluate the perceptions of spine surgeons on MISS identified technical difficulty and lack of convenient training opportunities as the top two barriers for the adoption of MISS techniques [42]. It is important for surgeons inexperienced with MISS to know that this learning curve can be overcome with experience and education. The field of MISS continues to grow which has resulted in numerous courses, cadaver labs, webinars, etc., with expert faculty that can serve as invaluable learning resources for any surgeon wishing to add MISS techniques to his or her armamentarium.

Conclusion

In this chapter, we have described our method for intradural spinal tumor resection via unilateral laminotomy through a non-expandable tubular retractor. The existing body of literature supports that such MISS techniques for spinal tumor resection are safe and effective, with high rates of gross total tumor resection and low complication rates. As has been demonstrated in the lumbar decompression and fusion literature, the small operative footprint left by MISS techniques results in faster patient recovery. This has many downstream effects, including increased patient satisfaction, earlier return to work, and increased cost-effectiveness of MISS procedures compared to their open counterparts without compromising in regard to complications. Larger studies directly comparing MISS techniques to the traditional open laminectomy for tumor resection are required to better define the advantages and disadvantages of the application of MISS to intradural tumor resection. As surgeons continue to advance MISS techniques and gain further comfort in performing such procedures, and as more surgeons become adept at such techniques, one would expect outcome studies to continue to highlight the benefits of MISS.

References

1. Foley KT, Smith MM. Microendoscopic discectomy. Tech Neurosurg. 1997;3:301–7.
2. Palmer S, Turner R, Palmer R. Bilateral decompressive surgery in lumbar spinal stenosis associated with spondylolisthesis: unilateral approach and use of a microscope and tubular retractor system. Neurosurg Focus. 2002;13:E4.
3. Palmer S. Use of a tubular retractor system in microscopic lumbar discectomy: 1 year prospective results in 135 patients. Neurosurg Focus. 2002;13:E5. https://doi.org/10.3171/foc.2002.13.2.6.
4. Hernandez RN, Wipplinger C, Kirnaz S, Härtl R. Minimal access techniques using tubular retractors for disc herniations and stenosis. In: Bridwell KH, Gupta M, editors. Bridwell and DeWald's textbook of spinal surgery. 4th ed: Wolters Kluwer, Philadelphia, PA; 2020.
5. Eggert HR, Scheremet R, Seeger W, Gaitzsch J. Unilateral microsurgical approaches to extramedullary spinal tumours. Operative technique and results. Acta Neurochir. 1983;67:245–53.
6. Chiou SM, Eggert HR, Laborde G, Seeger W. Microsurgical unilateral approaches for spinal tumour surgery: eight years' experience in 256 primary operated patients. Acta Neurochir. 1989;100:127–33.
7. Yasargil MG, Tranmer BI, Adamson TE, Roth P. Unilateral partial hemi-laminectomy for the removal of extra- and intramedullary tumours and AVMs. Adv Tech Stand Neurosurg. 1991;18:113–32.
8. Tredway TL, Santiago P, Hrubes MR, Song JK, Christie SD, Fessler RG. Minimally invasive resection of intradural extramedullary spinal neoplasms. Neurosurgery. 2006;58:ONS52–8.
9. Haji FA, Cenic A, Crevier L, Murty N, Reddy K. Minimally invasive approach for the resection of spinal neoplasm. Spine (Phila Pa 1976). 2011;36:E1018–26.
10. Formo. Minimally invasive microsurgical resection of primary, intradural spinal tumors is feasible and safe: a consecutive series of 83 patients. Neurosurgery. 2018;82:365–71.
11. Soriano Sanchez JA, Soto Garcia S, Rodriguez Garcia M, et al. Microsurgical resection of intraspinal benign tumors using non-expansile tubular access. World Neurosurg. 2020;133:e97–e104.
12. Boukebir MA, Berlin CD, Navarro-Ramirez R, Heiland T, Schöller K, Rawanduzy C, Kirnaz S, Jada A, Härtl R. Ten-step minimall invasive spine lumbar decompression and dural repair through tubular retractors. Oper Neurosurg (Hagerstown). 2017;13:232–45.
13. Hernandez RN, Wipplinger C, Navarro-Ramirez R, Soriano-Solis S, Kirnaz S, Hussain I, Schmidt FA, Soriano-Sánchez JA, Härtl R. Ten-step minimally invasive cervical decompression via unilateral tubular laminotomy: technical note and early clinical experience. Oper Neurosurg (Hagerstown). 2020;18:284–94.
14. Tan LA, Takagi I, Straus D, O'Toole JE. Management of intended durotomy in minimally invasive intradural spine surgery. J Neurosurg Spine. 2014;21:279–85.
15. Mannion RJ, Nowitzke AM, Efendy J, Wood MJ. Safety and efficacy of intradural extramedullary spinal tumor removal using a minimally invasive approach. Neurosurgery. 2011;68:208–16.
16. Turel MK, D'Souza WP, Rajshekhar V. Hemilaminectomy approach for intradural extramedullary spinal tumors: an analysis of 164 patients. Neurosurg Focus. 2015;39:E9.
17. Pompili A, Caroli F, Crispo F, Giovannetti M, Raus L, Vidiri A, Telera S. Unilateral laminectomy approach for the removal of spinal meningiomas and schwannomas: impact on pain, spinal stability, and neurologic results. World Neurosurg. 2016;85:282–91.
18. Tredway TL, Santiago P, Hrubes MR, Song JK, Christie SD, Fessler RG. Minimally invasive resection of intradural-extramedullary spinal neoplasms. Neurosurgery. 2006;58:ONS52–8.
19. Dahlberg D, Halvorsen CM, Lied B, Helseth E. Minimally invasive microsurgical resection of primary, intradural spinal tumours using a tubular retractor system. Br J Neurosurg. 2012;26:472–5.
20. Gandhi RH, German JW. Minimally invasive approach for the treatment of intradural spinal pathology. Neurosurg Focus. 2013;35:E5.
21. Nzokou A, Weil AG, Shedid D. Minimally invasive removal of thoracic and lumbar spinal tumors using a nonexpendable retractor. J Neurosurg Spine. 2013;19:708–15.
22. Tredway TL. Minimally invasive approaches for the treatment of intramedullary spinal tumors. Neurosurg Clin N Am. 2014;25:327–36.
23. Lee SE, Jahng TA, Kim HJ. Different surgical approaches for spinal schwannoma: a single surgeon's experience with 49 consecutive cases. World Neurosurg. 2015;84:1894–902.
24. Raygor KP, Than KD, Chou D, Mummaneni PV. Comparison of minimally invasive transspinous and open approaches for thoracolumbar intradural-extramedullary spinal tumors. Neurosurg Focus. 2015;39:E12.
25. Wong AP, Lall RR, Dahdaleh NS, Lawton CD, Smith ZA, Wong RH, Harvey MJ, Lam S, Kosko TR, Fessler RG. Comparison of open and minimally invasive surgery for intradural-extramedullary spine tumors. Neurosurg Focus. 2015;39:E11.
26. Fontes RBV, Wewel JT, O'Toole JE. Perioperative cost analysis of minimally invasive vs open resection of intradural extramedullary spinal cord tumors. Neurosurgery. 2016;78:531–9.
27. Dhandapani S, Karthigeyan M. "Microendoscopic" versus "pure endoscopic" surgery for spinal intradural mass lesions: a comparative study and review. Spine J. 2018;18:1592–602.
28. Krüger MT, Steiert C, Gläsker S, Klingler JH. Minimally invasive resection of spinal hemangioblastoma: feasibility and clinical results in a series of 18 patients. J Neurosurg Spine. 2013;31:880–9.

29. Soriano Sánchez JA, Soto García ME, Soriano Solís S, Rodríguez García M, Trejo Huerta P, Sánchez Escandón O, Flores Soria ER, Romero-Rangel JAI. Microsurgical resection of Intraspinal benign tumors using non-Expansile tubular access. World Neurosurg. 2020;133:e97–e104.

30. Ogden AT, Fessler RG. Minimally invasive resection of intramedullary ependymoma: case report. Neurosurgery. 2009;65:E1203–4.

31. Lu DC, Chou D, Mummaneni PV. A comparison of mini-open and open approaches for resection of thoracolumbar intradural spinal tumors. J Neurosurg Spine. 2011;14:758–64.

32. Winkler EA, Lu A, Rutledge WC, Tabani H, Rubio RR, Mummaneni PV. A mini-open transspinous approach for resection of intramedullary spinal cavernous malformations. J Clin Neurosci. 2018;58:210–2.

33. Bresnahan L, Ogden AT, Natarajan RN, Fessler RG. A biomechanical evaluation of graded posterior element removal for treatment of lumbar stenosis: comparison of a minimally invasive approach with two standard laminectomy techniques. Spine (Phila Pa 1976). 2009;34:17–23.

34. Ogden AT, Bresnahan L, Smith JS, Natarajan R, Fessler RG. Biomechanical comparison of traditional and minimally invasive intradural tumor exposures using finite element analysis. Clin Biochem (Bristol, Avon). 2009;24:143–7.

35. Xie T, Qian J, Lu Y, Chen B, Jiang Y, Luo C. Biomechanical comparison of laminectomy, hemilaminectomy and a new minimally invasive approach in the surgical treatment of multilevel cervical intra-

dural tumour: a finite element analysis. Eur Spine J. 2013;22:2719–30.

36. Ho YH, Tu YK, Hsiao CK, Chang CH. Outcomes after minimally invasive lumbar decompression: a biomechanical comparison of unilateral and bilateral laminotomies. BMC Musculoskelet Disord. 2015;16:208.

37. Goldstein C, Phillips FM, Rampersaud YR. Comparative effectiveness of economic evaluations of open versus minimally invasive posterior or transforaminal lumbar interbody fusion: a systematic review. Spine (Phila Pa 1976). 2016;41:S74–89.

38. Phan K, Hogan JA, Mobbs RJ. Cost-utility of minimally invasive versus open transforaminal lumbar interbody fusion: systematic review and economic evaluation. Eur Spine J. 2015;24:2503–13.

39. Al-Khouja LT, Baron EM, Johnson JP, Kim TT, Drazin D. Cost-effectiveness analysis in minimally invasive spine surgery. Neurosurg Focus. 2014;36:E4.

40. Ahn J, Iqbal A, Manning BT, Leblang S, Bohl DD, Mayo BC, et al. Minimally invasive lumbar decompression-the surgical learning curve. Spine J. 2016;16:909–16.

41. Parikh K, Tomasino A, Knopman J, Boockvar J, Härtl R. Operative results and learning curve: microscope-assisted tubular microsurgery for 1- and 2-level discectomies and laminectomies. Neurosurg Focus. 2008;25:E14.

42. Webb J, Gottschalk L, Lee YP, Garfin S, Kim C. Surgeon perceptions of minimally invasive spine surgery. SAS J. 2008;2:145. https://doi.org/10.1016/SASJ-2008-0006-MIS.

Index

© Springer Nature Switzerland AG 2021
S. Hanft, P. C. McCormick (eds.), *Tumors of the Spinal Canal*,
https://doi.org/10.1007/978-3-030-55096-7

Printed in the United States
by Baker & Taylor Publisher Services